124 Anaesthesiologie und Intensivmedizin Anaesthesiology and Intensive Care Medicine

Neue Aspekte in der Regionalanaesthesie 1

Wirkung auf Herz, Kreislauf und Endokrinium. Postoperative Periduralanalgesie

Herausgegeben
von H. J. Wüst und M. Zindler

Mit 97 Abbildungen

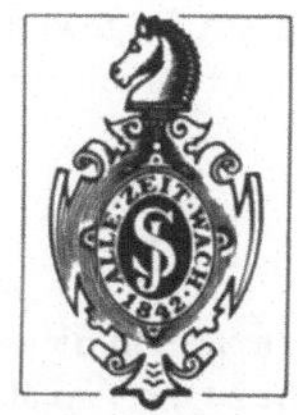

Springer-Verlag
Berlin Heidelberg New York 1980

Dr. med. Hans Joachim Wüst
und
Professor Dr. med. Martin Zindler
Institut für Anaesthesiologie
der Universität
Moorenstraße 5, 4000 Düsseldorf

ISBN-13: 978-3-540-09500-2 e-ISBN-13: 978-3-642-67384-9
DOI: 10.1007/978-3-642-67384-9

CIP-Kurztitelaufnahme der Deutschen Bibliothek.
Neue Aspekte in der Regionalanaesthesie / hrsg. von H.J. Wüst und M. Zindler. – Berlin, Heidelberg, New York: Springer.
NE: Wüst, Hans-Joachim [Hrsg.]
1. Wirkung auf Herz, Kreislauf und Endokrinium, postoperative Peridualanalgesie. – 1980.
(Anaesthesieologie und Intensivmedizin; 124)
ISBN 3-540-09500-4 (Berlin, Heidelberg, New York)
ISBN 0-387-09500-4 (New York, Heidelberg, Berlin)

Vorwort

Die Entwicklung langwirksamer, gering toxischer Lokalanaesthetika sowie die Weiterentwicklung der Kathertechnik haben in den letzten Jahren eine Renaissance der großen rückenmarksnahen Leitungsanaesthesien bewirkt.

Dieses ständig wachsende Interesse führte im Juni 1978 internationale Experten zu einem ersten Symposium in Düsseldorf zusammen, um über neue Aspekte in der Regionalanaesthesie zu diskutieren.

In diesem Band sind die 24 Vorträge zusammengefaßt, die zu den drei Themenkreisen über die Wirkung der Epiduralanaesthesie auf Herz und Kreislauf, über den Einfluß der Epiduralanaesthesie bzw. der Allgemeinnarkose auf Stressreaktionen während der Operation sowie über die postoperative Fortsetzung der Epiduralanaesthesie in ihrer Auswirkung auf die Atemfunktion und die Häufigkeit von Lungenkomplikationen gehalten wurden.

Anhand der weitgehend neuen Erkenntnissen wurden die Vor- und Nachteile der Epiduralanaesthesie im Vergleich zur Allgemeinnarkose, insbesondere beim Risikopatienten, herausgearbeitet.

Den Erfolg dieses Symposiums danken wir den informativen und interessanten Beiträgen der Referenten und Diskussionsteilnehmer sowie der großzügigen Unterstützung durch die Firma Astra Chemicals, Wedel/Holst.

Die vorgetragenen Ergebnisse dieses Symposiums werden den praktisch tätigen Anaesthesisten in der Hoffnung zugänglich gemacht, daß sie aus den neuesten Erkenntnissen der internationalen Forschung Anregungen zur Verbesserung der täglichen Routine erhalten.

Düsseldorf, im Juni 1979

Dr. H.J. Wüst
Prof. Dr. M. Zindler

Inhaltsverzeichnis

II. Herzkreislauffunktion bei Risikopatienten während Periduralanaesthesie
Vorsitz: J. Lassner, Paris und J.O. Arndt, Düsseldorf

III. Stress und Endokrinium während Narkose und Operation
Vorsitz: T. Tammisto, Helsinki und H. Lennartz, Marburg

Referentenverzeichnis

Arnold, G., Prof. Dr. med., Direktor des Instituts für Experimentelle Chirurgie der Universität Düsseldorf, Universitätsstr., 4000 Düsseldorf

Arndt, J.O., Prof. Dr. med., Leiter der Abteilung für experimentelle Anaesthesiologie der Universität Düsseldorf, Universitätsstr., 4000 Düsseldorf

Böhmer, G., Laborant, Institut für Anaesthesiologie der Universität Düsseldorf, Moorenstr. 5, 4000 Düsseldorf

Brandt, M.R., M D., Surgical Department of Anaesthesiology, Rigshospitalet, 2100 Copenhagen, Denmark

Engberg, G., M D., University Hospital, Department of Anaesthesiology, 75014 Uppsala 14, Sweden

Falke, K., Prof. Dr. med., Oberarzt am Institut für Anaesthesiologie der Universität Düsseldorf, Moorenstr. 5, 4000 Düsseldorf

Florack, G., Dr. med., Chirurgische Klinik A. der Universität Düsseldorf, Moorenstr. 5, 4000 Düsseldorf

Fournell, A., Dr. med., Institut für Anaesthesiology der Universität Düsseldorf, Moorenstr. 5, 4000 Düsseldorf

Godehardt, E., Institut für Biomathematik und medizinische Dokumentation der Universität Düsseldorf, Universitätsstr., 4000 Düsseldorf

Günther, D., Prof. Dr. med., Institut und Klinik für medizinische Strahlenkunde der Universität Düsseldorf, Moorenstr. 5, 4000 Düsseldorf

Hack, G., Priv. Doz., Oberarzt am Institut für Anaesthesiologie Venusberg, 5300 Bonn

Jynge, P., Department of Physiology, University of Tromsö, 9012 Tromsö, Norwegen

Katz, J., M D., Prof. and Vice Chairman, Department of Anesthesiology, Veterans Administration Hospital, 3350 La Jolla Village Drive, San Diego, California 92161

Kehlet, H., M D., Chief Ass. Surgeon, Rigshospitalet, University Hospital, 9 Blegdamsvej, 2100 Copenhagen, Denmark

Kern, F., Dr. med., Chefarzt am Institut für Anaesthesiologie Kantonspital, 9006 St. Gallen, Schweiz

Knitza, R., Dr. med., Universitäts-Frauenklinik, 6650 Homburg/Saar

Korttila, K., M D., Assoc. Prof., University if Iowa, Department of Anaesthesia, Iowa City, Iowa 52242, USA

Lassner, J., Prof. Dép. d'Anesthésiologie, 123 Bd. Port Royal, F 75674 Paris Cedex 14, Frankreich

Lehmacher, W., Rechenzentrum der Universität Düsseldorf, Universitätsstr., 4000 Düsseldorf

Lennartz, H., Prof. Dr. med., Direktor des Anaesthesiezentrums der Universitäts-Kliniken, Robert-Koch Str. 8, 355 Marburg a.d. Lahn

Levänen, J., Department of Anaesthesia, Helsinki University, Central Hospital, Haartmaninkatu 4, 00290 Helsinki 29, Finland

Liebau, W., cand. med., Insitut für Biomathematik und medizinische Dokumentation der Universität Düsseldorf, Universitätsstr., 4000 Düsseldorf

Lutz, H., Prof. Dr. med., Direktor des Instituts für Anaesthesiologie und Reanimation der Städt. Krankenanstalten Mannheim, Postfach 23, 6800 Mannheim

Modig, J., M D., Ass. Prof., Department od Anaesthesia, University Hospital, 75014 Uppsala, Schweden

Naumann, C., Dr. med., Abt. für Intensivbehandlung des chirurg. Departements, Kantonspital, 9007 St. Gallen, Schweiz

Nolte, H., Prof. Dr. med., Chefarzt des Instituts für Anaesthesiologie, Zweckverband Stadt- und Kreiskrankenhaus, Bismarckstr. 6, 4950 Minden/Westf.

Ottesen, St., M D., Med. avd. B, Rikshospitalet i Oslo, Oslo 1, Norwegen

Pontoppidan, H., M D., Prof. Chief Respiratory Unit and Respiratory Care Department, Massachusetts General Hospital, Boston, Massachusetts 02114, USA

Raiss, G., Dr. med., Institut für Anaesthesiologie und Reanimation der Städt. Krankenanstalten Mannheim, Postfach 23, 6800 Mannheim

Renck, H., M D., Prof., Department of Anaesthesia, Regionssjukhus, Linköping, Schweden

Richter, O., Dr. phil., Institut für Biomathematik und medizinische Dokumentation der Universität Düsseldorf, Universitätsstr., 4000 Düsseldorf

Sandmann, W., Priv. Doz., Oberarzt an der Chirurgischen Klinik A der Universität Düsseldorf, Moorenstr. 5, 4000 Düsseldorf

Siepmann, H.P., Priv. Doz., Oberarzt am Institut für Anaesthesiologie der Universität Düsseldorf, Moorenstr. 5, 4000 Düsseldorf

Stanton-Hicks, M.d', M D., Prof. and Chairman, Department of Anaesthesia, University of Maasachusetts, 55 Lake Avenue North, Worcester 01605, USA

Striebel, J.P., Dr. med., Institut für Anaesthesiologie und Reanimation, Städt. Krankenanstalten Mannheim, Postfach 23, 6800 Mannheim

Tammisto, T., M D., Prof. and Chairman, Department of Anaesthesia, Helsinki Central Hospital, Haartmaninkatu 4, 00290 Helsinki 29, Finland

Tolksdorf, W., Dr. med., Institut für Anaesthesiologie und Reanimation der Städt. Krankenanstalten Mannheim, Postfach 23, 6800 Mannheim

Vik-Mo, H., Department of Physiology, University Tromsö, 9012 Tromsö, Norwegen

Vetter, H., Priv. Doz., Medizinische Poliklinik der Universität Bonn, Venusberg, 5300 Bonn

Wiklund, L., M D., Doc. Department of Anaesthesia, University Hospital, 75014 Uppsala 14, Schweden

Wilhelmy, B., cand. med., Institut für Anaesthesiology der Universität Düsseldorf, Moorenstr. 5, 4000 Düsseldorf

Wüst, H.J., Dr. med., Institut für Anaesthesiologie der Universität Düsseldorf, Moorenstr. 5, 4000 Düsseldorf

Zindler, M., Prof. Dr. med., Direktor des Instituts für Anaesthesiologie der Universität Düsseldorf, Moorenstr. 5, 4000 Düsseldorf

Zumfelde, L., Dr. med., Chirurgische Klinik A der Universität Düsseldorf, Moorenstr. 5, 4000 Düsseldorf

I. Kreislauffunktion während rückenmarksnaher Regionalanaesthesie

Vorsitz: G. Arnold und H.P. Siepmann, Düsseldorf

Haemodynamic Effects of Regional Anaesthesia

M. Stanton-Hicks

In a discussion of the haemodynamic effects of regional anaesthesia it is convenient firstly to look at the cardiovascular effects of local anaesthetics, both direct and indirect and then to see how these arise during the course of regional anaesthetic procedures.

It is now understood that local anaesthetics effect the myocardium by interfering with the sodium conductance in much the same manner as they affect a nerve membrane. If we remind ourselves of the cardiac action potential (Fig. 1) we can identify the terms which will be

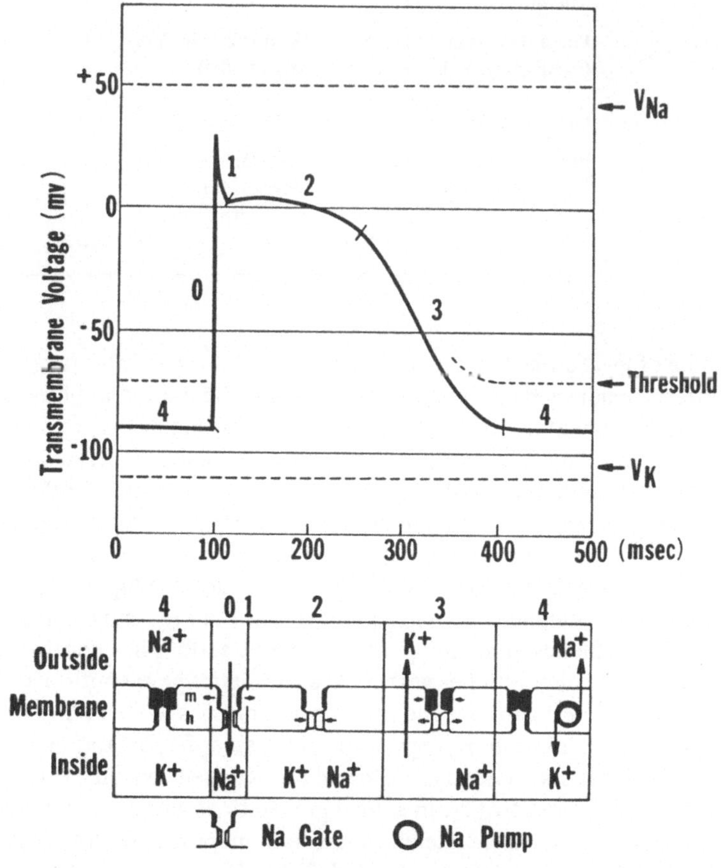

Fig. 1. Cardiac action potential, the resting potential of about −85 mV is recorded during diastole or relaxation. The rapid rise following stimulation, is phase 0 depolarization (rapid phase). Phase 1 shows membrane voltage declining from a positive voltage to a plateau or Phase 2. Phase 3 is repolarization and Phase 4 is again the resting plateau. Associated ion movements are shown below

used to describe the effects of local anaesthetics on normal depolarization and therefore cardiac activity. Of all the local anaesthetics, lidocaine has been most extensively investigated and in doses of 1-2 mg/kg, it shortens the action potential duration, reduces phase 4 depolarization, reduces the effective refractory period and increases the conduction velocity (Table 1). As the

Table 1. Cardiac alterations with increasing dose of lidocaine

Blood Level	Cardiac Effects Of Lignocaine			
	Electrophysiology		Haemodynamic	
μg/ml				
	Phase 4 Depol.	↓	Cardiac Rate	↑→
2-5	Apd.	↓	End Diastolic Volume	→
	Erp	↓		
	Conduction Vel.	↑	C.O.	→↑↓
	Phase 0 Depol.	↓	End Diastolic Vol.	↑
3-7	Conduction Vel.	↓	Myocardial Contraction	↓
	Qrs. Duration	↑	C.O.	↓
	Phase 0 Depol.	↓	End Diastolic Vol.	↑
	Conduction Vel.	↓	Myocardial Contraction	↓
> 10				
	A.V. Block		C.O.	↓

dose of local anaesthetic increases, the stimulatory effects are replaced by cardio-depressant effects manifested electrophysiologically by a reduction in phase 0 depolarization, a reduction in action potential amplitude and finally, a slowing of the conduction velocity leading to asystole [2, 6]. Clinically, these effects are seen as first an increase in heart rate, stroke volume and cardiac output. Then with higher doses through the antiarrhythmic range, we see a rise in end diastolic volume, reduction in myocardial force and a fall in cardiac output.

Other local anaesthetics also share the same biphasic properties, but do so at higher dosage. The vascular effects of local anaesthetics are also biphasic in nature and depend on many factors. In a number of in vitro preparations Blair [3] showed that in low concentrations all local anaesthetics stimulate spontaneous contractions in smooth muscle (Table 2, Fig. 2). Both human and animal studies with local anaesthetics have confirmed the stimulatory effects following both intra-arterial and intravenous infusion while at higher doses vasodilatation is seen. Intra-arterial infusion of mepivacaine decreased the forearm blood flow in human volunteers. Similar studies with lidocaine showed an increased tone in capacitance vessels indicated by a decreased blood flow [7]. In animal preparations whose sympathetic control was abolished by spinal section or adrenergic blockade, both mepivacaine and procaine caused an increase in hind limb vascular resistance [1, 12] (Table 3).

Generally therefore, the circulatory effects seen with increasing dosage of local anaesthetics are an increase or no change in blood pressure due to the increased sympathetic tone and direct myogenic stimulatory activity. There is likewise an increase in myocardial activity resulting from the same mechanism. As the dose increase, however, the negative inotropic effects

Table 2. Biphasic peripheral vascular effects of different local anaesthetics

Biphasic Peripheral Vascular Effect Of Various Local Anesthetic Agents

Agent	Isolated Rat Portal Vein % Increase (constriction) Spontaneous contractions	Basal tone	Canine Femoral Blood Flow % Increase (dilation)
Lidocaine	173	68	25
Mepivacaine	228	162	36
Prilocaine	293	163	42
Tetracaine	237	82	38
Bupivacaine	184	37	45
Etidocaine	147	–	44

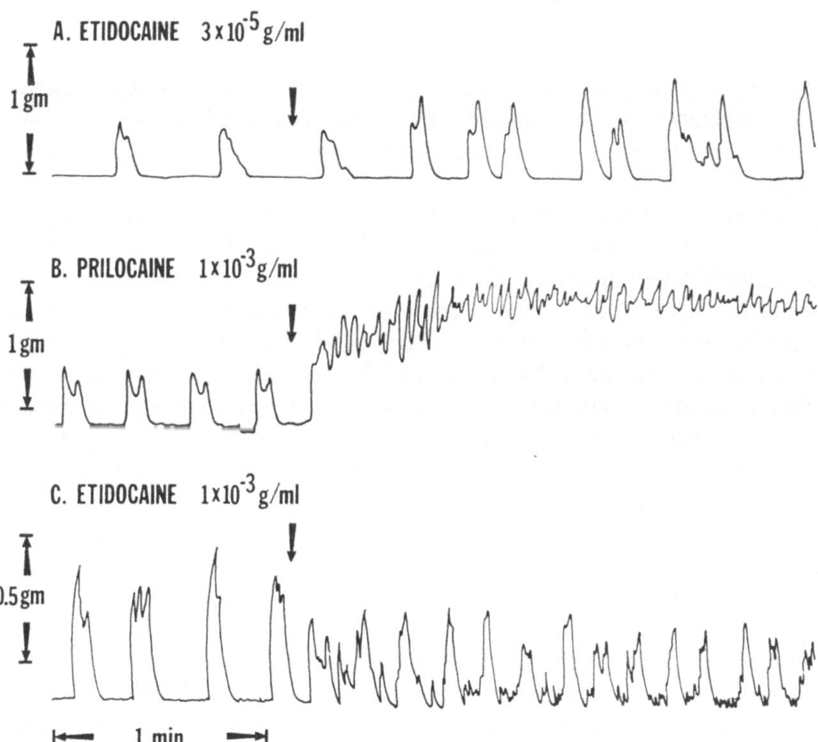

Fig. 2. Biphasic effects of different concentrations of etidocaine on the spike height of the spontaneously contracting portal vein. The effect of prilocaine is also shown (Blair)

on the myocardium and the fall in peripheral vascular resistance combine to produce a fall in systemic blood pressure. Before discussing the indirect haemodynamic effects of regional anaesthesia due to the particular procedure, mention must be made of those indirect effects of the local anaesthetics themselves to which I have just alluded. The increase in sympathetic tone which is seen at certain local anaesthetic blood levels has been shown to be a direct result of hypothalamic stimulation [8, 11].

Table 3. Some of the more important peripheral vascular effects at different ranges of local anaesthetic concentration

Blood Level μg/ml	Peripheral Vascular Effects of L.A.'S
Low Dose	Vasoconstriction
5-10	Vasodilatation B.P. ↓
> 10	Vasodolatation B.P. ↓ Circulatory Collapse

The local and systemic effects of added vasoconstrictors will now be discussed. The importance of these substances on the circulatory parameters has already been well established by the numerous data obtained from studies in human volunteers performed in Seattle during the past 15 years [5, 13, 14].

Adrenaline has been used as an α agonist both to prolong the duration of local anaesthetic action to reduce the systemic toxicity from absorption of the local anaesthetic. Not generally appreciated however, are the wide-ranging effects which accompany the commonly employed doses of adrenaline (100-200 μg). These effects have profound implications on the haemodynamic adjustments which attend many regional anaesthetic procedures, such as major conduction anaesthesia and coeliac block. Both spinal and epidural anaesthesia interrupt the thoracolumbar preganglionic autonomic outflow and, depending on how many spinal segments are involved, the haemodynamic effects may be slight or profound. Anaesthesia affecting any of the first three thoracic segments will interfere with the cardiac nerves thereby removing in part or completely this positive inotropic influence. Another important factor determining block is the much greater sensitivity of the preganglionic β fibres which are the most sensitive to local anaesthetics. Therefore the sympathetic block will always be more extensive than somatic analgesia: in the case of epidural anaesthesia, one to two spinal segments higher, and in subarachnoid block, three to four segments higher. Obviously, this must be taken into consideration with all extensive blocks of the spinal outflow.

Although the haemodynamic responses to sympathetic block are similar in both cases (an increase in leg blood flow, reduction in arm blood flow, fall in total peripheral resistance and compensatory increase in the cardiac output), whether or not a fall in mean arterial pressure occurs, will ultimately be determined by a number of factors not least of which will be the ability of the circulatory readjustments to cope with these changes. Table 4 shows the changes associated with epidural anaesthesia with and without adrenaline and subarachnoid block to a level of T_5. It should be noted that the fall in mean arterial pressure was greater when the local anaesthetic solution contained adrenaline. The reason for this is the widespread β effects which add to the vasodilatation in the lower limbs and counteract the compensatory vasoconstriction in the upper limbs (Fig. 3). The cardiotonic effects are not great enough in normovolaemic man to compensate for these peripheral vascular effects, a situation which is quite the reverse as we will see when we discuss the effects of added vasoconstrictors in the

Table 4. Cardiovascular changes associated with spinal anaesthesia, epidural anaesthesia with and without adrenaline to T_5 in a group of healthy human subjects (after Ward et al. [14])

	Mean % Change From Control				
	MAP	CR	SV	CO	TPR
Spinal Anesthesia	−21.3	+ 3.7	−25.4	−17.7	− 5.0
Epidural Plain	− 8.9	+ 6.7	−10	− 5.4	− 2.9
Epidural + Epinephrine	−22	+15.8	+ 7.9	+30.2	−39.6

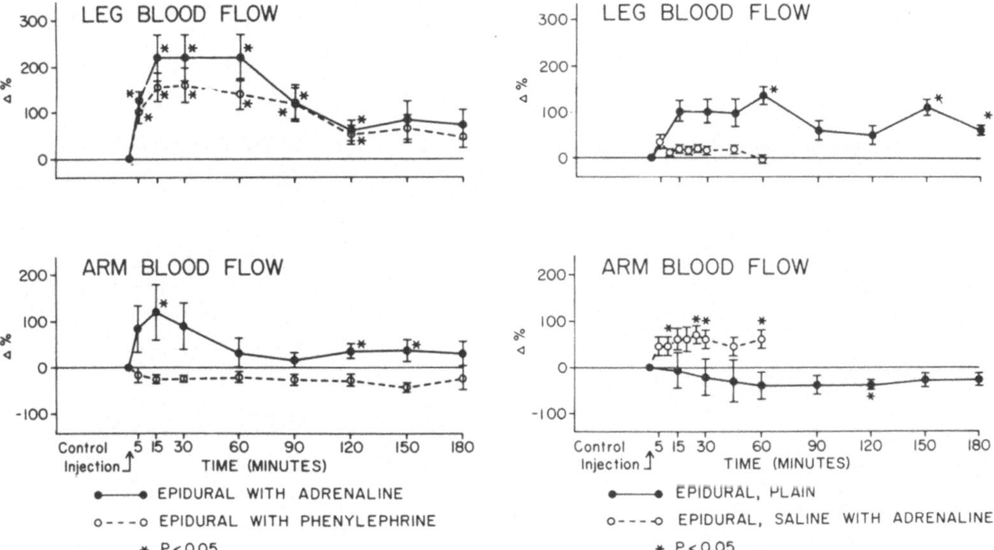

Fig. 3. Arm and leg blood flows during epidural block to T_5 in four situations. Lidocaine plain, with adrenaline 5 μ/ml, with phenylephrine 50 μg/ml, and saline in the same volume with adrenaline 5 μg/ml. Lidocaine dose, 20 ml 2%

presence of hypovolaemia and shock [4]. While adrenaline has been traditionally used as the vasoconstrictor of choice, the above systemic effects can be undesirable under most circumstances. Vasoconstrictors having predominantly α stimulatory effects such as phenylephrine and felypressin, have been used in conjunction with local anaesthetic solutions. Stanton-Hicks et al. [13] understook a study of the cardiovascular changes attending epidural anaesthesia in a group of human volunteers in which the local anaesthetic solution contained either phenylephrine or adrenaline. Some of the data relating to limb blood flow is shown in Fig. 3 and the other cardiovascular changes are shown in Fig. 4. One unexpected aspect related to the apparent negative inotropic effect seen during block with the anaesthetic containing phenylephrine. In spite of this however, the circulatory status was maintained within control limits. Without appropriate data regarding the use of a predominantly α agonist as a vasoconstrictor in hypovolaemic states it would appear to be imprudent to do so as far as cardiac performance, renal

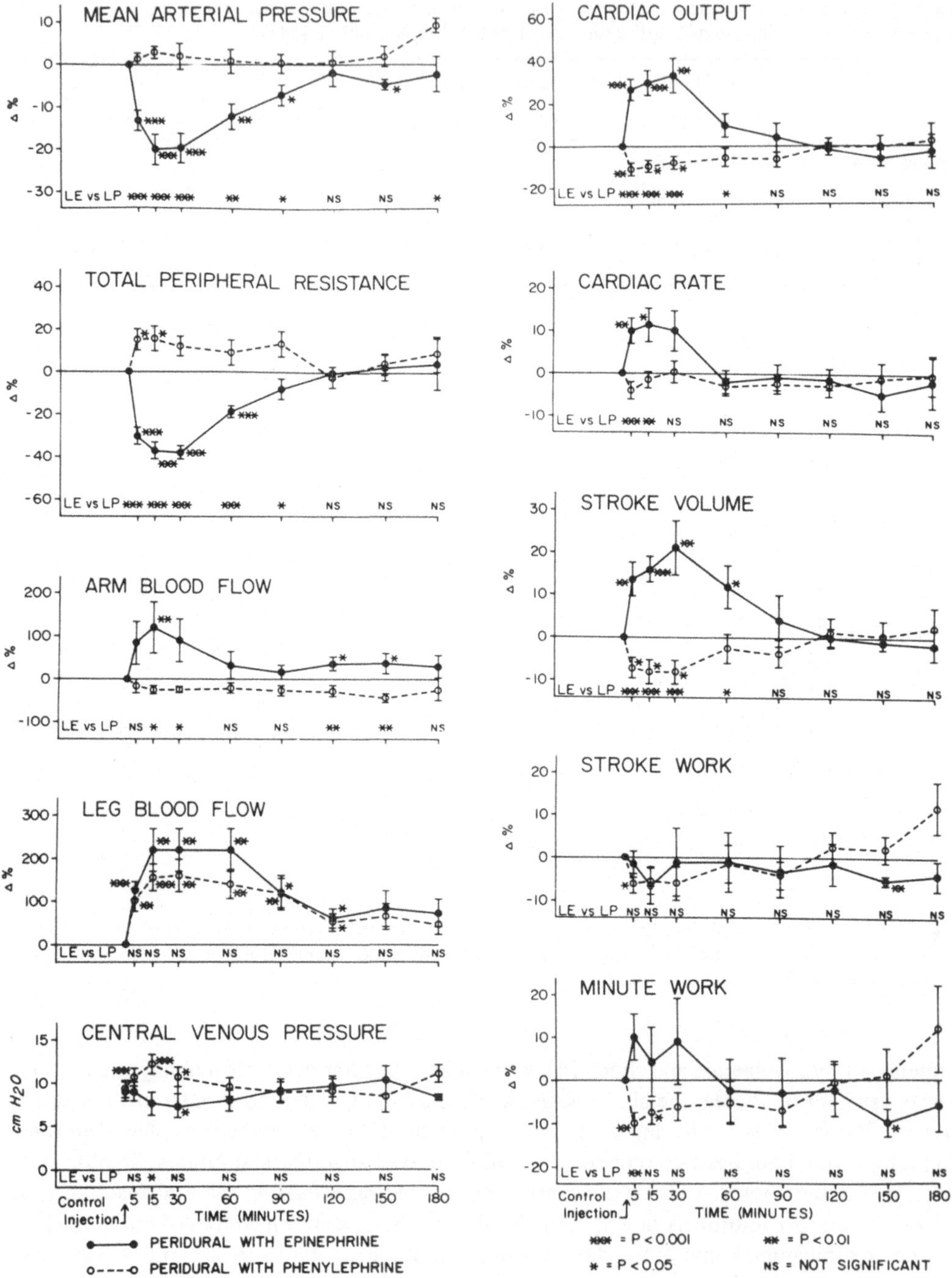

Fig. 4. Comparison of the cardiovascular effects of epidural anaesthetic solutions containing adrenaline or phenylephrine

and hepatic function are concerned although it would not appear to be contraindicated in normovolaemic man and might be the agent of choice under certain circumstances.

Although the haemodynamic responses to sympathetic block are similar in both cases the similarities cease once other factors, for example the effect of adsorbed local anaesthetics on the central nervous system and direct effects on the cardiovascular system, are considered. High blood levels of local anaesthetics occur following intercostal block, caudal block, epidural block, and brachial plexus block in this order (Fig. 5). It is possible for very high levels

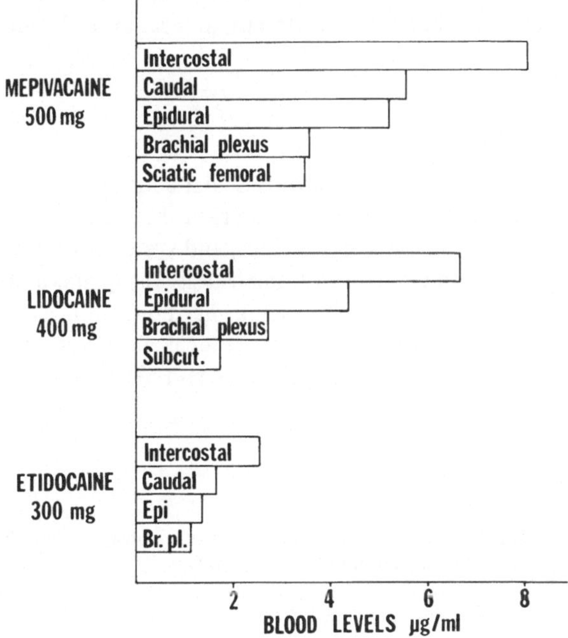

Fig. 5. Comparitive peak blood levels of various local anaesthetics after their use in the sites indicated

to attend a Bier block from premature sudden release of the tourniquet. A potentially hazardous situation exists when these high local anaesthetic blood levels react with hypnotic and sedative drugs. At best, it must be reasembered that the effects of CNS depressants on the hypothalamus may counteract the stimulatory effects of local anaesthetics, thereby aggravating the circulatory depression which can occur with regional anaesthesia.

Other haemodynamic effects of central neural blockade can influence both renal and hepatic function. Kennedy et al. [9. 10] studied these effects in human volunteers. Their results showed that the glomerular filtration rate (GFR) and effective renal plasma flow (ERPF) fell only 7% and 10% respectively with minimal change in systemic pressure. Similar results were obtained from another study in which spinal anaesthesia was used. When adrenaline was included in the local anaesthetic solution, more significant falls in the GFR and ERPF of 11% and 26% respectively were observed. Here the mean arterial pressure fell 21%. Changes in the renal vascular resistance were minimal and those changes seen were attributed to the systemic pressure changes. In studies of hepatic function during epidural anaesthesia to T_5, a reduction in the effective hepatic blood flow (EHBF) was attributed to an increase in splanchnic vascular resistance (SVR) of 30% with the plain lidocaine solution. When, however, a solution containing adrenaline was used, the increase in SVR was replaced by a decrease of 16%, the net result of which was to maintain the EHBF within control levels initially but this too fell to 20% of control after 30 min. It is possible that the difference in EHBF between the two epidural anaesthetics is due to the higher circulating lidocaine blood level associated with the plain solution causing a greater SVR and therefore lower EHBF.

The implication of these two situations on the metabolism and excretion of amide-type local anaesthetics will be to reduce their clearence and possibly augment their circulatory actions. Lastly, the physical status of the patient, while directly influencing the choice of a regional anaesthetic technique, may mitigate against such a choice, as for example when severe hypovolaemia or shock is present, at least until this has been corrected by volume replacement.

Summary

The direct and indirect cardiovascular actions of local anaesthetics and the relationship of these to the haemodynamic effects of the regional anaesthetic procedures themselves is presented. Also stressed are the local and systemic effects of added vasoconstrictors and their importance to circulatory homeostasis. Using major conduction block as an example, the very complicated interplay between the haemodynamic changes consequent upon sympathetic block and the circulating blood levels of local anaesthetic and vasoconstrictor is discussed. Particular reference is made to the splanchnic and renal circulations and their role in the excretion of local anaesthetics.

References

1. Aberg G, Dhunér K-G (1972) Effects of mepivacaine (Carbocaine®) on femoral blood flow in the dog. Acta Pharmacol Toxicol (kbh) 31:267
2. Bigger JT, Mandel WJ (1970) Effect of lidocaine on the electrophysiological properties of ventricular muscle and purkinje fibres. J Clin Invest 49:63
3. Blair MR (1975) Cardiovascular pharmacology of local anaesthetics. Br J Anaesth 47:247
4. Bonica JJ, Berges PU, Morikawa K (1970) Circulatory effects of peridural block I: Influence of level of analgesia and dose of lidocaine. Anesthesiology 33:619
5. Bonica JJ, Akamatsu TJ, Berges PU, Morikawa K, Kennedy WF Jr (1971) Circulatory effects of peridural block II: Effects of epinephrine. Anesthesiology 34:514
6. Davis LD, Tenite JV (1969) Electrophysiological actions of lidocaine on canine ventricular muscle and purkinje fibers. Circ Res 24:639
7. Jorfeldt L, Löfström B, Pernow B, Persson B, Wahren J (1970) The effect of mepivacaine and lidocaine on forearm resistance and capacitance vessels in man. Acta Anaesthesiol Scand 14:183
8. Kao FF, Jaiar VH (1959) The central action of lignocaine and its effect on cardiac output. Brit J Pharmacol 14:522
9. Kennedy WF, Jr, Sawyer TK, Gerbershagen HU, Cutler RE, Allen GD, Bonica JJ (1969) Systemic cardiovascular and renal hemodynamic alterations during peridural anesthesia in normal man. Anesthesiology 31:414
10. Kennedy WF, Everett GB, Cobb LA, Allen GD (1971) Simultaneous systemic and hepatic hemodynamic measurements during high peridural anesthesia in normal man. Anesth Analg (Cleve) 50:1069
11. McWhriter W, Frederickson E, Steinhaus J (1972) Interactions of lidocaine with general anesthetics. South Med J 65:796
12. Sanders HD (1965) Vasoconstrictor and vasodilator properties of procaine. Can J Physiol Pharmacol 43:39
13. Stanton-Hicks M, Berges PU, Bonica JJ (1973) Circulatory effects of peridural block IV: Comparison of the effects of epinephrine and phenylephrine. Anesthesiology 39:308

14. Ward RJ, Bonica JJ, Freund FG, Akamatsu TJ, Danziger F, Engelsson S (1965) Epidural and subarachnoid anesthesia: Cardiovascular and respiratory effects. JAMA 191:275

Diskussion

Frage: Sie haben deutliche Unterschiede im Verhalten des Kreislaufverhaltens während Epiduralanaesthesie mit Bupivacaine mit und ohne Adrenalinzusatz gezeigt. Würden diese Kreislaufveränderungen Sie veranlassen, Adrenalin der Lösung zuzusetzen?

Stanton-Hicks: Einen Adrenalinzusatz in der Regel: nein. Nur wenn hohe Dosen von Lokalanaesthetika wie bei der Kaudalanaesthesie verwandt werden oder wenn aus Zeitgründen eine Beschleunigung des Wirkungseintrittes erwünscht ist. Sonst nicht.

A Comparison of the Cardiovascular Effects of Neurolept-, Halothane or Continuous Thoracic Epidural Anaesthesia in Patients Undergoing an Aorto-Femoral Bypass Operation. A Prospective Randomized Study

H.J. Wüst, G. Florack, W. Sandmann, O. Richter und W. Lehmacher

Maintaining an adequate perfusion of vital organs is a central problem in the management of anaesthesia in poor risk patients. The first criterion for choosing an anaesthetic method for these patients is that as few changes as possible in the cardiovascular function are produced [11, 12]; the second criterion is that the defence mechanisms mediated via the sympathetic nervous system stay intact.

However, Page et al. [23] showed back in 1955 the beneficial effects of lowering the pressure and resistance work done by the left side of the heart in patients with a cardiac failure. This therapeutic measure can be applied either with the aid of ganglionic blocking agents, alpha-blockers or by specific vasodilatory drugs [4, 7, 31]. Theoretically continuous epidural anaesthesia also has this effect, due to concomitant sympathicolysis [3].

It was therefore asked firstly, if this therapeutic feature can be realized only by means of the anaesthetic regimen, and secondly, if poor risk patients better tolerate risky operations when the pressure and resistance work done by the left side of the heart is lowered.

Patients and Method

1. The patients, scheduled for major elective vascular surgery, were selected for three reasons:

a) The higher risks involved in the operation and anaesthesia for them due to arteriosclerotic disease in comparison with healthy patients. [9, 35, 38].
b) The enormous and acute changes in the cardiovascular function, induced by clamping and declamping the aorta. [1, 12, 19, 39].
c) The pulmonary risks in the postoperative course, due to the site of the operation. [24, 33, 38].

2. The effects of the three different anaesthetic methods on the cardiovascular function were evaluated in 68 patients undergoing an elective aorto-femoral bypass operation.

In randomized order the patients were anaesthetized either with neuroleptanaesthesia type II (NLA), halothane or a continuous thoracic epidural anaesthesia in combination with diazepam sleep.

The comparison was only justified if two basic claims were fulfilled: that the biometric data in the three groups were homogenous and that the therapy during and after the operation were as similar as possible.

The first condition was fulfilled as the biometric data, such as age, height and anaesthetic risk group show (Table 1). The second condition regarding similar therapy was met regarding:

a) Volume replacement during operation (Table 2);
b) Minute ventilation applied by controlling the respiration (Table 3);
c) Analgetic regimen for postoperative pain release.

The only differences between the three groups were the specific drugs necessary for NLA, halothane or continuous thoracic anaesthesia (Table 4).

Table 1. Biometric data in the three anaesthetic groups

	NLA		SD	Halothane		SD	Epidural		SD
Number of patients	23			22			23		
Age (years)	59.32	±	9.30	60.41	±	6.89	57.49	±	7.46
Weight (kg)	70.13	±	7.77	70.99	±	8.90	71.35	±	11.85
Duration of anaesthesia (h)	5.45	±	0.99	5.47	±	1.18	4.94	±	1.07
Risk group (ASA)									
1.	1			1			2		
2.	6			10			10		
3.	15			10			10		
4.	1			1			1		

Table 2. Volume replacement and infusion therapy in the three anaesthetic groups

	NLA		SD	Halothane		SD	Epidural		SD
Electrolytes ml	4059	±	1254	3918	±	1475	4828	±	1612
Volume replacement ml	2182	±	882	2140	±	846	2007	±	639

Table 3. Inspiratory oxygen concentration and minute ventilation in the three anaesthetic groups

	NLA	Halothane	Epidural
$N_2O : O_2$	50	50	50
Respiratory rate	10	10	10
Minute ventilation ml/kg ($\bar{x} \pm S_X$)	108 ± 9.3	108.1 ± 9.7	108.6 ± 9.1

Table 4. Duration of operation and medication in the three anaesthetic groups

	NLA		SD	Halothane		SD	Epidural		SD
Number of patients	23			22			23		
Duration of anaesthesia (h)	5.45	±	0.99	5.47	±	1.18	4.94	±	1.07
Total dose Fentanyl (mg)	3.43	±	0.99						
% Halothane in the vapour				0.91	±	0.54			
Total dose Diazepam (mg)							68.77	±	20.43

The anaesthetic technique, the procedures of measurement and the methods of statistical evaluation were recently described in detail [39].

Results

Haemodynamics During Aorto-Femoral Bypass Operation

a. Total Peripheral Resistance

It is possible to influence the total peripheral resistance in two ways: by decreasing the viscosity [14, 15, 34] and by changing the diameter of the resistance vessels. In this study both possibilities were used.

Viscosity. As the circulating blood volume in patients with arteriosclerotic disease was reduced [2, 6, 8, 35] and the patients were substituted intraoperatively with 4200 ml electrolyte solution and 2000 ml blood and protein solution. This led to a decrease of haemoglobin concentration from 15 g% to 12 g%.

Vasodilatory Effects of Anaesthesia. During anaesthesia and operation there were two characteristic response patterns of the total peripheral resistance. The mean rank transformed curves exhibited the following features: an increase in the NLA group and a decrease in the halothane and epidural groups (N : H $p < 0.04$; N : E $p < 0.06$) (Fig. 1).

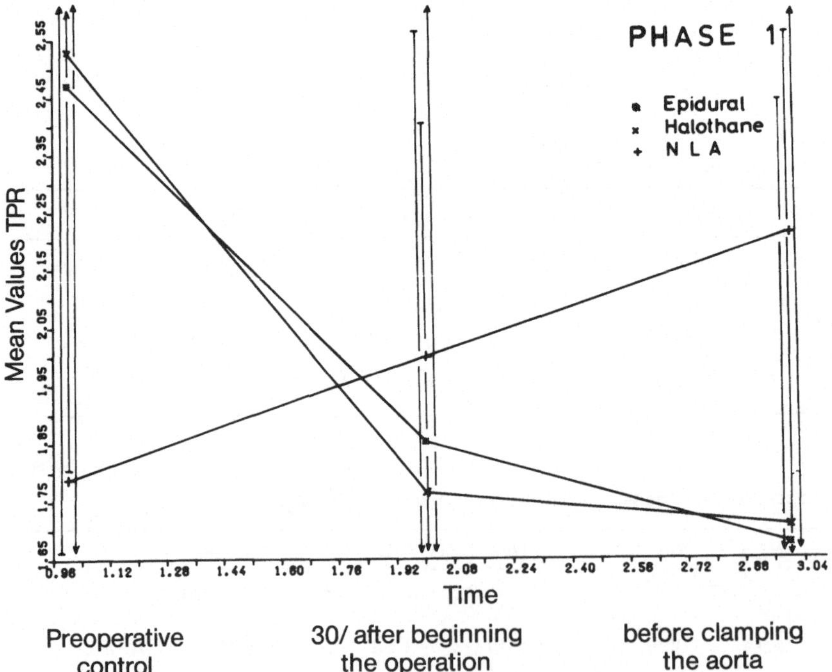

Fig. 1. Response patterns of total peripheral resistance (anaesthesia and operation)
In the means of the rank transformed curves there were two different reactions:
1. an increase in the NLA group
2. a decrease in the halothane and epidural group (N : H $p < 0.04$; N : E $p < 0.06$)
Tested by the Lehmacher-Wall test

Effects of Surgical Manipulation on the Total Peripheral Resistance. Clamping the aorta counteracted the lowered resistance in the halothane and epidural groups and enhanced the vasoconstriction under NLA. Thus the resistance was elevated by 20% in the NLA group in comparison with the preoperative control. In the halothane and epidural groups the total peripheral resistance increased to the preoperative control values again (Fig. 2). Because of the wide variations in the reaction under NLA (range from +1691 to –440 dyn sec cm^{-5}) there were no significant differences in the levels of the means (Fig. 3).

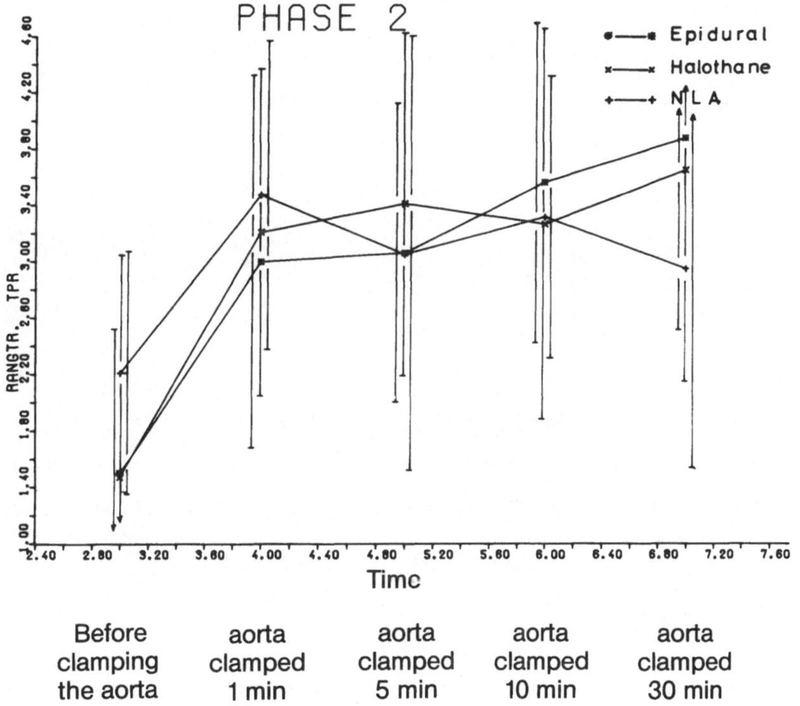

Fig. 2. Response of the total peripheral resistance to clamping the aorta.
There were no significant differences in the reactions between the three anaesthetic groups

Declamping the Aorta. The total peripheral resistance in all three groups was reduced by declamping the aorta.

While the effect was evident in the two phases of declamping under halothane and epidural anaesthesia, the total peripheral resistance increased again 5 min after the manoeuvre under NLA (see Fig. 3).

b. Arterial Mean Pressure

The changes in the total peripheral resistance influenced the level of the arterial mean pressure (Fig. 4). The parameter was nearly unchanged under NLA. There was a marked decrease in the other two groups, both in comparison with the preoperative control and with the NLA.

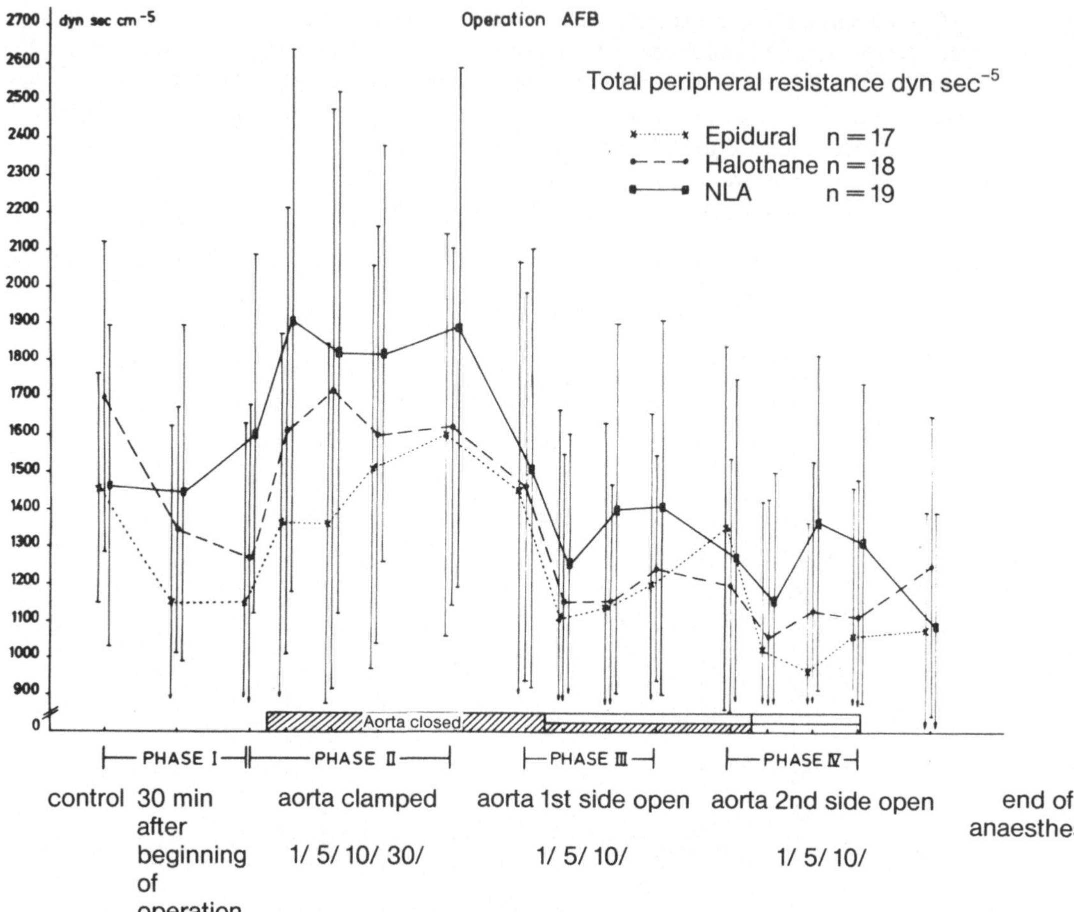

Fig. 3. Means ($\overline{x}$) and standard deviation (S_x) of the total peripheral resistance in the phase I-IV. The total peripheral resistance decreased after the induction of halothane and epidural anaesthesia and remained unchanged under neuroleptanaesthesia. These differences between the groups were abolished by the wide variance of individual reactions to clamping the aorta

Independent of the surgical manipulation the changes from the control were: under NLA –7.3 ± 7.7%; under halothane –19.4 ± 4.7%; and under epidural anaesthesia –23.8 ± 5.9%.

Effects on the Arterial Mean Pressure of Clamping the Aorta. The arterial mean pressure showed two characteristic responses to this surgical manoeuvre. The mean course of rank transformed showed (Fig. 5):

a) An initial increase with a following decrease under halothane and NLA,
b) No reaction in the epidural group (N : E $p < 0.009$).

c. Cardiac Index ($1 \ min^{-1} \ m^{-2}$)

The cardiac index was similar in the three groups during anaesthesia and operation (Fig. 6). When clamping the aorta the cardiac index decreased by 20% to the same degree in the three different anaesthetic groups.

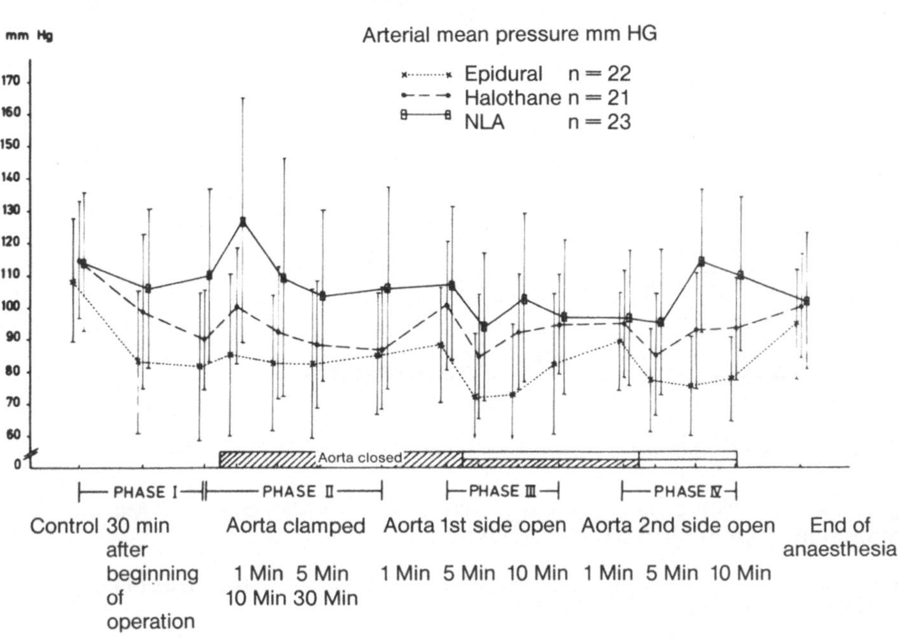

Fig. 4. Means ($\bar{x}$) and standard deviations (S_x) of the arterial mean pressure in the phases I-IV.
In the NLA group the mean arterial pressure was throughout the operation significantly higher than under halothane and epidural anaesthesia

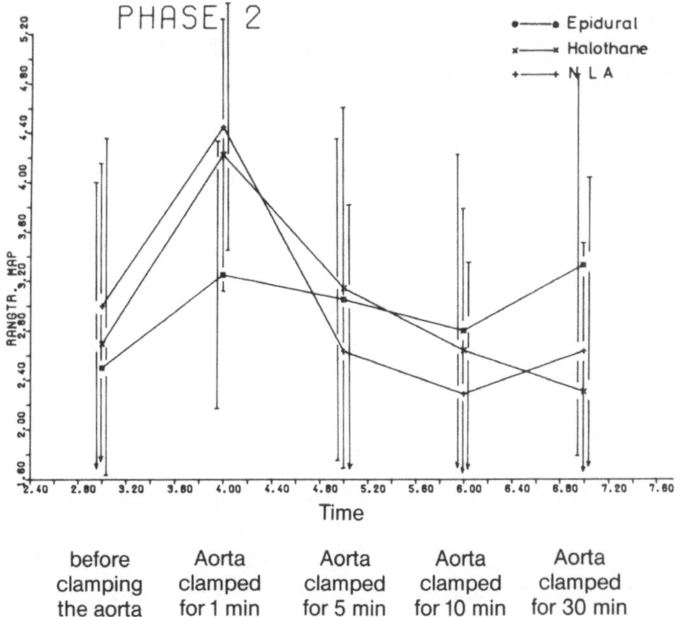

Fig. 5. Means of rank transformed curves of the arterial mean pressure in phase II (clamping the aorta).
There were two characteristic responses:

1. an initial increase with a following decrease under halothane and NLA,
2. no reaction in the epidural group (N : E $p < 0.009$)

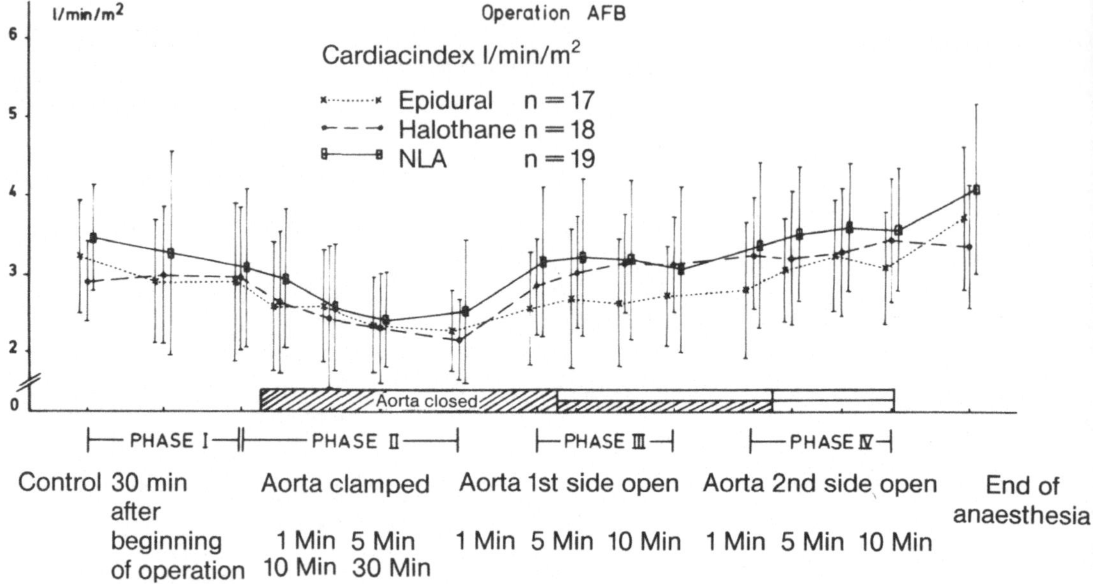

Fig. 6. Means $(\bar{x})$ and standard deviation $(S_{\bar{x}})$ of the cardiac index $1\ min^{-1}\ m^{-2}$ in the phases I-IV. There were no differences between the three groups

After releasing the two clamps the cardiac index increased slowly to the preoperative control again.

Frank-Starling Law Under Clamping of the Aorta. Alterations in the pressure-volume relation of the left ventricle by increasing the left arterial filling pressure give some information about the left ventricular function. To counteract the hypotension due to the release of the clamps, all patients were infused with 1 litre protein solution (human albumin 5% and/or plasma) when the aorta was still clamped (Fig. 7).

This induced a change in the preload of the left ventricle in all anaesthetic groups. Only under halothane anaesthesia however, as there a direct relation between the changes in the preload and the cardiac index (r = 0,61). No relation between the changes of the two parameters in the epidural group (r = 0.1) were shown, indicating the influence of other factors on this relationship, while NLA showed a tendency to an inverse relationship (r = –0.4).

d. Intraoperative Arterial PO_2, PCO_2 and Acid Base Balance

The arterial PO_2 increased intraoperatively to the same degree under the three anaesthetic regimens when the inspiratory oxygen concentration was increased to 50% (Fig. 8).

The PCO_2 in the arterial blood showed a different response due to the controlled ventilation. Under NLA and halothane anaesthesia the $PaCO_2$ was kept in the normocapnic range. In the epidural group on the other hand the $PaCO_2$ was significantly lowered by ventilating the patients with the same minute-volume per kg body wt. with which the respiration was maintained in the NLA group (Fig. 8).

The pH in the arterial blood was unchanged in the halothane and epidural groups until the declamping of the first anastomosis. This decreased the pH from 7.39 ± 0.08 to 7.31 ± 0.08 ($p < 0.01$) in the halothane group and from 7.39 ± 0.06 to 7.36 ± 0.07 in the epidural group.

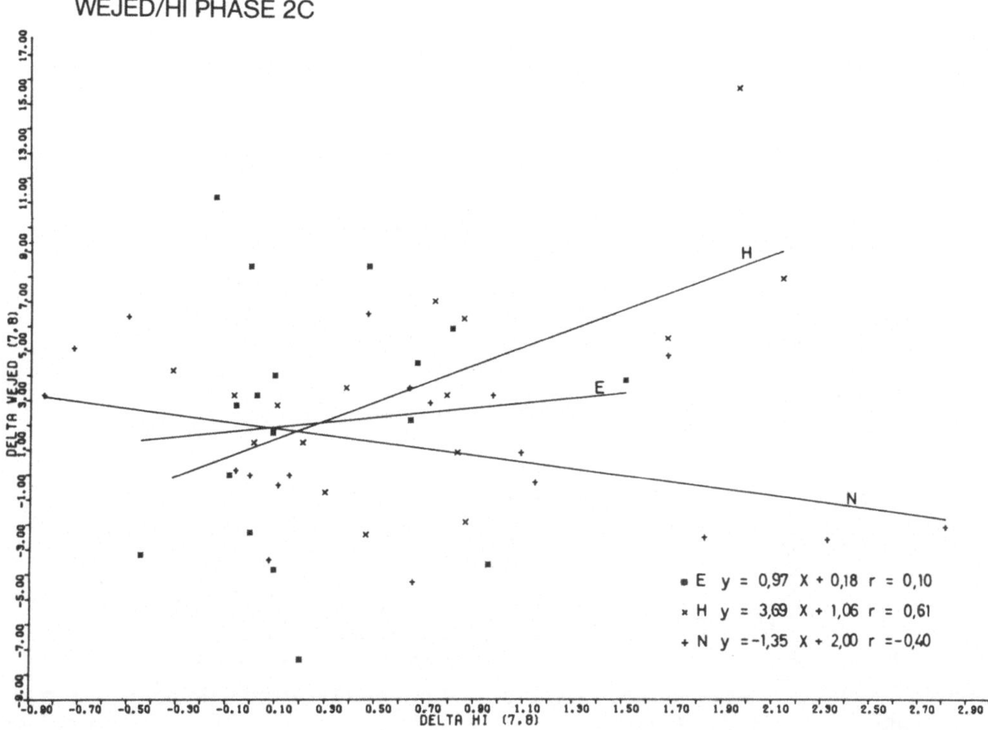

Fig. 7. Pressure-volume relationship between the changes of the left arterial pressure and the cardiac index, induced by rapid infusion of 1000 ml protein solution in three anaesthetic groups, the aorta still clamped (phase 2 c). By increasing the pressure load of the left ventricle the cardiac index increased also only under halothane. In the NLA group there was a tendency to an inverse relationship between the changes of the two parameters. In the epidural group the parameters changed independently of each other, making the influence of other factors evident

Declamping the second anastomosis enhanced this tendency to an acidosis only in the epidural group (pH 7.34 ± 0.07; n.s.), but it finally increased again. At the end of the operation the pH was in the normal range (pH 7.37 ± 0.06) only in the epidural group.

Discussion

Comparing the effects of three different anaesthetics – NLA, halothane and continuous thoracic epidural anaesthesia – on blood pressure, total peripheral resistance and heart rate, striking differences between the groups were found. By the significantly lower arterial mean pressure and total peripheral resistance both under halothane and thoracic epidural anaesthesia in comparison to NLA the hypothesis was supported that it is possible to lower the pressure and resistance work done by the left heart only by means of the anaesthetic regimen.

On the other hand, the cardiac index was not influenced by the different anaesthetics. These results were in contrast with some other investigations which showed under different anaesthetics a direct relationship between the arterial mean pressure and the cardiac index, while the total peripheral resistance was unchanged [2, 5, 22, 25, 26]. While in these studies

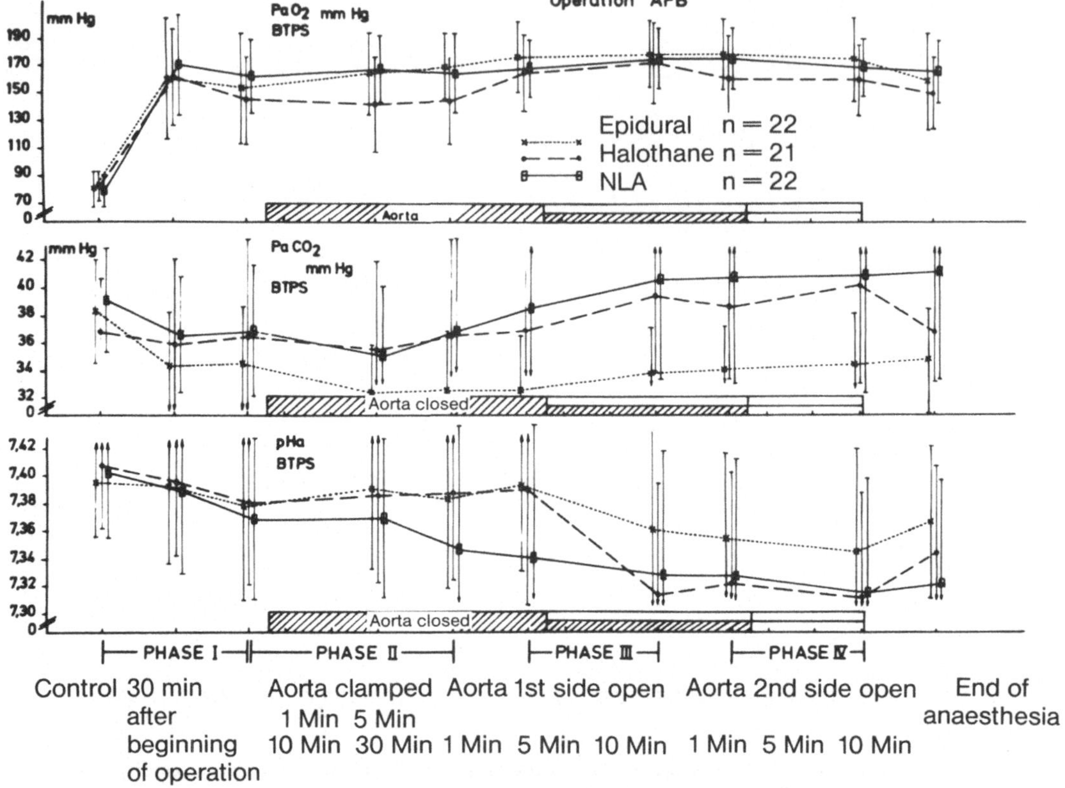

Fig. 8. Means ($\bar{x}$) and standard deviation (S_x) of arterial PO_2, PCO_2 and pH in the three anaesthetic groups in the phases I-IV.
The PCO_2 indicated in the halothane- and neuroleptanaesthesia normoventilation, in the epidural group hyperventilation.
While the pH was maintained in the normal range under halothane and epidural anaesthesia, showing after the release of the aortic clamps a "wash out" effect, the pH in the neuroleptic group fell continuously

an infusion therapy was not mentioned, it has to be considered that in patients suffering from hypertension or from arteriosclerotic disease, the blood volume is reduced [2, 8, 35, 36]. The negative effects of hypovolaemia on the haemodynamics were already pointed out by Renck et al. [28] for epidural anaesthesia and by Morse et al. [18] for halothane anaesthesia.

Taking this fact into account in the present study, a fluid replacement with 1000 ml cristalloid solution was started before the induction of anaesthesia. In accordance with the recommendations of Thompson et al. [35, 36] this was completed with a total amount of 4200 ml electrolyte solution and 2000 ml blood and protein solution during the operation.

By doing so while the aorta was clamped, a direct relationship between the preload and the cardiac index could be shown under halothane, indicating an intact Frank-Starling mechanism.

This does not exclude a myocardial depression by halothane in this study [17, 25, 26, 27], since a decrease in the afterload increased the stroke volume in the insufficient heart [37]. Although the afterload was reduced to the same degree by epidural anaesthesia as by halothane, no relationship between the preload and cardiac index could be found in contrast with other investigations [21, 28, 32]. It should be mentioned however, that our patients were hypocapnic. Therefore an impairment of the left ventricular function by respiratory alcalosis [13, 16] has to be considered.

Under NLA however, the arterial PCO_2 was kept within the normal range, the cardiac index tended to decrease, while the preload was increased. Thus some of these patients were unable to increase the stroke volume against the unchanged or increased aortic mean pressure [29, 30, 31].

This is in agreement with Attia et al. [1] who pointed out that patients with coronary heart disease did not tolerate increases in the afterload by clamping the aorta with an unchanged or already increased arterial mean pressure. Attia et al. [1] suggested therefore, that these patients would not develop a myocardial insufficiency, if the afterload was decreased prior to the clamping manoeuvre.

The results in our halothane group support this suggestion, although it seems doubtful in the presence of epidural anaesthesia and hypocapnia. Hyperventilation should therefore be avoided in these patients.

Declamping the aorta reduced the afterload by a decrease in the total peripheral resistance. At the same time the cardiac index increased stepwise again, indicating a restoration of the myocardial function.

Independent of the fact that the haemodynamic parameters in the NLA group showed the least changes, the pH decreased continuously from 7.40 preoperatively to 7.32 at the end of the operation, indicating a metabolic acidosis in this anaesthetic group [10, 11]. In the two other groups however, the pH was maintained in a normal range, while blood pressure and total peripheral resistance were reduced. The "wash-out" acidosis after declamping the aorta was at the end of the operation nearly compensated for in the epidural group. This indicates both under halothane and epidural anaesthesia the maintenance of an adequate tissue perfusion [20], while the absence of a wash-out effect and the continuous drop in pH under NLA indicates the contrary.

Conclusion

The results supported the hypothesis that it is possible to lower the pressure and resistance by means of halothane and thoracic epidural anaesthesia, maintaining an adequate tissue perfusion. By doing so, the haemodynamic changes, due to clamping the aorta, were better tolerated than in a group of patients where the blood pressure and the peripheral resistance were maintained at the high level of the preoperative control. These results furthermore show that blood pressure under NLA was kept stable by increasing the peripheral resistance rather than by increasing the cardiac output. Thus the trend in pH indicates an inadequate perfusion.

Diskussion

Frage: Es war mir nicht ganz klar, ob die Beatmung in den drei Gruppen wirklich gleich war oder warum die Patienten der Epiduralgruppe hyperventiliert waren.

Wüst: Alle Patienten wurden mit im Mittel 108 ± 9 ml/kg/m/min beatmet. Aus den niedrigeren Werten für das PCO_2 in der Epiduralgruppe muß auf eine verminderte CO_2-Produktion in dieser Gruppe geschlossen werden. Hierfür dürfte die deutlich niedrigere Körpertemperatur unter der Epiduralanaesthesie eine der Ursachen gewesen sein.

Frage: Sie empfehlen, mit dem Abklemmen der Aorta rasch 1000 ml Proteinlösung zu infundieren.

Wüst: Ja, und zwar am Ende der Abklemmphase kurz vor Eröffnen der Aorta. Dies ist eine allgemein anerkannte Maßnahme um exzessive Hypotensionen bei der Freigabe der Strombahn zu verhindern.
Frage: Warum beschränken Sie sich auf Proteinlösung, wo wir doch wissen, daß der Risikopatient ja einen erhöhten Bedarf vielleicht an Sauerstoffträgern hat, so daß doch die Gabe von Blutkonserven wichtiger wäre?
Wüst: Wir wählen deshalb Proteinlösung, da die Patienten schon im Verlauf der Operation einen sehr hohen Eiweißverlust haben. Dies ist einmal erklärlich aus den großen Wundflächen und der Beeinträchtigung der Zirkulation des Darmes durch die Eventeration. Bei der Rückverlagerung ist die Darmwand ödematös und das Darmlumen mit reichlich eiweißhaltigem Exsudat gefüllt. Selbstverständlich wird der Blutverlust mit Vollblut bzw. Erykonzentrat ersetzt, so daß der Hämatokrit nicht unter 30% bzw. der Hämoglobingehalt nicht unter 10 g% absinkt.
Frage: Sie haben bei der Neuroleptanaesthesie 12,5 mg Dehydrobenzperidol gegeben. Glauben Sie nicht, daß diese Dosis relativ niedrig ist und daß diese niedrige Dosierung eine relativ starke Zunahme des peripheren Widerstandes nicht verhindert. Ich denke da an die sehr hohen Dosen, die de Castro gegeben hat, bei denen es zu starken Abfällen des Blutdrucks und auch des peripheren Widerstandes gekommen ist.
Wüst: Sicher ist es möglich, durch hohe Dosen von Dehydrobenzperidol eine noch deutlichere Verminderung des peripheren Widerstandes zu erreichen, aber eine Dosiserhöhung verlängert nicht zwingend die Dauer der Kreislaufwirkung. Sie ist auf etwa 20 Minuten begrenzt, d.h. die Wirkung des Medikamentes hört dann auf, wenn wir sie am dringendsten benötigen, nämlich während der Operation. Auf der anderen Seite haben sie einen langen sedativen Effekt, der 6 bis 12 Stunden anhalten kann.
Frage: Herr Wüst, wenn ich Sie noch einmal kurz um Erläuterung zur Methodik in der Epiduralanaesthesie bitten dürfte. Wenn ich Sie recht verstanden habe, wurde auch die Periduralgruppe künstlich beatmet. In welcher Höhe haben Sie bei diesen abdominellen Eingriffen die Periduralanaesthesie gesetzt und in welcher Weise haben Sie die Intubation und die Bewußtseinssituation kontrolliert?
Wüst: Wir sind bei diesen Patienten bei TH8/9 eingegangen und haben einen Periduralkatheter 5 cm nach kranial geschoben. Dann wurden 5 ml Testdosis gegeben. Nachdem festgestellt worden war, daß keine Perforation oder eine Spinalanaesthesie vorlag, wurden 15 ml, also insgesamt 20 ml Buvivacain 0,5%ig ohne Adrenalinzusatz injiziert, und nach 30 Minuten Wirkdauer wurden die Patienten unter Gabe von Valium bis zum Erlöschen des Lidreflexes unter Zuhilfenahme von Succinylcholin (1 mg/kg) intubiert und dann anschließend mit einem Sauerstoff-Lachgasgemisch im Verhältnis von 1:1 beatmet.
Frage: Glauben Sie tatsächlich, daß die dabei angewendeten Valiumdosierungen keine Wirkung auf die Kreislaufreaktion hatten?
Wüst: Nein, selbstverständlich hat Diazepam eine Wirkung auf die Herz-Kreislauffunktion. Mit einer anderen Adjuvans sind andere Kreislaufreaktionen durchaus möglich. Wir haben z.B. Etomidate als Adjuvans verwendet. Dann ergibt sich im Verhalten des Blutdruckes etc. ein ganz anderes Bild. Das beschriebene Verfahren mit Diazepamsedierung ist im Moment unser Standardverfahren bei diesen Eingriffen.
Frage: Mich interessiert der postoperative Zustand dieser Patienten. Sie haben eine Gesamtdosis von etwa 60 mg genannt, bei der Neuroleptanaesthesie habe ich ja ein Antidot in der Hand, bei Diazepam nicht.
Wüst: Nach dem Eingriff, der etwa 5 Stunden dauert, wurden die Patienten extubiert und wach auf die Intensivstation gelegt. Sie verblieben dort in der Regel 3 Tage.
Frage: Wie war der Zustand dieser drei Gruppen, vor allem der Epiduralgruppe, postoperativ? Schlechter als bei den Vergleichsgruppen?
Wüst: Die Patienten, die intraoperativ eine Halothan- oder Epiduralanaesthesie erhalten hatten, waren in einem deutlich besseren Allgemeinzustand als die Patienten der Neuroleptgruppe. Die letztgenannte Gruppe hatte am 1. postoperativen Tag einen deutlich niedrigeren PO_2 im arteriellen Blut, der Abfall gegenüber der präoperativen Kontrolle betrug in der Neuroleptgruppe im Durchschnitt 28%, in der Halothan- und Epiduralgruppe maximal 12%. Außerdem fanden sich in der Neuroleptgruppe bei 16 von 23 Patienten Infiltrationen im Röntgenbild der Lunge, während diese Veränderungen in der Epiduralgruppe nur bei 5 von 23 Patienten zu beobachten war.
Frage: Warum wird bei Extremitäteneingriffen die thorakale Epiduralanaesthesie bevorzugt?
Wüst: Bei Extremitäteneingriffen wird im Lumbalbereich, d.h. bei L2-L5, bei Oberbaucheingriffen wird im Thorakalbereich, d.h. bei Thorakale 8-12 punktiert. Dadurch kommen wir immer mit 20 ml Bupivacain ohne Adrenalin aus. Wir erreichen bei Wiederholung der halben Einleitungsdosis gleicher Konzentration eine Analgesie von 5-6 Stunden, so daß wir in dieser Zeit mit einer Maximaldosis von insgesamt 30 ml Bupivacain 0,5% auskommen.

Frage: Sie haben die These aufgestellt, daß die Widerstandsentlastung durch die Periduralanaesthesie besser ist als bei den anderen Kollektiven mit Halothan oder Neuroleptanaesthesie. Aber ist sie nun auch besser als die Widerstandsentlastung bei Herzinsuffizienten, die man durch Natriumnitroprussid machen könnte oder auch macht?

Wüst: Wir haben keine vergleichenden Untersuchungen gemacht. Wir haben nur drei Patienten mit Nierenarterienstenosen, die in Epiduralanaesthesie und Hypothermie operiert wurden, zusätzlich Natriumnitroprussid gegeben, da die Widerstands- und Drucksenkung durch die Epiduralanaesthesie nicht ausreichte. Dabei wurde ein synergistischer Effekt mit Natriumnitroprussid festgestellt, aber ein direkter Vergleich wurde nicht angestellt.

Frage: Ist das nicht eine sehr hohe Dosis, 15 ml Bupivacain bei Th8, wenn man mit 8 ml denselben Effekt erreichen kann?

Wüst: Intraoperativ brauchen wir Muskelentspannung und das können wir mit 8 ml nicht erreichen. Postoperativ sind wir bemüht, den Block wirklich nur segmentär zu halten, so daß wir eine maximale Blockade zwischen Th5 als oberster Grenze und einer unteren Grenze bei L3/4 maximal haben. Dadurch hat der Patient die volle Sensibilität in den Beinen, er kann sie bewegen und auch zur Not laufen. Dies kann mit 8 ml einer 0,125%igen Lösung erreicht werden.

Frage: Für die Operation kann man mit Etidocain eine ausgezeichnete Muskelrelaxation erreichen. Sie brauchen dann eine geringere Dosis, machen keine totale Sympathikusblockade und postoperativ können Sie dann mit einer kleineren Dosis Bupivacain weitergehen.

Wüst: Da hier eine randomisierte Studie durchgeführt wurde, sind konstante Voraussetzungen notwendig und ein Wechsel von Medikamenten und Techniken unerwünscht. Man kann dies durchaus in der Praxis machen, aber wir haben dies hier nicht getan.

References

1. Attia RR, Murphy JD, Snider M, Lappas DG, Darling RC, Lowenstein E (1976) Myocardial ischemia due to infrarenal aortic crossclamping during aortic surgery in patients with severe coronary artery disease. Circulation 53:961
2. Brismar B, Borgenwald L, Cronestrand R, Jorfeldt L, Jublin-Dannfeldt A (1977) The cardiovascular effects of neuroleptanaesthesia. Acta Anaesthesiol Scand 21:100
3. Bromage PR (1969) The physiology and pharmacology of epidural blockade. Regional Anesthesia. Clin Anesth 2:45
4. Cohn JN (1973) Blood pressure and cardiac performance. Am J Med 55:351
5. Cullen DJ, Eger II EJ, Gregory GA (1969) The cardiovascular effects of carbondioxide in man, conscious and during cyclopropane anesthesia. Anesthesiology 31:407
6. Dintenfass L (1971) The rheology of blood in vascular disease. J R Coll Physicicans Lond 5:231
7. Forrester JS, Da Luz PL, Chatterje K (1975) Peripheral vasodilators in low cardiac output states. Surg Clin North Am 55:531
8. Guyton AC, Young DB, De Clue JW, Ferguson JD, Mc Caa RE, Cevese A, Tripodo NC, Hall JE (1975) The role of the kidney in hypertension. In: Berglund G, Hanssen L, Werkö L (eds) Pathophysiology and management of arterial hypertension. Lingren u. Söner, Mölndal
9. Keats AS, Jackson L (1963) Anesthesia for emergency cardio-vascular surgery. Clin Anesth 2:48
10. Lewis DG, Mackenzie A (1972) The effect of mild hypothermia and hyperventilation on acid/base balance in major vascular surgery. Br J Anaesth 40:1085
11. Lewis DG, Mackenzie A (1972) Cooling during major vascular surgery. Br J Anaesth 44:859
12. Lutz H, Müller C (1967) Erfahrungen mit der Neuroleptanalgesie bei Gefäßoperationen. In: Henschel WF (ed) Neuroleptanalgesie, Klinik und Fortschritte. Bericht über das III. Bremer NLA-Symposium. Schattauer, Stuttgart, S. 107
13. McElroy WT, Gerdes AJ, Brown EB (1958) Effects of CO_2, bicarbonate and pH on the performance of isolated perfused guinea pig heart. Am J Physiol 195:412
14. Messmer K (1970) Grundlagen der modernen Schocktherapie. Münch Med Wochenschr 9:357
15. Messmer K, Sunder-Plassmann L (1974) Hemodilution. Progr Surg 13:208
16. Monroe RG, French G, Whittenberger JL (1960) Effects of hypocapnia and hypercapnia on myocardial contractility. Am J Physiol 199:1121

17. Moran JE, Rusy BF, Verigvisces P, Luttanand S (1972) Effects of halothane-oxygen and innovar[R] – nitrous-oxygen on the maximum acceleration of the left ventricular ejection and tension time index in dogs. Anesth Analg (Cleve) 51:350
18. Morse HT, Linde HW, Mishalove RD, Price HL (1963) Relation of blood volume and hemodynamic changes during halothane anesthesia in man. Anesthesiology 24:790
19. Nobbe F, Dölp R (1976) Risikofaktoren in der Gefäßchirurgie. In: Ahnefeld FW, Bergmann H, Burri C, Dick W, Halmágyi M, Rügheimer E (Hrsg) Der Risikopatient in der Anaesthesie. 1. Herzkreislauf-System. Klinische Anaesthesiologie und Intensivtherapie, Bd. 11. Springer, Berlin Heidelberg New York, S. 89
20. Norden J (1974) The influence of anaesthesia on systemic vascular resistance during cardiopulmonary bypass. Scand J Thor Cardiovasc Surg 8:81
21. Ottesen S, Renck H, Vik-Mo H, Jynge P (1980) Koronare Durchblutung bei lumbaler und thorakaler Periduralanaesthesie (Schaf). Neue Aspekte in der Regionalanaesthesie. Wirkung auf Herz, Kreislauf und Endokrinium. Postoperative Peridural-Analgesie, Düsseldorf. In: Wüst HJ, Zindler M (Hrsg) Anaesthesiologie und Intensivmedizin, Bd. 124. Springer, Berlin Heidelberg New York
22. Otton PE, Wilson EJ (1966) Cardiocirculatory effects of upper thoracic epidural analgesia. Can Anaesth Soc J 13:541
23. Page JH, Corcorab AC, Duston HP, Koppanyi T (1955) Cardiovascular actions of sodium nitroprusside in animals and hypertensive patients. Circulation 11:188
24. Palmer KNV, Gardiner AJS (1964) Effect of partial gastrectomy on pulmonary physiology. Br Med J I:347
25. Prys-Roberts C, Kelman GR, Greenbaum R, Kain ML, Bay J (1968) Hemodynamics and alveolar-arterial PO_2 differences at varying $PaCO_2$ in anesthetised man. J Appl Physiol 25:80
26. Prys-Roberts C, Meloche R, Foex P (1971) Studies of anaesthesia in relation to hypertension I. Cardiovascular responses of treated and untreated patients. Br J Anaesth 43:122
27. Prys-Roberts C, Lloyd JW, Fisher A, Kerr JH, Patterson TJS (1974) Deliberate profound hypotension induced with halothane: Studies of haemodynamics and pulmonary gas exchange. Br J Anaesth 46:105
28. Renck H, Ottesen S, Jynge P (1976) Lumbal epidural analgesi på får – modifikationer av den hemodynamiska responsen av volymexpansion alt. adrenalin-tillförsel. Acta Soc Med Sued 85:65
29. Sarnoff SJ, Berglund E (1954) Ventricular function. I. Starlings law of the heart studied by means of simultaneous right and left ventricular function curves in the dog. Circulation 9:706
30. Sarnoff SJ, Case RB, Berglund E, Sarnoff LC (1954) Ventricular function. V. The circulatory effects of aramine: mechanism of action of vasopressor drugs in cardiogenic shock. Circulation 10:84
31. Siegel JH (1969) The myocardial contractile state and its role in the response to anesthesia and surgery. Anesthesiology 30:519
32. Sjögren S, Wright B (1972) Circulation, respiration and lidocaine concentration during continuous epidural blockade. Acta Anaesthesiol Scand [Suppl] 46:
33. Spence AA, Smith G, Harris R (1968) The influence of continuous extradural analgesia on lung function in the postoperative period. Br J Anaesth 40:801
34. Störmer B, Wüst HJ, Sandmann W, Kremer K (1978) Der Effekt von Operation, Narkose und Blutviskosität auf die Haemodynamik während der aorto-femoralen Bypassoperation. Anaesthesist 27:76
35. Thompson JE, Vollman RW, Austin DJ, Kartchner MM (1968) Prevention of hypotensive and renal complications of aortic surgery using balanced salt solution. Thirteen-year experience with 670 cases. Ann Surg 167:767
36. Thompson JE, Hollier LH, Patman RD, Persson AV (1975) Surgical management of abdominal aortic aneurysms: Factors influencing mortality and morbidity – A 20-year experience. Ann Surg 181:654
37. Urschel CW, Covell JW, Sonnenblick EH, Ross J, Braunwald E (1968) Myocardial mechanics in aortic and mitral valvular regurgitation. The concept of instantaneous impedance as a determinant of the performance of the intact heart. J Clin Invest 47:867
38. Wüst HJ, Zumfelde L, Sandmann W, Lennartz H (1975) Kardiorespiratorische Komplikationen nach aorto-femoralen Bypassoperationen. Vortrag auf dem Nordwestdeutschen Chirurgen-Kongreß, Hamburg
39. Wüst HJ, Sandmann W, Richter O, Godehardt E, Günter D (1978) Effects of neuroleptanaesthesia on haemodynamics and postoperative respiratory function in patients undergoing minor and major vascular surgery. Proc R Soc Med Intern Congr Ser Suppl 3:75

Koronare Durchblutung bei lumbaler und thorakaler Periduralanalgesie

S. Ottesen, H. Renck, H. Vik-Mo und P. Jynge

Der koronare Gefäßwiderstand wird durch ein internes Kontrollsystem gesteuert, das mit sogenannter metabolischer Vasodilatation antwortet [5]. Diese kann z.B. aus dem mit zunehmender Herzarbeit verbundenen, erhöhten Herzstoffwechsel resultieren oder von reduzierter Sauerstoffzufuhr zum Herzen, wie bei der Hypoxie, verursacht werden. Dieser Regulationsmechanismus bleibt nach chirurgischer Denervation des Herzens ungestört [10]. Als verantwortlich für diese koronare Vasodilatation scheinen Adenosin und Prostaglandine zu sein [6].

Vieles spricht dafür, daß es auch einen neurogenen Steuerungsmechanismus gibt. Es hat sich gezeigt, daß neurogene sympathische Reizung beim Hund koronare Vasokonstriktion verursacht [12], während cholinerge Stimulation in einer Dilatation resultiert [9]. Die Vasokonstriktion wird über koronare Alfarezeptoren vermittelt, die mittels Phentolamin blockiert werden können [17]. Koronare Betarezeptoren [4, 12] und dopaminerge Rezeptoren [2] sind wahrscheinlich auch vorhanden. Eine hormonelle Stimulation dieser Rezeptoren ist auch möglich, z.B. mit Sympathomimetika wie Noradrenalin [17], Isoprenalin [12] und Dopamin [16]. Es muß aber hinzugefügt werden, daß während der Allgemeinnarkose eine sympathische Reizung nur geringe Wirkung auf die Koronargefäße hat [15].

Bekanntlich kann die Periduralanalgesie (PA) sowohl die sympathische Innervation des Herzens beeinflussen, wie bei hohen Periduralblockaden [7], als auch die Arbeitsbelastung des Myokards herabsetzen, z.B. durch Reduktion der Herzfrequenz, des arteriellen Blutdrucks und der Kontraktilität [14]. Zur Behandlung der durch Periduralanalgesie induzierten Hypotension werden verschiedene Vasopressorsubstanzen verwendet. Wie schon erwähnt, sind dies alles Faktoren, die die Koronarzirkulation direkt oder indirekt beeinflussen können. Aus diesem Grunde waren Studien der Myokarddurchblutung (MBF) in Relation zum Sauerstoffverbrauch ($M\dot{V}O_2$) und zur Arbeitsbelastung des Herzens während lumbaler und thorakaler PA (LPA und TPA) von Interesse.

Methode

27 künstlich beatmete Tiere mit offenem Thorax wurden in Allgemeinnarkose untersucht. 8 Hunde und 10 Schafe wurden während der TPA studiert. 9 Schafe wurden während der LPA untersucht. Nach Induktion der PA kam es zur Entwicklung von arterieller Hypotension und Bradykardie bei allen Tieren.

Die Wirkung auf die durch die PA verursachten Herz-Kreislauf-Veränderungen wurde untersucht von:

1. 0,05 μg/kg/min Isoprenalin intravenös während der TPA beim Schaf,
2a. 10 ml/kg Dextran 70,
2b. plus nachfolgender Infusion von 0,01 bis 0,1 μg/kg/min Adrenalin während der LPA beim Schaf,
3. Phenylephrin plus Vorhofstimulation bis zum Erreichen der Leerversuchswerte von Herzfrequenz (HR) und systolisch arteriellen Blutdrucks (SABP) während der TPA beim Hund.

Die Wirkung von sowohl der PA allein als auch von den nachfolgenden Interventionen auf den MBF wurde bei allen Tieren mittels der Wasserstoffdesaturationstechnik untersucht, wie von Aukland et al. [3] beschrieben. Die Bestimmung der Wasserstoffkonzentration im Sinus Coronarius-Blut erfolgte polarographisch mit einer Platinelektrode, montiert auf der Spitze eines Sinus Coronarius-Katheters. Der MBF wurde von der Halbwertzeit der monoexponentiellen Desaturationskurve berechnet nach der Formel: MBF = $69{,}3/\frac{T}{2}$ ausgedrückt als ml/100 g/Min (Abb. 1).

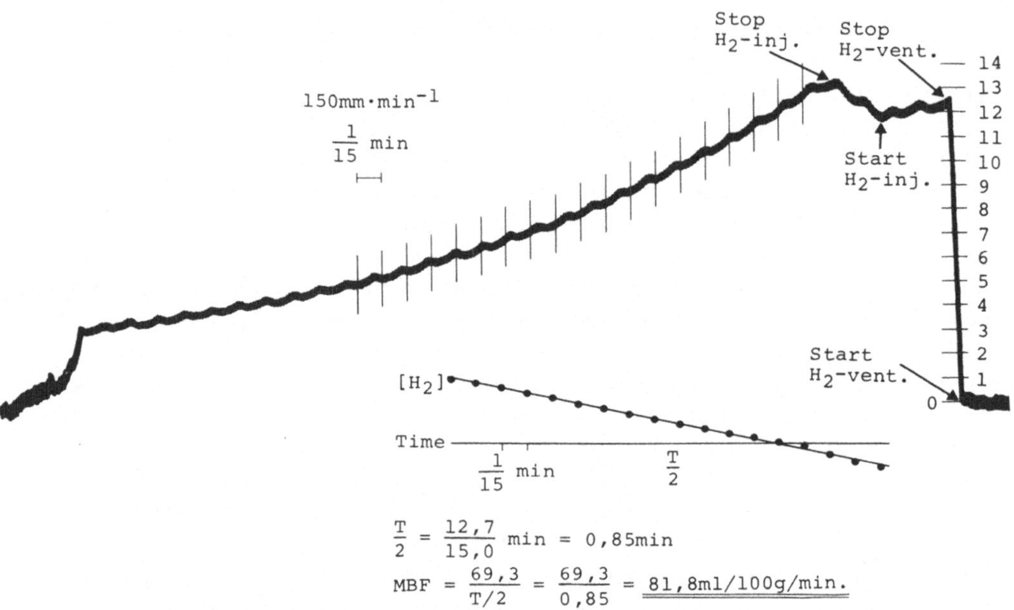

Abb. 1. Messung der Koronardurchblutung mit Wasserstoffdesaturationstechnik

Nach Bestimmung der Sauerstoffdifferenz zwischen Arterie und Sinus-Coronarius konnte der $M\dot{V}O_2$ berechnet werden.

Als Index der Herzmuskelkontraktilität wurde das links-ventrikuläre (LV) dP/dt max von der Druckkurve des LV abgeleitet.

Ergebnisse

Tabelle 1 zeigt prozentuelle Werte im Verhältnis zum Leerversuch von sowohl $M\dot{V}O_2$ und MBF als auch von HR, SABP und LV dP/dt max nach der Induktion der PA.

In dieser Untersuchung wurden allgemein während der PA sowohl der MBF als auch der $M\dot{V}O_2$ in engem Verhältnis zur Herzarbeit reduziert. Die prozentuelle Sauerstoffextraktion blieb unverändert. Die beste Übereinstimmung zeigten MBF und SABP als Indikator der Spannung des Herzmuskels. Nachfolgende Administration von alpha- und betastimulierenden Katecholaminen veränderte dieses Muster nicht. Dementsprechend bewirkte die Wiederherstellung von SABP und HR zu den Leerversuchswerten durch Gabe von Dextran plus Adrenalin

Tabelle 1. Verhalten von myokardialem Sauerstoffverbrauch, Myokarddurchblutung, Herzfrequenz, arteriellem Blutdruck und Myokardkontraktilität nach Anlegen einer thorakalen bzw. lumbalen Periduralanaesthesie im Tierversuch. (Angaben in % des Ausgangswertes)

	$M\dot{V}O_2$	MBF	HR	SABP	LV dP/dt max
TPA_{Schaf}	40	46	75	47	33
TPA_{Hund}	73	72	80	72	63
LPA_{Schaf}	57	63	79	68	60

während der LPA eine Restitution von MBF und $M\dot{V}O_2$. Das gleiche Ergebnis zeigte auch Phenylephrin und Vorhofstimulation während der TPA. Die Zufuhr von Isoprenalin während der TPA dagegen, welche zu einer Überkompensation der HR führte, aber einen bloß geringen Anstieg des SABP verursachte, restituierte MBF und $M\dot{V}O_2$ nicht. Eine schnelle Infusion von Dextran während der LPA, aus der nur eine geringe Zunahme des Blutdrucks resultierte, bewirkte gleichfalls bloß einen nichtsignifikanten Anstieg des MBF und des $M\dot{V}O_2$. Gleichzeitig wurde eine leichte Zunahme der Sauerstoffextraktion des Herzmuskels gemessen.

Diskussion

Ein paralleler Abfall des MBF und des $M\dot{V}O_2$ bei gleichzeitiger Reduktion des arteriellen Blutdrucks ist sowohl von Hackel et al. [8] während der Spinalanästhesie beim Menschen als auch von Amory et al. [1] während der LPA bei Rhesusaffen beschrieben worden. Lynn et al. [11] konnten keine kardiologischen Folgen nach höhergradiger arterieller Hypotension (etwa 40 mm Hg Mitteldruck) bei hoher Spinalanästhesie nachweisen; und dies trotz Erlöschen der Autoregulation des Koronarkreislaufes bei etwa 70 mm Hg [13].

Die Resultate unserer Untersuchung zeigten, daß sowohl die von der LPA als auch der TPA in Allgemeinnarkose verursachte Reduktion der Arbeitsbelastung des Herzens in einer entsprechenden Abnahme des MBF und $M\dot{V}O_2$ resultiert. Eine direkte Wirkung der PA auf die Koronargefäße schien weniger bedeutungsvoll zu sein. Die Zunahme der Herzarbeit und damit des $M\dot{V}O_2$, die eine metabolische Vasodilatation der Koronargefäße verursacht, scheint für die ansteigende Koronarperfusion während Katecholaminzufuhr bei der PA hauptverantwortlich zu sein.

Literatur

1. Amory DW, Sivarajan M, Lindbloom LE (1977) Systemic and regional blood flow during epidural anesthesia with epinephrine in the rhesus monkey. Acta Anaesthesiol Scand 21:423
2. Armour JA, Randall WC, Sinha S (1975) Localized myocardial responses to stimulation of small cardiac branches of the vagus. Am J Physiol 228:141
3. Aukland K, Bower BF, Berliner RW (1964) Measurement of local blood flow with hydrogen gas. Circ Res 14:164
4. Baron GD, Speden RN, Bohr DF (1972) Betaadrenergic receptors in coronary and skeletal arteries. Am J Physiol 223:878
5. Berne RM (1964) Regulation of coronary flow. Physiol Rev 44:1
6. Berne RM (1974) The coronary circulation. In: Langer GA, Brady AJ (eds) The mammalian Myocardium. Wiley, New York, p. 251-281

7. Bromage PR (1967) Physiology and pharmacology of epidural analgesia. Anesthesiology 28:592
8. Hackel DB, Sancetta SM, Kleinerman J (1956) Effect of hypotension due to spinal anesthesia on coronary blood flow and myocardial metabolism in man. Circulation 13:92
9. Higgins CB, Vatner SF, Braunwald E (1973) Parasympathetic control of the heart. Pharmacol Rev 25:119
10. Kent KM, Cooper T (1974) The denervated heart. A model for studying autonomic control of the heart. N Engl J Med 291:1017
11. Lynn RB, Sancetta SM, Simeone FA, Scott RW (1952) Observations on the circulation in high spinal anesthesia. Surgery 32:195
12. McRaven DR, Mark AL, Abboud FM, Mayer HE (1971) Responses of coronary vessels to adrenergic stimuli. J Clin Invest 50:773
13. Mosher P, Ross J Jr, McFate PA, Shaw RF (1964) Control of coronary blood flow by an autoregulatory mechanism. Circ Res 14:250
14. Otton PE, Wilson EJ (1966) The cardiocirculatory effects of upper thoracic epidural analgesia. Can Anaesth Soc J 13:541
15. Vatner SF, Braunwald E (1975) Cardiovascular control mechanisms in the conscious state. N Engl J Med 293:970
16. Vatner SF, Millard RW, Higgins CB (1973) Coronary and myocardial effects of dopamine in the conscious dog: Parasympatholytic augmentation of pressure and inotropic actions. J Pharmacol Exp Ther 187:280
17. Vatner SF, Higgins CB, Braunwald E (1974) Effects of norepinephrine on coronary circulation and left ventricular dynamics in the conscious dog. Circ Res 34:812

Diskussion

Frage: Haben Sie eigene tierexperimentelle Befunde dafür, daß Noradrenalin tatsächlich an den Koronargefäßen eine Vasokonstriktion macht?
Ottesen: Diese Untersuchungen sind von Vatner et al. (1974) gemacht worden. Das große Problem bei diesen Untersuchungen ist, daß nach Noradrenalin auch die Herzarbeit ansteigt. Um diesen Anstieg zu verhindern, wurde eine Betarezeptorenblockade gemacht und wurden in dieser Weise die Befunde erhoben.
Frage: Nach den Untersuchungen, die mir bekannt sind, gibt es im Koronargebiet überhaupt keine Alpharezeptoren, sondern ausschließlich Betarezeptoren. Und wenn Sie Noradrenalin intrakoronar geben, tritt keine Vasokonstriktion auf. Es ist richtig, daß die Herzarbeit ansteigt. Wir müssen ja bei der Koronardurchblutung die intravasale und die extravasale Komponente beachten.
Ottesen: Nach McRaven et al. (1971) macht Noradrenalin diese Konstriktion, aber die Alpharezeptoren haben für die Koronargefäße geringe, während die Betarezeptoren eine große Bedeutung haben. Aber ich meine, daß die metabolische Situation eine entscheidende Bedeutung für die Koronardurchblutung hat, d.h. wenn der Sauerstoffbedarf des Herzens ansteigt, dann steigt auch sekundär die Koronardurchblutung an.
Frage: Würden Sie sagen, daß die psychische Ausgangssituation des Patienten, d.h. eine Katecholaminausschüttung, einen Einfluß auf die Kreislaufsituation hat? Müßte man den Patienten mehr sedieren?
Ottesen: Das habe ich nicht untersucht. Beim Schaf ist das wahrscheinlich ein bißchen schwierig. Aber ich glaube, daß auch beim Menschen diese metabolische Vasodilatation wichtig ist, aber das sollte kein Grund sein, die Patienten mehr zu sedieren.
Frage: Herr Ottesen, wie erklärt sich der Unterschied zwischen Hund und Schaf bezüglich zweier wichtiger Parameter. Einmal des Sauerstoffverbrauchs und der Kontraktilität. Sind das Speziesunterschiede, die man nicht erklären kann, oder gibt es dafür Erklärungsmöglichkeiten?
Ottesen: Die Schafe haben hämodynamisch stärker reagiert als die Hunde. Beide Tiere hatten einen offenen Thorax. Bei offenem Thorax resultiert ein erhöhter Sympathikustonus, also der Sympathikustonus in der Ausgangssituation ist hoch und dann sind auch die hämodynamischen Wirkungen der Periduralanalgesie bekanntlich stärker. Aber es kann schon sein, daß es einen Speziesunterschied gibt.

The Effects of Regional Anesthesia on the Brain

J. Katz

There are three factors that have to be considered when discussing the effects of regional anesthesia on the brain. [1] The sequelae of blocking the sympathetic activity to the cerebral vasculature. [2] The effects of the regional technique on systemic blood pressure, and hence on cerebral perfusion. [3] The direct effects of local anesthetics on cerebral perfusion and cerebral metabolism.

It is practical to discuss the first two components together, i.e., the blocking of the sympathetics to the cerebral vasculature and the effects of the anesthetic on blood pressure, since that is what is usually produced in the experimental and clinical situation. There are, however, multiple studies in which stellate ganglion block alone, either unilateral or bilateral, have been performed in various subjects both on an experimental basis as well as therapy for the treatment of cerebral ischemic attacks or stroke. The preponderance of evidence is that when blood pressure is maintained, block of the stellate ganglion produces an increase in blood flow to the cerebral cortex. Although the percentage varies, an average of 15%-25% increase in blood flow has been reported by several investigators. Interpreted from a different point of view, one can state that a proportion of the cerebral circulation is under sympathetic control. In fact, the estimates of 15%-25% of neurocontrol over cerebral blood flow are compatable with available evidence. This should not be interpreted to mean that these procedures are beneficial to patients who have had strokes. In fact, the literature on this topic is quite controversial. The current opinion in the United States is that the use of stellate blocks for the management of stroke patients is of little clinical benefit.

If in the performance of a regional technique, only sympathetics which eventually join the sympathetic ganglion on their way to the brain are blocked (as in a cervical epidural), an increase in cerebral blood flow could be anticipated. However, the usual and common occurrence is a total disruption of sympathetic activity.

Cerebral blood flow is maintained over a range of perfusion pressures which vary from 60 to 150 torr. All authors agree that unless there is a profound reduction in cardiac output and blood pressure, the effects on cerebral circulation are minimal. When low spinal or epidural are performed, hemodynamic changes are almost nil. If however, the level is raised to T_1 certain changes are noted.

In Table 1 note the difference in the effects of a T_1 spinal sensory level versus a T_1 epidural sensory level. The epidural was performed with lidocaine without epinephrine. It is noteworthy that there are decreases in magnitude in arterial blood pressure and cardiac output with both T_1 spinal and T_1 epidural. The magnitude of the change was greatest with epidural. Concentrating on the cerebral blood flow, note that there was a smaller and nonsignificant change with T_1 spinal, whereas there was a 33% change with the T_1 epidural which was significantly different from control.

If one contrasts the effects of a T_4 epidural to a T_1 epidural, and compares the information in Table 1 with previous works [1, 2, 7], changes in cardiac output and blood pressure are reported to be smaller and less significant with the T_4 epidural.

Table 1. Comparison of peak effects of T_1 spinal anesthesia and T_1 epidural anesthesia without epinephrine (mean per cent change fron control)

	T_1 Spinal	T_1 Epidural
Mean arterial pressure	–23[a]	–47[a]
Cardiac output	–22[a]	–32[a]
Coronary blood flow	–19	–52[a]
Cerebral blood flow	–18	–33[a]
Renal blood flow	–36[a]	–37[a]
Hepatic blood flow	–23[a]	–40[a]

[a] Statistically significant change compared with the control for the same group (modified from Sivarajan et al. [6]

Sympathetic block after an epidural is, in essence, the same as the sensory level of the epidural. In other words, a T_4 epidural produces a T_4 sympathetic block in contrast to a T_4 spinal which might produce a total.sympathetic block. Obviously, a T_1 epidural which produces a total sympathectomy, also blocks the cardiac accelerator nerves, which come primarily from T_1 and T_2. Block of the cardiac accelerator fibers do not allow baro-receptor reflex activity to occur in response to systemic hypotension. Therefore, the effects of systemic hypotension which do occur at both levels of the block are better compensated for at the lower (T_4) level. Compensatory responses tend to return the blood pressure toward normal and maintain organ perfusion.

Another factor abbeeting organ blood flow may be the effects of the local anesthetics themselves. The literature says that local anesthetics have cardiac stimulatory properties. The usual blood level achieved after an epidural anesthetics is, on average, 1-2 μg/cc when lidocaine is used. Evidence in the literature suggests that small to moderate doses of lidocaine produce cardiovascular stimulation, whereas larger doses of lidocaine may depress the circulation. Our work in this area indicates that even large doses of local anesthetic do not significantly affect a large variety of cardiovascular parameters (J. Katz, unpublished work).

An additional factor is the presence of epinephrine in the solution used to perform an epidural. Epinephrine can have two effects: a direct effect on the heart which increases cardiac output and a peripheral effect which produces decrease in peripheral vascular resistance. This primary beta effect is reported with the low dose of epinephrine used during a regional technique. In one instance, blood pressure would be increased and in the other, the decrease in peripheral vascular resistance would tend to produce hypotension. There are papers which support both effects of epinephrine in human subjects. The consensus of opinion is that cardiac effects of epinephrine counterbalance the decrease in peripheral vascular resistance and tend to stabilize the vascular response to the block. A recent paper [3] takes issue with this stating that the hypotensive effects of epidural anesthetic performed with local anesthetic plus epinephrine tend to be greater than those performed wihtout epinephrine.

Of importance also is the direct action of the systemic concentration of local anesthetic on cerebral function. There is indirect evidence to indicate that when lidocaine levels are in the 2-4 gamma range, the effect on cerebral metabolic rate is minimal. Only when local anesthetic concentrations were maintained above 10 gamma/cc were any physiologically significant decreases in oxygen consumption noted [5].

In another study, Japanese researchers noted that a 40% decrease in blood pressure did not affect cerecral circulation or oxygenation. They did note that there was a slight shift in the lactate: pyruvate ratio indicating that at this level of hypotension some cerebral metabolic alterations occurred [4].

In summary, the effects of regional anesthesia on the cerebral circulation are minimal. Only when certain extreme conditions are reached, which involve suppression of whole body circulatory responses, does the brain appear to be adversely affected. A word of caution, however: Almost all studies that have been reported are in animals or humans with normal cerebral circulation. The same factors, if measured, in patients with compromised cerebral blood supply might be altered. For one to be anything less than ultra-cautious in the use of regional anesthesia in this group of patients would be to tread on unknown ground.

References

1. Bonica JJ, Kennedy WF, Ward RJ, et al. (1966) A comparison of the effects of high subarachnoid and epidural anesthesia. Acta Anaesthesiol Scand [Suppl] 23:429-437
2. Kennedy WF, Sawyer TK, Gerbershagen HU, Cutler RE, Allen GD, Bonica JJ (1969) Systemic cardiovascular and renal hemodynamic alterations during peridural anesthesia in normal man. Anesthesiology 31:414-421
3. Kennedy WF, Everett GB, Cobb LA, Allen DG (1971) Simultaneous systemic and hepatic hemodynamic measurements during high peridural anesthesia in normal man. Anesth Analg (Cleve) 50:1069-1078
4. Kusumoto H (1971) Effects of hypotension on cerebral function during epidural anesthesia. Jap J Anesthesiol 20:821-832
5. Sakabe T, Mackawa T, Ishikawa T, et al. (1974) The effects of lidocaine on canine cerebral metabolism and circulation related to the electroencephalogram. Anesthesiology 40:433-441
6. Sivarajan M, Amory DW, Lindbloom LE (1976) Systemic and regional blood flow during epidural anesthesia without epinephrine in the Rhesus monkey. Anesthesiology 15:300-310
7. Wahba WM, Craig DB, Don HF, et al. (1972) The cardiorespiratory effects of thoracic epidural anesthesia. Can Anaesth Soc J 19:7-19

The Effect of Sympathetic Block on Splanchnic and Renal Blood Flow

L. Wiklund

The greater part of the innervation of the abdominal viscera originates in the thoracic portion of the spinal cord. The sympathetic nerve fibres leave the spinal cord via the anterior horn. Here they are of the B type, that is, about 2-4 μ in diameter, and myelinated. The terminal neuron, which is adrenergic, has its ganglion cell in the sympathetic trunk or the coeliac ganglion. Through the coeliac plexus traverse numerous parasympathetic fibres in addition to sensory (afferent) fibres from the abdominal viscera. The ganglion cells of these sensory neurons are generally found at the site of entry of the dorsal root into the spinal cord. Conduction blockade of the sympathetic or sensory nerve fibres that pass to the abdominal organs can, in principle, be performed on two levels – either as an epidural or spinal block that attacks the nerves in their course of passage into or out of the spinal cord, or more peripherally, when the anaesthetic agent is deposited around the peripheral ganglia and nerve fibres. These peripheral nerve fibres are non-myelinated. From anatomical and etymological aspects it should be pointed out that blockade of the sensory innervation of the abdominal viscera cannot be called "coeliac ganglion blockade", since as far as is known this ganglion does not contain any ganglion cells of afferent nerves. Thus from this point of view the term "splanchnic blockade" or "coeliac plexus blockade" is more appropriate.

After Lennander [6, 7, 8] established at the beginning of this century that the sensory afferents and sympathetic efferents run alongside one another, surgeons of that time began to inject procaine around the coeliac plexus. Kappis [2] used an injection technique in which the needle was inserted through the patient's back, whereas Braun, somewhat later [1], described a method of performing the blockade through the open abdomen. It soon became known that splanchnic blockade lowered the arterial blood pressure. One result of this observation was that attempts were made to reduce the blood pressure therapeutically in hypertensive patients by dividing the coeliac plexus. Wilkins et al. [13] showed, however, that after a time the blood pressure rose again to the original level, but that during the time when it was decreased the hepatic blood flow was augmented. In the light of these results, and also of other findings in shock research on experimental animals, it came as a surprise when Kennedy et al. [3, 4, 5] published results indicating that epidural or spinal blockade induced with lidocaine without addition of adrenaline increased the vascular resistance both in the region of the intestines and liver and in the kidneys. This effect seemed even more paradoxical against the background of the reduction of the total vascular resistance in investigated human volunteers. There was indeed reason to ask what the difference was between sympathetic blockade of the abdominal viscera and the extremities.

In an attempt to find out how a more selective blockade affects the hepatic blood flow, a few years ago I began to study the physiological effects of splanchnic blockade in patients who had undergone elective cholecystectomy [10, 11, 12]. After the operation, before the patients woke up, catheters were inserted to the coeliac plexus, and were then used for postoperative analgesia. The effects of the blockade were evaluated by comparing measurement data after induction of the blockade both with preoperative findings and with postoperative data obtained before the blockade. During the latter postoperative measurements the patients thus had pain (Table 1). In addition, the results obtained from this group of patients were compared with those from another group who were given a morphine-like drug (fentanyl) for postoperative pain relief.

Table 1. Investigation programme

Periods	
I	60-90 minutes preoperatively
II	80-100 minutes after surgery (Blockade 100 minutes after surgery)
III	10-20 minutes after splanchnic blockade or fentanyl
IV	20-35 minutes after splanchnic blockade or fentanyl
V	45-60 minutes after splanchnic blockade or fentanyl

The results showed that the cardiac output, mean arterial blood pressure, total peripheral resistance and heart work all decreased immediately after induction of the blockade, whereas fentanyl had very little influence on these variables (Fig. 1). The already increased hepatic blood flow was maintained despite a reduced mean arterial blood pressure, and the ratio between the estimated hepatic blood flow (EHBF) and cardiac output increased – about 30% of the cardiac output going to the liver after the blockade (Fig. 2).

The blockade had no effect on the blood gases, in contrast to the morphine-like drug. On closer analysis of the results from the fentanyl group it was found that the pH decrease was not due solely to an increase in $PaCO_2$ but also to a slight metabolic acidosis (Fig. 3).

An important question for the clinician is whether the splanchnic blockade reaches the sympathetic trunk, so that the patient also has a sympathetic blockade in the legs. This question was examined by means of a galvanic skin response test, i.e. measurement of the skin's electrical resistance, which is affected by the sympathetic nervous system via the secretion of sweat. This test revealed that a partial sympathetic blockade had occurred in about 50% of the patients with a splanchnic blockade, and plethysmography showed that this sympathetic blockade had resulted in some increase of the calf blood flow (Fig. 4). In other words the splanchnic blockade is not completely selective.

Splanchnic blockade used in this way had a very pronounced clinical effect. Immediately after injection of lidocaine through the previously inserted catheters, the patient became calm almost immediately, whereas it took a longer time for fentanyl to have the same effect. Oxygen uptake decreased, and measurements of the splanchnic exchange of energy metabolites showed, among other things, that the glycerol concentration in the arterial blood decreased considerably (Fig. 5). As it is known that free glycerol in the blood comes from lipolysis initiated by noradrenaline from the sympathetic nervous system, and that noradrenaline release is increased in the presence of pain, these results indicate that splanchnic blockade has an analgesic effect of the same order of magnitude as that of the fairly large dose of fentanyl which we gave to the other group of patients. Thus, there is good reason in clinical practice to use splanchnic blockade as a complement to an intercostal block when good analgesia is required immediately after an upper laparotomy.

Yet another investigation of the physiological effects of splanchnic blockade has been undertaken, this time in collaboration with the Departments of Diagnostic Radiology and Inter-

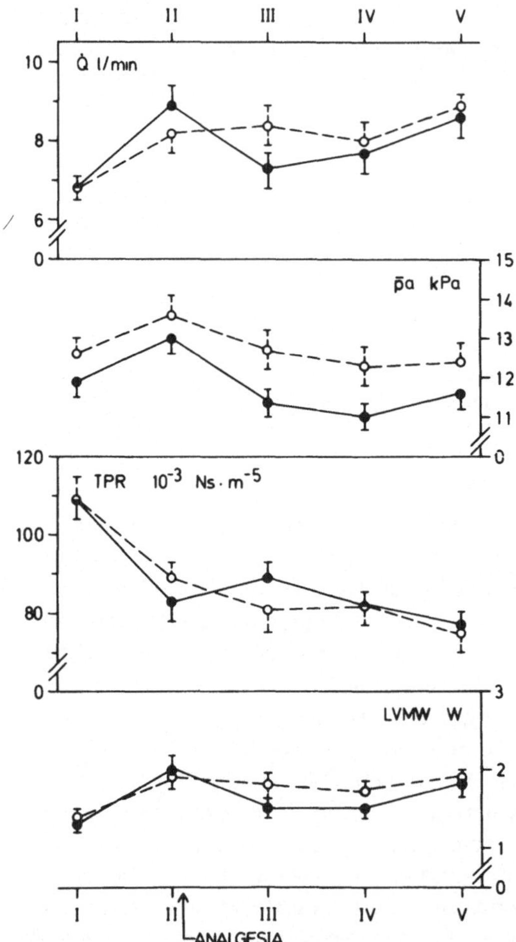

Fig. 1. Cardiac output ($\dot{Q}$), mean arterial blood pressure ($\bar{pa}$), total peripheral resistance (TPR) and left ventricular minute work (LVMW) during periods I-V in the blockade group (– • –) and in the fentanyl group (– ○ –). The values are presented as means ± the standard error. By courtesy of Acta anaesth. scand.

nal Medicine at our hospital [9]. Eigtheen patients were investigated in connection with selective renal angiography, which was being performed to establish whether their refractory hypertension had a renal origin. Catheters were inserted to the coeliac plexus under short general anaesthesia on the day before the haemodynamic investigation. Before the blockade the aortic blood pressure and renal blood flow were measured and blood was taken from the renal vein for determination of renin activity. After injecting 40 ml 0.25% bupivacaine (plain) through the catheters, all determinations were repeated.

Radiographic signs of renal arterial stenosis were found in nine of the patients. For analysis of the results these patients comprised one group, while the other patients, who were considered to have essential hypertension, made up a control group. As expected, the renal vascular resistance was correlated to the mean arterial blood pressure in both groups (Fig. 6). In both groups a minor fall in blood pressure was noted after the blockade, but the renal blood flow was not significantly affected. In other words the renal vascular resistance decreased. This decrease varied in magnitude, however, depending on the renal vascular resistance. The decrease was greatest in patients with a very high resistance before the blockade, and very small

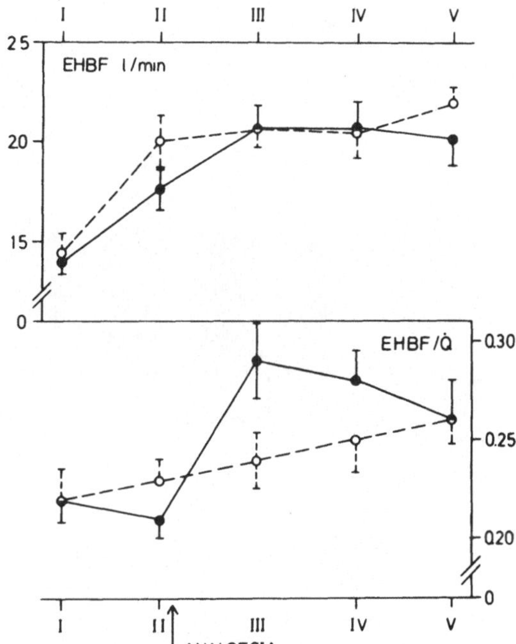

Fig. 2. Estimated hepatic blood flow (EHBF) and its fraction of the cardiac output (EHBF/$\dot{Q}$) in the blockade group (– ● –) and in the fentanyl group (– ○ –). The values are presented as means ± the standard error. By courtesy of Acta anaesth. scand.

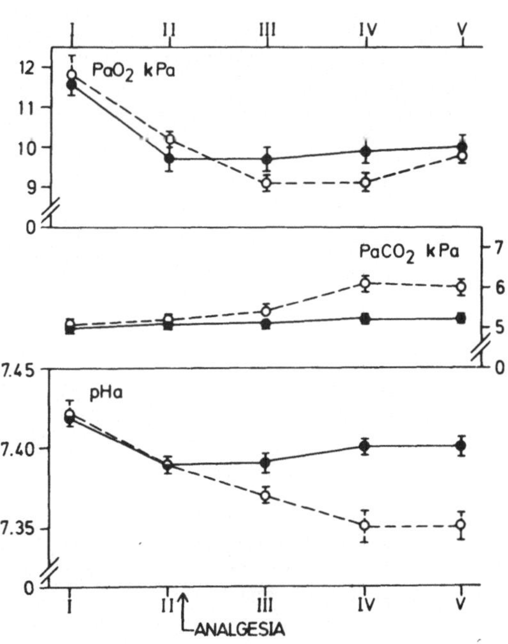

Fig. 3. Arterial oxygen tension (PaO_2), arterial carbon dioxide tension ($PaCO_2$) and pH in arterial blood (pHa) in the blockade group (– ● –) and in the fentanyl group (– ○ –). The values are presented as means ± the standard error. By courtesy of Acta anaesth. scand.

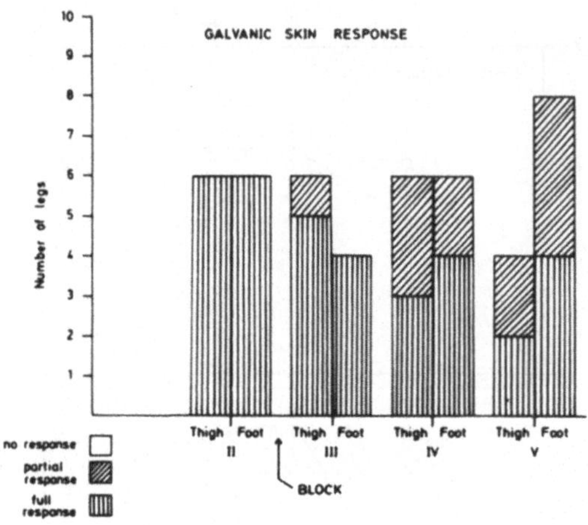

Fig. 4. Glavanic skin response in the legs before and after splanchnic blockade. Presence of galvanic skin response = no sympathetic blockade. By courtesy of Acta anaesth. scand.

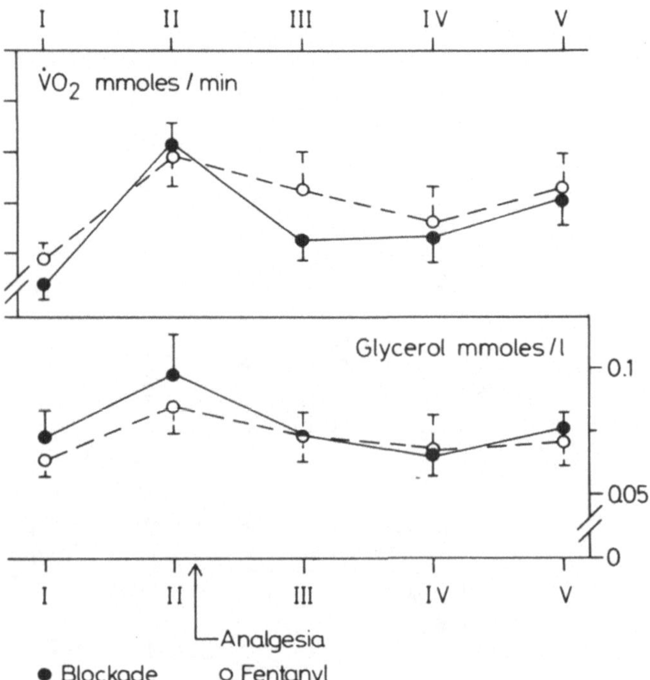

Fig. 5. The mean values and standard errors of systemic oxygen uptake ($\dot{V}O_2$) and arterial blood concentration of glycerol in the blockade group (– ● –) and in the fentanyl group (– ○ –) during periods I-V. By courtesy of Acta anaesth. scand.

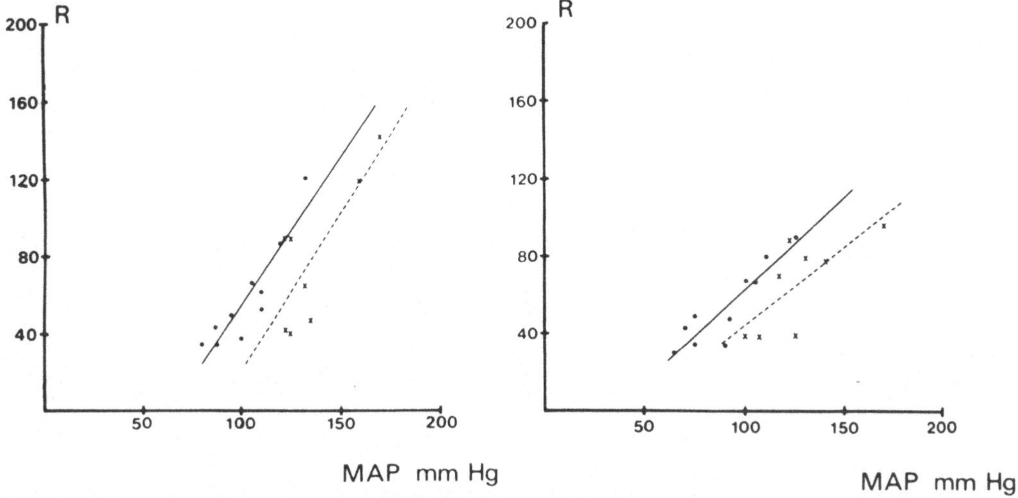

Fig. 6. Relation between renal vascular resistance R and mean arterial pressure MAP, left drawing presenting data before and right after splanchnic block. x = kidney with arterial stenosis; o = kidney without arterial stenosis; dotted line = line of linear regression kidney with arterial stenosis; bold line = line of linear regression kidney without arterial stenosis. Reproduced by permission of Scand. J. clin. Lab. Invest.

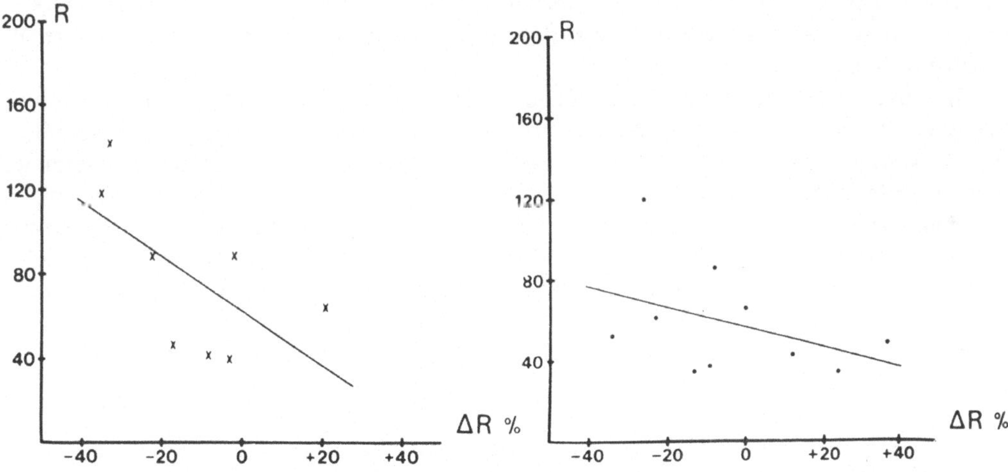

Fig. 7. Relation between initial renal vascular resistance R and relative change in resistance after splanchnic block ΔR (%). Left drawing showing kidneys with arterial stenosis and right kidneys without arterial stenosis. Bold line indicates linear regression. Reproduced by permission Scand. J. clin. Lab. Invest.

or absent in those with a low pre-blockade resistance (Fig. 7). Before the blockade the blood flow in the most rapid of the renal compartments – the compartment corresponding most closely to the renal cortex – showed a negative correlation to the mean arterial blood pressure in both groups; i.e. the renal cortical blood flow was lowest at the highest mean arterial blood pressures. This correlation disappeared after the blockade (Fig. 8). It may also be mentioned that the renin activity in the renal vein blood decreased in relation to the reduction of the

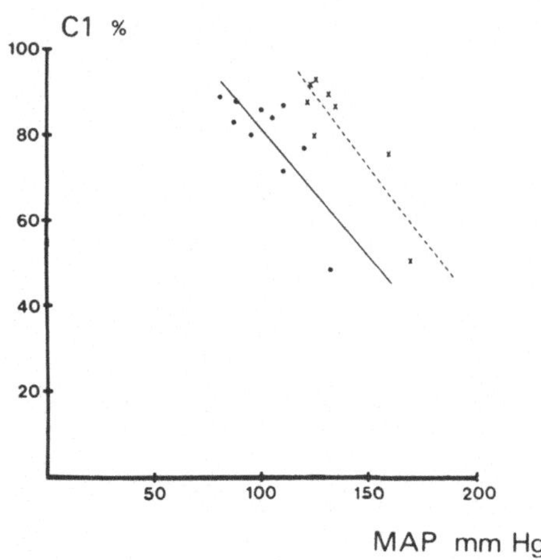

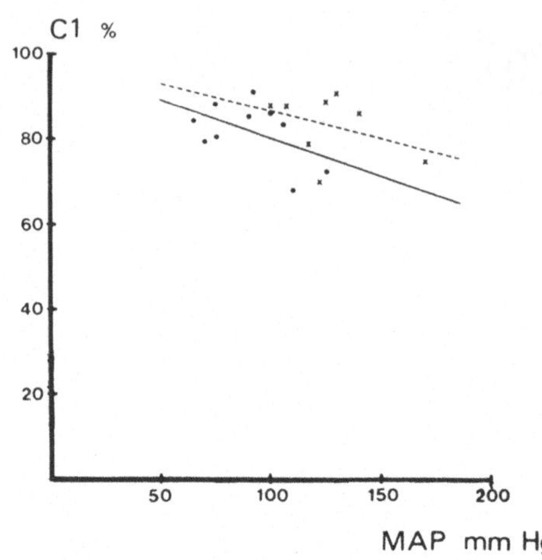

Fig. 8. Relation between relative proportion of the flow in compartment 1, C1%, and mean arterial pressure MAP. Left drawing before and right after splanchnic block. Reproduced by permission of Scand. J. clin. Lab. Invest.

total renal vascular resistance. Thus we found that the renal vascular resistance is influenced by the nerves passing through the coeliac plexus and that elimination of this nervous function results in an increase of the cortical blood flow in the kidney and a decrease of the total renal vascular resistance when this is elevated.

In summary, it may be stated that splanchnic blockade results in a decreased vascular resistance in the intestinal, hepatic and renal areas when this resistance is raised. Furthermore, this blockade provides a degree of analgesia which early after a cholecystectomy, for example, is comparable to that resulting from a relatively large dose of a morphine-like drug. In contrast to epidural and spinal blockade, splanchnic blockade does not cause a reduction of the hepatic and renal blood flows. Epidural and spinal blockade should not therefore be used therapeutically when it is the aim to increase or maintain the blood flow in the visceral organs by lowering vascular resistance.

References

1. Braun H (1921) Ein Hilfsinstrument zur Ausführung der Splanchnicusanaesthesie. Zentralbl Chir XLVIII:1544-1545
2. Kappis M (1914) Erfahrungen mit Localanästhesie bei Bauchoperationen. Verh Dtsch Ges Chir 43:87
3. Kennedy WF Jr, Sawyer TK, Gerbershagen HU, Cutler RE, Allen GD, Bonica JJ (1969) Systemic cardiovascular and renal hemodynamic alterations during peridural anesthesia in normal man. Anesthesiology 31:414
4. Kennedy WF, Everett GB, Cobb LA, Allen GD (1970) Simultaneous systemic and hepatic hemodynamic measurements during high spinal anesthesia in normal man. Anesth Analg Curr Res 49:1016
5. Kennedy WF, Everett GB, Cobb LA, Allen GD (1971) Simultaneous systemic and hepatic hemodynamic measurements during high peridural anesthesia in normal man. Anesth Analg Curr Res 50:1069
6. Lennander KG (1902) Beobachtungen über die Sensibilität in der Bauhhöhle. Mitt Grenzgeb Med Chir 10, 38
7. Lennander KG (1906) Über lokale Anästhesie und über Sensibilität in Organ und Gewebe, weitere Beobachtungen II. Mitt Grenzgeb Med Chir 15:465

8. Lennander KG (1906) Leibschmerzen, ein Versuch, einige von ihnen zu erklären. Mitt Grenzgeb Med Chir 16:24
9. Lörelius LE, Löfroth P-O, Mörlin C, Wiklund L, Åberg H (1978) Renal hemodynamics before and after splanchnic block in patients with hypertension. Scand J Clin Lab Invest 38:233
10. Wiklund L (1975) Postoperative hepatic blood flow and its relation to systemic circulation and blood gases during splanchnic blockade and fentanyl analgesia. Acta Anaesthesiol Scand [Suppl] 58:5
11. Wiklund L (1975) Splanchnic oxygen uptake in relation to systemic oxygen uptake during postoperative splanchnic blockade and postoperative fentanyl analgesia. Acta Anaesthesiol Scand [Suppl] 58:29
12. Wiklund L, Jorfeldt L (1975) Effects of abdominal surgery under general anaesthesia and of postoperative analgesic therapy on splanchnic exchange of some blood borne energy metabolites. Acta Anaesthesiol Scand [Suppl] 58:41
13. Wilkins RW, Culbertson JW, Ingelfinger FJ (1951) The effect of splanchnic sympathectomy in hypertensive patients upon estimated hepatic blood flow in the upright as contrasted with the horizontal position. J Clin Invest 30:312

Das quantitative Verhalten der Blutströmung in rekonstruierten Arterien in Abhängigkeit von Narkose- und Analgesie-Verfahren

W. Sandmann und H.J. Wüst

Einleitung

Die medikamentöse Blockierung der Leitung in den Nerven umfaßt bei der Peridural-Anaesthesie auch die Fasern des sympathischen Systems. Durch die Sympathikolyse kommt es zu einer Gefäßerweiterung im Blockadegebiet mit einer entsprechenden Volumenverschiebung. Wird der dadurch eintretende Abfall des arteriellen Blutdrucks durch rechtzeitige Volumengabe aufgefangen – und dies ist bei den Patienten mit arterieller Verschlußerkrankung aus vielerlei Gründen besonders wichtig – so resultiert eine erhebliche Mehrdurchströmung in allen arteriellen Segmenten, welche durch die Leitungsanaesthesie erfaßt werden. Da wir bei den Operationen an den Arterien ohnehin intra- oder postoperativ die Stromstärke durch die wiederhergestellte Strombahn mit dem elektromagnetischen oder mit dem gepulsten Doppler-Ultraschall-Verfahren messen, um den Operationserfolg haemodynamisch zu kontrollieren, konnte der Effekt der verschiedenen Analgesieformen auf die Durchströmung miterfaßt werden.

Material und Methode

Schon McDonald [5] hatte 1952 mit der Hochgeschwindigkeits-Kinematographie festgestellt, daß die Strömungsgeschwindigkeit in den Extremitäten-Arterien phasisch und bidirektionell ist: Er beschrieb systolische Vorwärtsgeschwindigkeit und diastolische Rückwärtsgeschwindigkeit (Abb. 1). Rückwärtsströmung in der Aorta in der frühen Diastole unmittelbar nach Klappenschluß als Ausdruck des Abstroms in die Koronararterien erscheint plausibel; aber Rück-

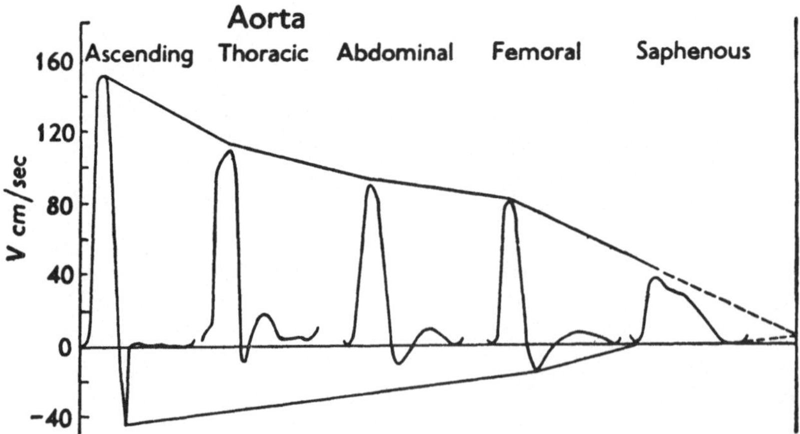

Abb. 1. Das Verhalten der pulsatilen Strömungsgeschwindigkeit in verschiedenen Abschnitten des arteriellen Systems. Der Rückwärtsfluß in der Femoralarterie ist besonders ausgeprägt (aus: Mc. Donald [5])

wärtsströmung in der Arteria femoralis des Menschen und dazu noch ausgeprägter als in der Aorta ascendens?

Das Phänomen war vor allem durch die Arbeitsgruppe um Wetterer [6, 9] am Hund längst näher untersucht worden. Extremitäten-Arterien sind Widerstandsarterien. Mit Zunahme des peripheren Widerstandes kommt es zur Reflexion der Flußwelle in der Peripherie und damit zum diastolischen Rückstrom.

Organarterien haben einen niedrigeren peripheren Widerstand (Abb. 2). Es gibt keine Rückflußwelle, wie die Beispiele von Messungen an der Arteria renalis und an einer RIOLAN'

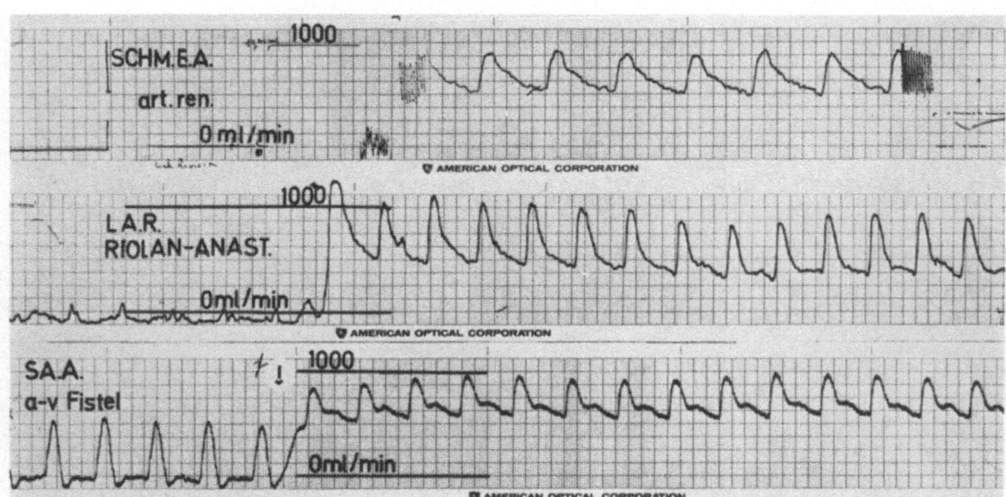

Abb. 2. Beispiele für niedrigen peripheren arteriellen Widerstand.
Obere Reihe Stromstärke in einer Arteria renalis (Pat. Schm. E.A., Arch.-Nr. 73/575),
mittlere Reihe Strömungsvolumen in einer RIOLAN'schen Arterie (Pat. La.R., Arch.-Nr. 74/2380),
untere Reihe Strömung in einer Arteria femoralis, welche zu einer arteriovenösen Fistel führte.
Im ersten Drittel der unteren Registrierung ist der arteriovenöse Kurzschluß geschlossen, es zeigt sich die normale biphasische Extremitäten-Widerstandskurve, die übrige Registrierung zeigt die Stromstärke bei geöffnetem Kurzschluß

schen Arterie zeigen. Wird durch einen Defekt in der Arterienwand, etwa bei einer traumatischen arteriovenösen Fistel, der periphere Widerstand gesenkt, so ist ebenfalls der systolische Vorwärtsstrom in der zur Fistel führenden Arterie hoch und der Rückfluß aufgehoben. Schließt man die Fistel, so ist die biphasische Stromstärkenkurve wieder meßbar.

Unter Ruhebedingungen und unter den Bedingungen der Allgemeinnarkose, das gilt besonders für die Neurolept-Analgesie in der Spätnarkose-Phase, ist der periphere Widerstand der Extremitäten-Arterien hoch. Eine Senkung des peripheren Widerstandes ist bei Gefäßerkrankungen zur Verbesserung der Perfusion der ischaemischen Gewebsbezirke und zur Erreichung einer höheren Stromstärke, welche einer Rethrombosierung operierter Gefäßabschnitte vobeugt, wünschenswert.

Zwei Behandlungsprinzipien finden zur Zeit Anwendung:

1. Verbesserung der Fließeigenschaften des Blutes zur Erreichung einer niedrigeren Viskosität und
2. die periphere Vasodilatation.

Letztere kann kurzfristig durch intraarterielle Injektion eines Vasodilatators, längerfristig durch die Leitungsanaesthesie und langandauernd durch die Sympathektomie erreicht werden.

Injeziert man in die Arteria femoralis Papaverin (0,5 mg pro kg Körpergewicht), so kommt es zu einer kurzfristigen, erheblichen Zunahme der Stromstärke (Abb. 3, hier von 300 ml pro Minute auf 1130 ml pro Minute). Die systolische Vorwärtsflußwelle vergrößert sich, und in der

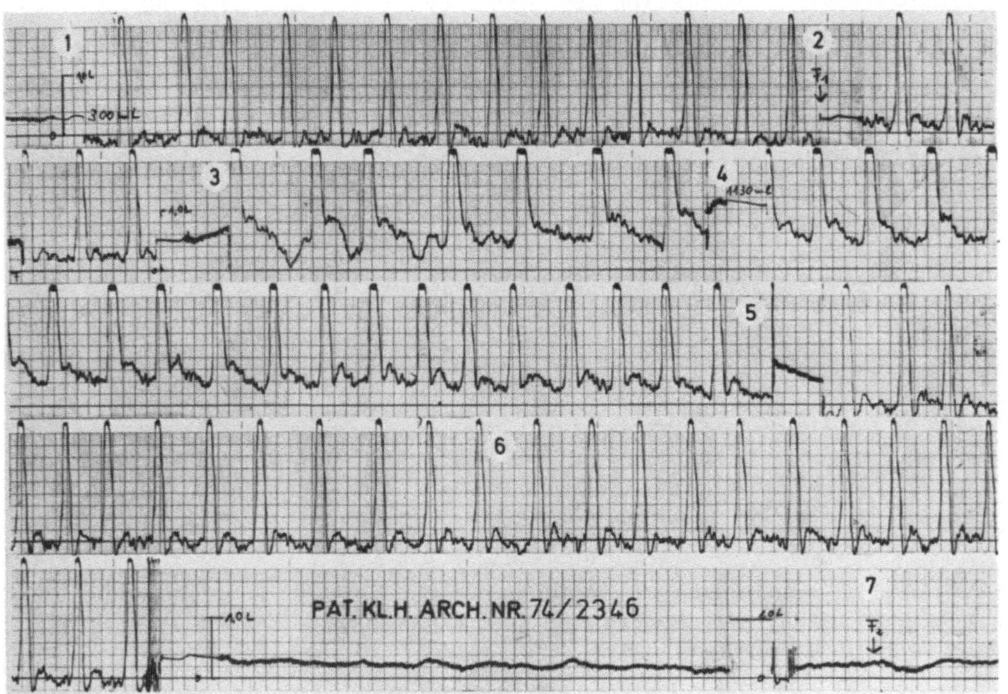

Abb. 3. Registrierung der pulsatilen Blutströmung in der linken Arteria femoralis eines 58-jährigen Mannes (Pat. Kl. H., Arch.-Nr. 74/2346),
15 cm Minuten nach Embolektomie in Lokalanaesthesie. (1) Unbeeinflußte Ruheströmung, (2) Injektion von 35 mg Papaverin in die linke Arteria femoralis, (3) Verlust der Rückflußwelle und Anstieg des diastolischen Strömungsvolumens sowie der systolischen Strömung, (4) maximale Mehrdurchströmung, (5) Abklingen der Papaverinwirkung, (6) Rückkehr der biphasischen Flußkurve, (7) Anzapfeffekt durch Injektion von 35 ml Papaverin in die rechte Femoralarterie

Diastole kommt es zur Strömungsumkehr mit Aufhebung des Rückflusses und ausgeprägter Vorwärtsströmung. Nach 5 Minuten ist der Effekt aufgehoben.

Wenngleich der Angriffspunkt von Papaverin und Leitungsanaesthetikum unterschiedlich ist, finden wir haemodynamisch eine gleichartige Reaktion. Während unter Allgemeinnarkose-Bedingungen entsprechend dem hohen peripheren Widerstand in der Diastole ein erheblicher Rückflußanteil in der Arteria femoralis besteht (Abb. 4), findet man unter Leitungsanaesthesie die monophasische Form der Flußkurve (Abb. 5). Auch während der Diastole liegt die Stromstärke deutlich über Null.

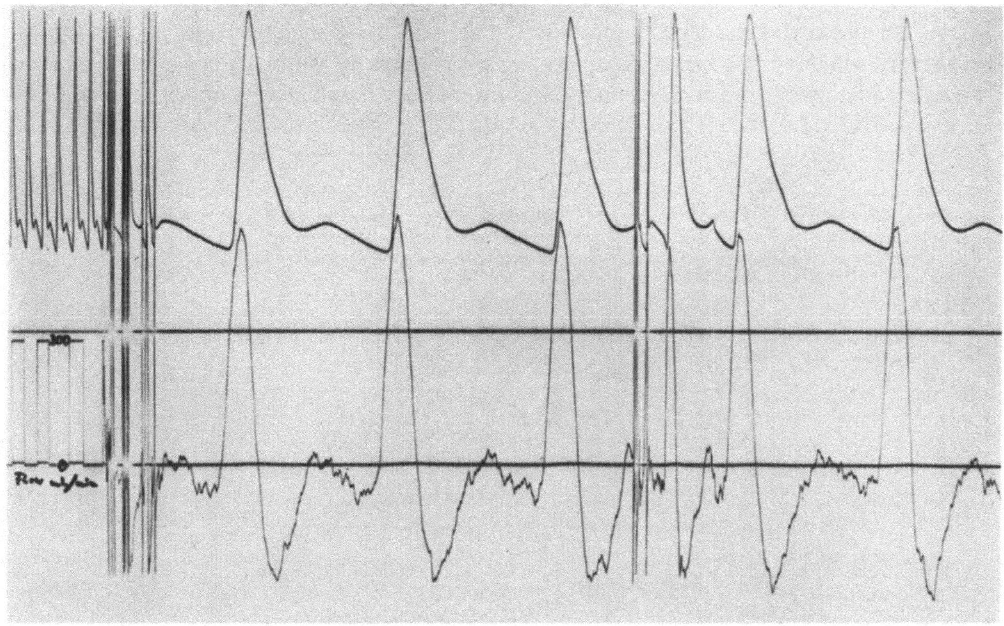

Abb. 4. Registrierung der pulsatilen Blutströmung (unten) und des phasischen Blutdruckes (oben) in der proximalen Arteria femoralis nach Anschluß eines distalen femorotibialen Bypass (Pat. Me. H., Arch.-Nr. 74/0164). Der effektive Vorwärtsfluß beträgt nur 40 ml/Min. Der hohe Rückflußanteil entspricht dem erhöhten peripheren Widerstand. Die Flußwelle erreicht vor der Druckwelle das Maximum

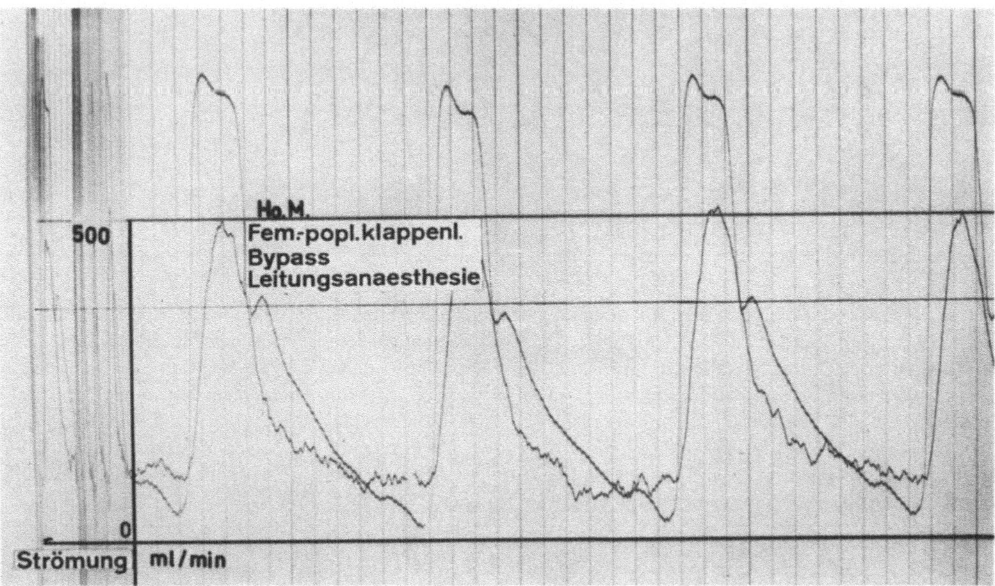

Abb. 5. Registrierung der pulsatilen Blutströmung (untere Kurve) in dem proximalen Drittel des femoropoplitealen klappenlosen Saphena-Bypass und des Blutdruckes in der Arteria radialis eines 65-jährigen Mannes (Pat. Ho.M., Arch.-Nr. 73/5010). Die Operation war in Leitungsanaesthesie durchgeführt worden, das diastolische Strömungsvolumen ist hoch, eine Rückflußwelle tritt nicht auf

Wie bei allen Effekten der Leitungsanaesthetika tritt die komplette Widerstandssenkung nicht sofort, sonderen in unserem Beispiel etwa nach 20 bis 30 Minuten ein (Abb. 6). Eine fortlaufende Registrierung des Systemdrucks (untere Kurve) und der Stromstärke (obere Kur-

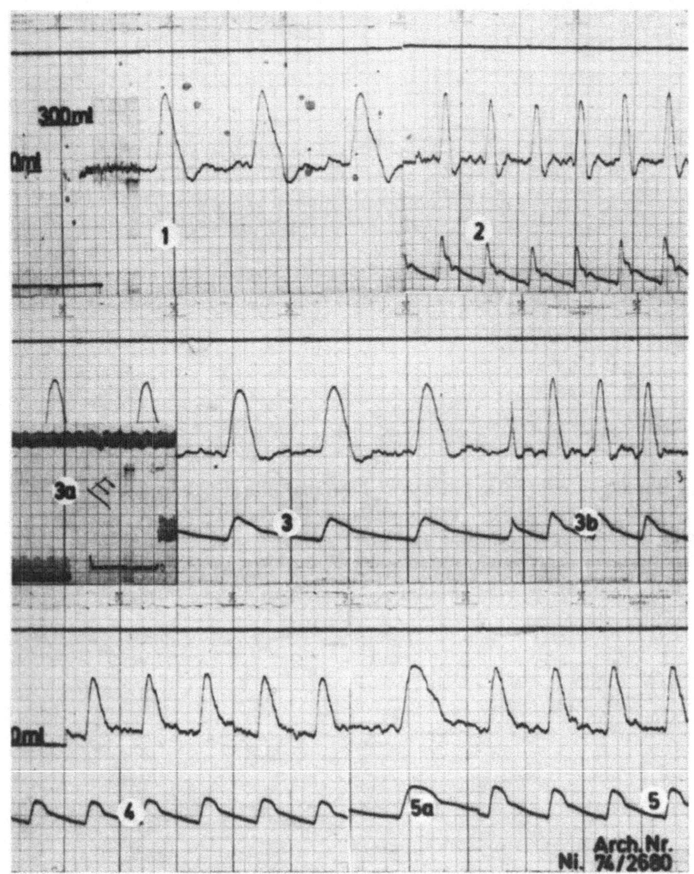

Abb. 6. Registrierung der pulsatilen Blutströmung und des phasischen Blutdruckes in der Art. femoralis bei einem 59-jährigen Mann (Pat. Ni.W., Arch.-Nr. 74/2680) nach aorto-femoraler Bypass-Operation beiderseits. (1) 20 Minuten nach Fertigstellung der Anastomose in Neurolept-Analgesie, (2) 5 Minuten nach Injektion des Anaesthetikums in den Periduralraum, (3) 15 Minuten nach Injektion eines Anaesthetikums, der Abfall des arteriellen Mitteldruckes um 28 mm Hg mach eine Anhebung des Meßbereiches auf dem Registrierpapier erforderlich. (3a) Die Rückflußwelle ist kleiner geworden, das diastolische Volumen steigt an, der Mittelfluß ist um 30% angestiegen. (4) 37 Minuten nach Injektion des Anaesthetikums: Deutlicher Anstieg des systolischen und diastolischen Volumens, Verlust der Rückflußwelle. Der Mittelfluß ist um 85% angestiegen, der Mitteldruck in der Femoralarterie liegt noch um 13% unter dem Ausgangswert vor der Periduralblockade. (5) 41 Minuten nach Injektion des Anaesthetikums ist der Ausgangsmitteldruck fast wiederhergestellt, der Mittelfluß liegt 132% über dem Ausgangswert. Der Abfall des arteriellen Mitteldruckes wurde mit 500 ml Ringer-Laktat-Lösung und 500 ml Macrodex ausgeglichen. Um die haematokritabhängige Anzeigen-Änderung am elektromagnetischen Strömungsmesser zu berücksichtigen, wurden mehrere Zwischen-Eichungen durchgeführt. (Beachte: (1), (3) und (5a) jeweils Registriergeschwindigkeit 5 cm/Sek., (2), (3b), (4) und (5) jeweils Registriergeschwindigkeit 2,5 cm/Sek.)

ve) in einer Arteria femoralis nach aorto-femoraler Bypassoperation zeigt, daß bei Ingangsetzen der Epidural-Blockade zunächst der Blutdruck abfällt und sodann die Zunahme der Stromstärke einsetzt. 15 Minuten nach Injektion des Anaesthetikums in den Periduralraum ist der arterielle Mitteldruck um 28 mm Hg gefallen. Gleichzeitig ist die Rückflußwelle kleiner geworden, das diastolische Volumen steigt an, der Mittelfluß nimmt um 30% zu. 41 Minuten nach Injektion des Anaesthetikums ist der Ausgangsmitteldruck fast wiederhergestellt, der Mittelfluß liegt 132% über dem Ausgangswert.

Für das gleiche Fallbeispiel ist der Verlauf von Systemdruck und Fluß während des Wirksamwerdens der Leitungsanaesthesie noch einmal graphisch aufgezeichnet (Abb. 7). Man erkennt zum einen die Wichtigkeit der rechtzeitigen, besser der vorzeitigen Volumengabe und zum anderen das inkongruente Verhalten von Blutdruck und Stromstärke. Obwohl der arterielle Mitteldruck noch fällt, steigt die Stromstärke breit an.

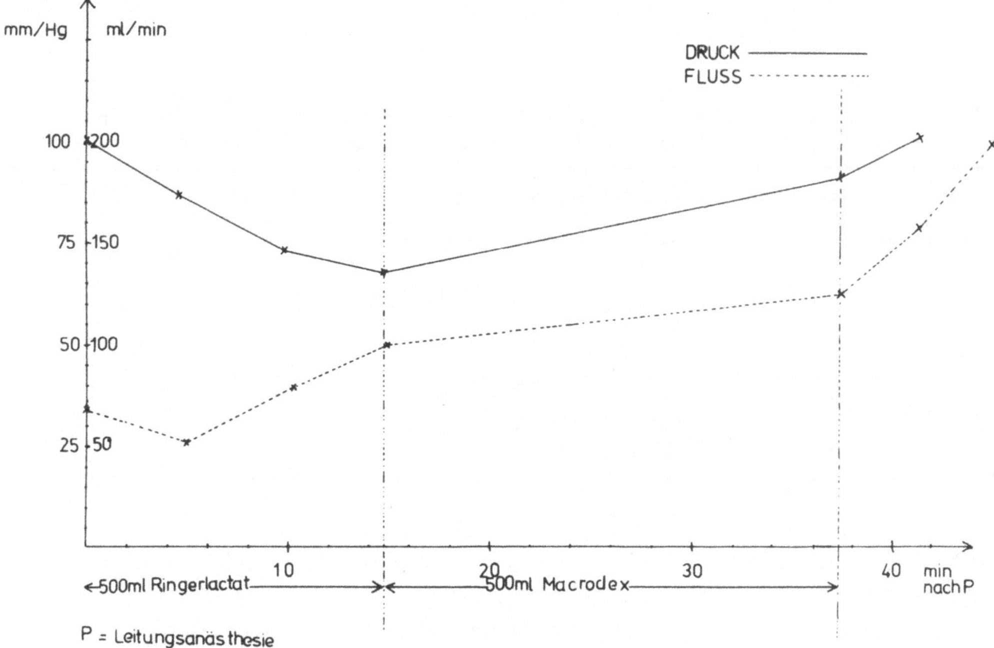

Abb. 7. Verhalten des Mitteldruckes und der mittleren Stromstärke in der Arteria femoralis des gleichen Patienten wie in Abb. 6. Beachte das inkongruente Verhalten der beiden Parameter während des Wirksamwerdens der Leitungsanaesthesie. Die lokale Senkung des peripheren Widerstandes macht eine Mehrdurchströmung auch bei erniedrigtem Mitteldruck möglich

Vergleicht man im nicht ausgewählten Kollektiv die Mittelwerte der Stromstärke nach arteriellen Wiederherstellungsoperationen am Bein, so ergibt sich zunächst ein deutlicher Einfluß der Kapazität der Unterschenkelperipherie (Tabelle 1). Bei drei offenen Unterschenkelarterien war eine deutlich höhere Stromstärke zu messen als bei einem offenen Anschlußgefäß.

Tabelle 1. Das quantitative Verhalten der sogenannten Ruheströmung in der Transplantatvene bei 30 funktionstüchtigen Transplantaten während der Operation in Allgemeinanaesthesie

Elektromagnetische Strömungsmessung (n. Kolin u. Wetterer)			
Allgemeinanästhesie		femoro-poplitealer Saphena-Bypass 30 funktionstüchtige Transplantate	
Gruppe Angio	Patienten N	$\bar{V}_{ruhe}$ ml/min	Bereich ml/min
III	14	152	80-230
II	10	122	70-220
I	6	71	65- 90

Tabelle 2. Das quantitative Verhalten der sogenannten Ruheströmung in der Transplantatvene bei 28 funktionstüchtigen Transplantaten während der Operation in Leitungsanaesthesie (siehe Text)

Elektromagnetische Strömungsmessung (n. Kolin u. Wetterer)			
Leitungsanästhesie		femoro-politealer Saphena-Bypass 28 funktionstüchtige Transplantate	
Gruppe Angio	Patienten N	$\bar{V}_{ruhe}$ ml/min	Bereich ml/min
III	10	162	120-250
II	12	144	110-240
I	6	98	87-120

Der Einfluß der Leitungsanaesthesie machte sich ebenfalls durch höhere Stromstärke bemerkbar, die Mittelwerte lagen im Durchschnitt um 20 ml pro Minute höher (Tabelle 2).
Daß neben dem anatomischen Zustand der peripheren Arterien auch die Narkoseform die Stromstärke in der zugehörigen Transportarterie beeinflußt, wird durch Messungen an aorto-femoralen Bypass-Transplantaten besonders deutlich (Tabelle 3). Wir kennen zwei Verschlußtypen. Im Falle A werden Stenosen oder Verschlüsse der Beckenstrombahn überbrückt, der Abstrom des Bypass kann in die Arteria femoralis und Arteria profunda femoris erfolgen, beide Gefäße sind offen.

Entsprechend ist die Stromstärke im Transplantat-Schenkel hoch. Im Falle AB steht für den Abstrom nur die Arteria profunda femoris zur Verfügung, die Arteria femoralis ist verschlossen, was ohne weiteres an den niedrigeren Stromstärkewerten kenntlich wird. Die Standardabweichung weist jedoch eine erhebliche Streuung aus. Die Kollektive werden erst homogener, wenn zusätzlich die Aufteilung in Patienten mit Allgemein- (A) oder Leitungsanaesthesie (L) erfolgt. Die mittlere Stromstärke für die Fälle, welche in Leitungsanaesthesie operiert wurden, liegt um 80% bzw. 130% höher als in der Vergleichsgruppe.

Auch in der postoperativen Phase hat die Analgesieform einen erheblichen Einfluß auf die Stromstärke im rekonstruierten Arterienabschnitt (Abb. 8). Im Rahmen der postoperativen Funktionskontrolle haben wir bei 50 Patienten mit femoro-poplitealem Venenbypass den Strö-

Tabelle 3. Im linken oberen Abschnitt der Tab. sind die von 39 Transplantaten gemittelten Ruheströmungsvolumina bei Patienten mit isoliertem Beckenarterienverschluß = Gruppe A und bei Patienten mit gleichzeitig bestehendem, zum Zeitpunkt der Messung nicht korrigiertem Verschluß der Arteria femoralis = AB dargestellt. Die Standardabweichung F zeigt die breite Streuung der Einzelwerte.
Im linken unteren Tab.-Abschnitt sind die gleichen Patienten jeweils nach Operation in Allgemeinanaesthesie „A" oder Leitungsanaesthesie „L" dargestellt. Die abnehmende Standardabweichung bestätigt die Annahme, daß die absoluten Ruheströmungswerte größere Aussagekraft haben, wenn neben der Gefäßperipherie gleichzeitig die Narkoseform mit berücksichtigt wird. Bei Operationen in Allgemeinanaesthesie ergaben sich deutlich niedrigere Stromstärkewerte.
Im re. Abschnitt der Tab. sind jeweils die Stromstärkewerte nach Injektion einer standardisierten Papaverindosis in die rekonstruierte Art. wiedergegeben. Auch zeigt sich, daß die erreichbare Mehrdurchströmung nicht nur von der Kapazität der Peripherie abhängig ist, sondern ebenfalls von dem Narkoseverfahren abhängig ist. Beachte die deutlich höheren Durchströmungswerte für Operationen in Leitungsanaesthesie. (Aus: Sandmann et al. [8])

Elektromagnetische Strömungsmessung (n. Kolin u. Wetterer)						
	aorto-femoraler Bypass Narkoseeinfluß					
Verschlußtyp	Ruheströmung $\bar{V}$(ml/min)	S(ml/min)	n	Mehrströmung $\bar{V}$(ml/min)	S(ml/min)	n
A	384	201	19	809	386	19
AB	195	98	20	309	157	20
A_A	291	144	8	589	256	8
A_L	453	214	11	901	403	11
AB_A	109	34	7	180	49	7
AB_L	241	89	13	378	152	13

mungsaufnehmer um das Transplantat bis zu 4 Tage belassen. Bei 12 Patienten war der Erfolg der Rekonstruktion durch das Auftreten kräftiger Fußpulse am Operationstag sofort eindeutig, der Strömungsaufnehmer wurde deshalb sofort entfernt. In 8 weiteren Fällen hatte sich der Strömungsaufnehmer versehentlich vom Bypass gelöst und wurde wegen Funktionsuntüchtigkeit entfernt. Bei 4 Patienten trat ein Frühverschluß ein. Bei der Zusammenstellung der Meßwerte von den 26 funktionstüchtig gebliebenen und mehrtägig gemessenen Transplantaten in Abhängigkeit von der Analgesieform – es handelte sich um 16 Patienten mit postoperativer kontinuierlicher Epidural-Blockade und um 10 Patienten mit Schmerzausschaltung durch Dolantin – ergaben sich für die Patienten mit Leitungsanalgesie deutlich höhere Stromstärken, hier ausgedrückt in Prozent der intraoperativ gemessenen Ruhedurchströmung.

Abschließend soll noch der Einfluß von Schmerz – und Volumenverlust an zwei Einzelbeispielen gezeigt werden. Im ersten Falle wird der Einfluß des postoperativen Wundschmerzes auf die Strömung im femoro-poplitealen Venenbypass am ersten postoperativen Tag demonstriert (Abb. 9). Die obere Kurve entspricht jeweils der pulsatilen Stromstärke, die untere Kurve jeweils der gemittelten Stromstärke, infolge der geringen Papiergeschwindigkeit ist eine Wischkurve entstanden. Bei ineffektiver kontinuierlicher Epiduralblockade war es zum Auftreten von Schmerzen verbunden mit deutlicher Abnahme der Bypass-Durchströmung gekommen, dieser Effekt ist nach Wiedereintritt der Analgesie verschwunden.

Der Einfluß des postoperativen Wundschmerzes in Kombination mit Volumenmangel auf die Strömung im femoro-poplitealen Venenbypass am Abend des Operationstages wird in

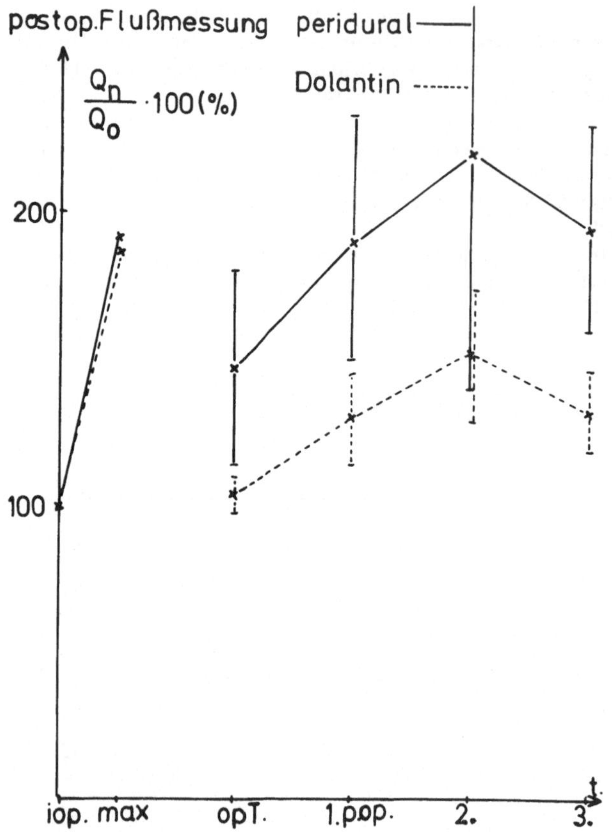

Abb. 8. Verhalten der postoperativen Ruheströmung (Basalströmung) in 26 funktionstüchtig gebliebenen femoro-poplitealen Venentransplantaten in Abhängigkeit von der postoperativen Analgesie. 16 Fälle mit Epiduralanalgesie und 10 Fälle mit Dolantinanalgesie. Beachte die deutlich höhere Ruheströmung bei Patientin mit Leitungsanalgesie. (Ordinate: Veränderung der Stromstärke ausgedrückt in % der Ruheströmung, welche intraoperativ gemessen wurde. Abszisse: zeitlicher Verlauf bis zum 3. postoperativen Tag)

Abb. 10 deutlich. Nach Beseitigung des Schmerzes kommt infolge Weitstellung der Gefäßperipherie der Volumenmangel erst recht zum Tragen. Nach Volumenausgleich steigt die Strömung im Transplantat deutlich an.

Diskussion

Es ist auffällig, daß in der Literatur keine systematischen Untersuchungen über das Verhalten der Blutströmung in Abhängigkeit vom Narkoseverfahren mitgeteilt wurden, obwohl das elektromagnetische Meßverfahren seit Anfang der 60-er Jahre auch für den klinischen Routinebetrieb zur Verfügung stand [3]. Die Ursachen dafür sind mannigfaltig: Zum einen befand sich die elektromagnetische Strömungsmessung in den Händen von Gefäßchirurgen, welche dem Narkoseverfahren keinen größeren Einfluß auf die Funktionstücjtigkeit rekonstruierter Arterienabschnitte beigemessen haben. Dieses Vorurteil kann insoweit bestätigt werden, als auch die

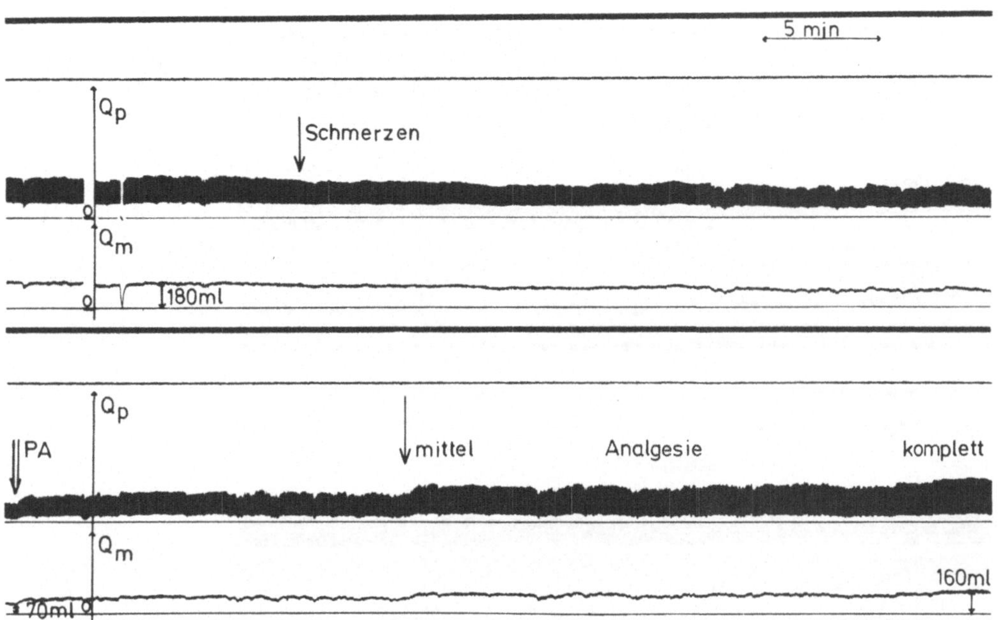

Abb. 9. Einfluß des postoperativen Wundschmerzes auf die Strömung im femoro-poplitealen Venenbypass am 1. postoperativen Tag. Infolge Ausfall der kontinuierlichen Epiduralblockade war es zum Auftreten von Schmerzen verbunden mit deutlicher Abnahme der Bypass-Durchströmung gekommen, dieser Effekt ist nach Wiedereintritt der Analgesie verschwunden (Ordinate: Q_p = obere Kurve: jeweils pulsatile Stromstärke, Q_m = gemittelte Stromstärke = untere Kurve; geringe Papiergeschwindigkeit = „Wischkurve"; Abszisse: Zeitlicher Verlauf)

beste Narkoseform nicht in der Lage ist, Frühthrombosen nach gefäßchirurgischen Eingriffen, welche auf dem Boden von technischen Fehlern entstanden sind, zu verhüten.

Der zweite Grund für das Fehlen solcher Untersuchungen mag darin zu sehen sein, daß der Indikationsbereich für das Spektrum der zur Verfügung stehenden Anaesthesieformen noch nicht klar abgesteckt ist. Ein solcher Indikationsbereich kann jedoch nur auf dem Boden von objektiven Daten, also durch Messung von kardiovaskulären und pulmonalen Parametern erarbeitet werden. Das Fehlen solcher Untersuchungen erstaunt aber auch deswegen, weil Einzelbefunde über das Verhalten der arteriellen Strömung vor allem aus skandinavischen Untersuchungen seit längerem bekannt sind. [3] Die intraoperativ gemessene Ruhestromstärke nahm bei den funktionstüchtigen Transplantaten bis zum zweiten postoperativen Tag deutlich zu, entsprechend dem klinischen Bild der postoperativen Hyperaemie. Die postoperativ gemessenen Stromstärkewerte konnten deutlich erhöht werden, wenn die Patienten Beinarbeit leisteten. Die hierdurch bewirkte periphere Widerstandssenkung erzeugte eine Mehrdurchströmung, welche etwa dem Stromstärkeanstieg nach intraarterieller Injektion von Papaverin während der Operation entsprach. Über das Narkoseverfahren sowie die Art der postoperativen Schmerzbekämpfung wird von Hall leider nichts mitgeteilt.

Cronenstrand u. Ekeström [1] fordern zurecht, daß es im Rahmen der Gefäßchirurgie besonders wichtig sei, den höchstmöglichen Fluß durch eine rekonstruierte Arterie intra- und postoperativ zu erzielen. Die Autoren stellen unter anderem einen Patienten vor, welcher infolge von Herzrhythmusstörungen und Hypovolaemie eine Bypass-Durchströmung von nur 30 ml

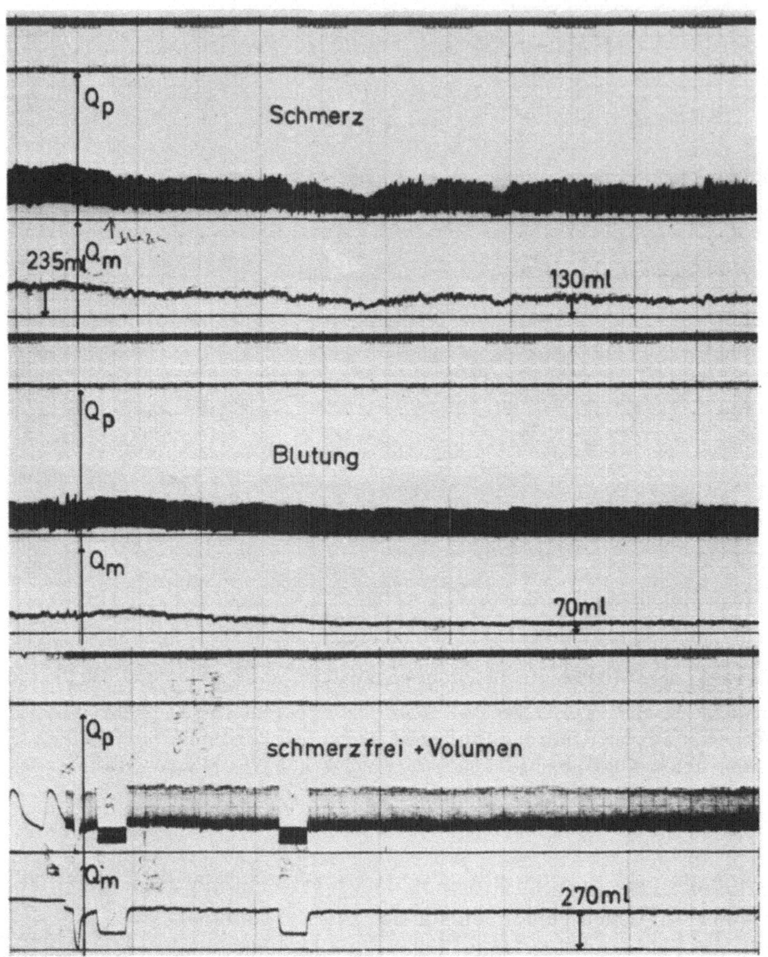

Abb. 10. Einfluß des postoperativen Wundschmerzes in Kombination mit Volumenmangel auf die Strömung im femoro-poplitealen Venenbypass am Abend des Operationstages. (Zeichenerklärung siehe Abb. 9). Nach Beseitigung des Schmerzes kommt infolge Weitstellung der Gefäßperipherie der Volumenmangel erst recht zur Wirkung. Nach Volumenausgleich steigt die Strömung im Transplantat deutlich an. (Auf dem unteren Maßpapierstreifen finden sich außerdem in der Reihenfolge von links nach rechts: Strömungs „0" nach Kompression der Art. poplitea sowie zwei kurzfristige Phasen, in welchen das Strömungssignal mit einer geringeren Verstärkung geschrieben wurde)

pro Minute aufwies. Dieser Wert liegt nach eigenen Untersuchungen in dem Bereich, welcher zur Frühthrombose führen kann [7].

Die Gefäßrekonstruktionen von Cronenstrand u. Ekeström [1] wurden ausnahmslos in Allgemeinnarkose durchgeführt. Eine postoperative Zunahme der Stromstärke wurde auch hier durch Beinarbeit erzielt. In der sehr umfangreichen Untersuchung von Dedichen [2] wird ebenfalls die Notwendigkeit einer ausreichenden Strömstärke in den rekonstruierten Arteriensegmenten betont, um einer frühen Rethrombosierung entgegenzuwirken. Volumenverlust und Blutdruckabfall führten bei zwei Patienten zu einem Verschluß der Bypass-Vene. Darüber hinaus war die Frühthrombose-Rate bei Patienten mit Stromstärkewerten unter 75 ml pro Minute 51,1%.

Zur Gewährleistung einer ausreichenden Stromstärke empfiehlt Dedichen [2] ein kontinuierliches Druckmonitoring mit ausreichendem Volumenersatz sowie postoperative frühzeitige Beinarbeit. Während Dedichen [2] das Verhalten der pulsatilen Stromstärkenkurve nur am Rande erwähnt, kommt Lee et al. [4] das Verdienst zu, eine quantitative Analyse der Stromstärkenkurve durchgeführt zu haben. Die Bedeutung der Rückflußwelle für den peripheren Widerstand in der Extremitätenarterie wurde analysiert, der Einfluß des Sympathikotonus konnte dabei herausgestellt werden. Die klinische Konsequenz war eine zusätzliche lumbale Sympathektomie der Arterienrekonstruktionen am Bein. Leider wird auch von Lee et al. [4] die Narkoseform nicht erwähnt, die Analyse der Strompulskurven läßt jedoch auf eine Allgemeinanaesthesie schließen. Unsere Untersuchungen haben nun ergeben, daß durch die Kombination von Leitungsanaesthesie und ausreichender Volumensubstitution eine signifikante Zunahme der arteriellen Strömung in den Gefäßbereichen erzielt werden kann, welche von der Leitungsblockade erfaßt werden.

Dabei darf man sich jedoch nicht von Absolutwerten leiten lassen, da die Extremitäten-Durchströmung neben dem peripheren Widerstand und dem Systemdruck besonders vom Herzzeitvolumen abhängig ist [10].

Dies ist bei Patienten in Leitungsanaesthesie von Bedeutung, da hier die arterielle Stromstärke überwiegend vom Herzzeitvolumen bestimmt wird und gilt auch für Patienten, welche mit kontinuierlicher Epiduralblockade postoperativ schmerzfrei gehalten wurden. Erwähnenswert ist noch, daß die Ausschaltung des Sympathikotonus nicht mit einem motorischen Block einhergehen muß, so daß Beinarbeit in der frühen postoperativen Phase durchaus zusätzlich geleistet werden könnte.

Frühe aktive Bewegungsübungen erscheinen uns jedoch weniger zur Gewährleistung einer ausreichenden Durchströmung in den operierten Arterien notwendig zu sein, da diese ja nachgewiesenermaßen durch die Leitungsblockade erreicht wird. Vielmehr ist eine frühe postoperative Mobilisierung zur Vermeidung von Venenthrombosen zu fordern. Welchen Einfluß die Leitungsblockade auf die venöse Strömung, insbesondere auf die Rückstromgeschwindigkeit, hat, bleibt in Zukunft zu untersuchen. Hier bietet sich besonders das gepulste Ultraschall-Verfahren mit seinen transkutanen Anwendungsmöglichkeiten an. Die Meßgenauigkeit entspricht dem elektromagnetischen Verfahren [8].

Zusammenfassung

Die Interpretation des gemessenen Strömungsvolumens in rekonstruierten Arterien muß in Abhängigkeit von der Gefäßperipherie und der benutzten Narkoseverfahren erfolgen. Bei Patienten mit Femoro-poplitealen Venentransplantaten wurde für die Gruppe, welche in Allgemeinnarkose operiert worden war, eine deutlich niedrigere Stromstärke gefunden als bei Patienten in Leitungsanaesthesie. Gleiche Befunde ergaben sich für die unterschiedlichen Narkoseformen bei Durchführung von aorto-femoralen Überbrückungs-Transplantaten, wobei hier gleichzeitig durchgeführte Untersuchungen des Herzzeitvolumens zeigten, daß die höhere Transplantat-Durchströmung bei Patienten, welche in Leitungsanaesthesie operiert worden waren, überwiegend auf ein erhöhtes Herzzeitvolumen zurückzuführen war. Die postrekonstruktive Hyperaemie war abhängig von der Art und Wirkung der Analgesiemethode. Bei Patienten mit Leitungsanaesthesie und Volumenausgleich wurde eine höhere Transplantat-Durchströmung gemessen als bei Verwendung von Morphinanalgetika. Somit richtet sich unser Interesse neben der Perfektionierung gefäßchirurgischer Technik auch auf die Möglichkeiten der Analgesie und der Sympathikolyse in der frühen postoperativen Phase.

Summary

The electromagnetic principle and the pulsed Doppler method were used to measure the blood flow rate during and after arterial reconstructive procedures. Patients with aorto-femoral grafts and those with femoro-popliteal vein grafts were studied. In patients with patent grafts it was found that the basal and hyperemic blood flow rate was dependent on the cardiac output and on the peripheral vascular resistance. The latter could be influenced significantly by the type of anesthesia. The sympaticolysis in patients with intra- and postoperative epidural analgesia caused a higher blood flow rate through the graft and an increase of the heart flow rate accordingly. Therefore this type of anesthesia seems to be the method of choice, but the typical arterial pressure drop has to be avoided by previous and simultaneous volume substitution. It has been measured, that pain and blood loss reduce the graft flow significantly. This implies a continuous analgesia like the epidural block even postoperatively for 3 or 4 days and adequate blood volume substitution.

Literatur

1. Cronenstrand R, Ekeström S (1970) Blood flow after peripheral arterial reconstruction. Scand J Thorac Cardiovasc Surg 4:159-171
2. Dedichen H (1976) Hemodynamics in arterial reconstructions of the lower limb. Acta Chir Scand 142: 213-220
3. Hall KV (1969) Postoperative blood flow measurements in man by the use of implanted electromagnetic probes. Scand J Thorac Cardiovasc Surg 3:135-144
4. Lee BY, Castillo HT, Madden JL (1970) Quantification of the arterial pulsatile blood flow waveform in peripheral vascular disease. Angiology 21:595-605
5. Mc Donald DA (1974) Blood flow in arteries, 2nd edn. Arnold, London
6. Pieper H, Wetterer E (1955) Die Beziehung zwischen Blutdruck und direkt gemessener diastolischer Stromstärke einzelner arterieller Gebiete bei künstlich herbeigeführten periodischen Druckänderungen. Verh Dtsch Ges Kreisl Forsch 88:439-447
7. Sandmann W, Kremer K, Florack B, Kovacicek S, Wüst H (1975) Das Verhalten der Blutströmung in rekonstruierten Arterien in Abhängigkeit von Gefäßperipherie und Narkoseverfahren. Kongr. Ber. 16. Tg. Österr. Ges. Chir., Wien, S. 543-550
8. Sandmann W, Peronneau P, Schweins G, Wildeshaus KH, Xhaard M, Kremer K (1978) Quantitative Strömungsmessung mit dem elektromagnetischen und dem gepulsten Doppler-Ultraschallverfahren in der Gefäßchirurgie. In: Kriessmann A, Bollinger A (Hrsg) Ultraschall-Doppler-Diagnostik in der Angiologie. Thieme, Stuttgart
9. Wetterer E, Kenner T (1968) Grundlagen der Dynamik des Arterienpulses. Springer, Berlin Heidelberg New York
10. Wüst HJ, Sandmann W, Florack B, Lennartz H (1976) Kreislaufveränderungen während und nach aorto-femoralen Bypass-Operationen unter kontinuierlicher Epiduralanaesthesie. Langenbecks Arch Klin Chir 342:594

Diskussion

Frage: Herr Sandmann, vielleicht können Sie uns ganz kurz sagen, wie der Unterschied gegenüber unserem früheren postoperativen Vorgehen, vorwiegend mit Papaverin, verglichen jetzt mit der Epiduralgruppe ist. Ist das etwa gleichwertig oder schneidet die Epiduralgruppe sogar günstiger ab?

Sandmann: Die Effekte, die durch das intraarterielle Papaverin erreicht werden, sind ganz kurzfristige Effekte. Im Bereich der Gefäßchirurgie verbietet sich natürlich die postoperative intraarterielle Injektion von Vasodilantien wegen eventuell auftretender Wundheilungsstörungen. Die intravenöse Applikation der sog. Vasodilatatoren führt natürlich auch zu einer Weitstellung in Gebieten, in denen wir eine bessere Durchströmung überhaupt nicht wünschen. Deshalb machen wir vom Papaverin und ähnlichen Medikamenten zu einer besseren Perfusion nach einer Arterienrekonstruktion nicht mehr Gebrauch, sondern wir wenden eben nur die Leitungsanaesthesie an, weil sie uns ganz gezielt für den Bereich, den wir operiert haben, eine höhere Stromstärke liefert; dabei ist ein genügender Volumenersatz natürlich vorausgesetzt.

Frage: Sie haben gesagt, daß die Stromstärke unter einer Neuroleptnarkose sich vermindert, da mit der Neuroleptanalgesie der periphere Widerstand erhöht wird. Das ist mir nicht bekannt. Droperidol bewirkt eine Alpharezeptorenblockade und senkt somit den peripheren Widerstand.

Sandmann: Bei allen diesbezüglichen Patienten ist dieses Phänomen aufgetreten. Da wir mittlerweile über Messungen bei 300 Patienten verfügen, glaube ich, selbst wenn andere Mitteilungen existieren, diese in Zweifel ziehen zu dürfen. Ich habe versucht, Ihnen mit dem Umgang über den Vergleich mit dem Papaverin zu zeigen, wie die hämodynamische Wirkung der Epiduralblockade und der Neuroleptanalgesie ist. Wir haben immer gefunden, daß der periphere Widerstand zumindest in dem Abschnitt, in dem wir gemessen haben, und das ist ja der Abschnitt der Rekonstruktion, unter dem Einfluß der Neuroleptanalgesie hoch war. Ich glaube, zu dieser Frage könnte Herr Wüst direkt antworten.

Wüst: Die alphablockierende Wirkung von Dehydrobenzperidol, und darauf wurde bereits hingewiesen, ist maximal 20 Minuten nachweisbar. Diese Messungen aber sind 5-8 Stunden nach der einmaligen Gabe von Dehydrobenzperidol erfolgt, so daß eine wesentliche Kreislaufwirkung von Dehydrobenzperidol nicht mehr zu erwarten war.

Frage: Die Weitstellung der Gefäße könnte u.U. zu einer Verminderung der Fließgeschwindigkeit führen und damit eine erhöhte Thrombosegefahr bedingen.

Sandmann: Wir selber haben das noch nicht untersucht. Eine erhöhte arterielle Stromstärke im Kreislaufgebiet einer Extremität könnte auch zu einem vermehrten Rückfluß in den tiefen Beinvenen führen. Wir würden deshalb unter Leitungsanaesthesie aus haemodynamischen Gründen ein geringeres venöses Thromboserisiko annehmen. Ich meine, vielleicht könnte man aus der Empirie der Klinik noch etwas dazu beitragen. Die Thromboserate und auch die Lungenarterienembolierate bei diesen vorbehandelten Patienten ist außerordentlich gering. Ich spreche jetzt also nur für den Sektor der Gefäßchirurgie und das ist erstaunlich, da wir bei unseren Manipulationen gar nicht vermeiden können, daß die eine oder andere Vene auch mal mit der Pinzette erfaßt wird und etwas hart auf die Seite geschoben wird. Man könnte also, ausgehend von einem Venenwandschaden, eine erhöhte Thromboserate erwarten. Dies ist bei diesen Patienten nicht der Fall und wir führen das darauf zurück, daß einfach eine höhere Stromstärke auch in den Venen zu finden ist. Aber zu Ihrer anfangs gestellten Frage zur Fließgeschwindigkeit in den Venen muß ich sagen, das bleibt noch zu untersuchen.

Frage: Wie steht es mit der Thrombosierungsrate in den frisch anastomosierten Gefäßabschnitten. Gibt es da Unterschiede zwischen den beiden Kollektiven?

Sandmann: Das wäre sozusagen die Quintessenz, wenn bei der höheren Stromstärke in den rekonstruierten arteriellen Gefäßen bei Periduralanalgesie auch die Häufigkeit der Thrombose geringer ist. Diese Antwort muß ich Ihnen noch schuldig bleiben, da das Kollektiv daraufhin noch nicht untersucht worden ist.

Kontinuierliche Messung der Sauerstoffaufnahme bei postoperativer Periduralanalgesie

A. Fournell, B. Wilhelmy, K. Falke, W. Sandmann und G. Böhmer

Die postoperative Periduralanalgesie bietet nach einigen Untersuchungen gegenüber der Schmerzbekämpfung mit Opiaten entscheidende Vorteile. So ist nach Spence u. Smith [6] die Häufigkeit postoperativer entzündlicher Lungenkomplikationen deutlich herabgesetzt. Die alveolär-arterielle Sauerstoffdruckdifferenz ist in ihren Untersuchungen signifikant niedriger bei postoperativer Periduralanalgesie als bei der Gabe von Morphin.

Besondere Bedeutung bei der Beurteilung von verschiedenen Verfahren zur Schmerzbekämpfung in der postoperativen Phase kommt ihrem Einfluß auf das kardiovaskuläre System zu. Einer der wichtigsten Parameter dieses Systems, der nach den Untersuchungen von Reeves et al. [4] linear mit dem Herzzeitvolumen korreliert, ist die Sauerstoffaufnahme. Die bisher veröffentlichten Daten über die Sauerstoffaufnahme wurden aus punktuellen Einzelmessungen [2, 5] gewonnen. Nach der Methode von Neuhof et al. [3] ist es möglich geworden, die Sauerstoffaufnahme kontinuierlich und nicht-invasiv zu messen. Ziel der vorliegenden Arbeit war es, den Einfluß der postoperativen Periduralanalgesie auf die kontinuierlich bestimmte Sauerstoffaufnahme festzustellen.

Untersuchungsgut und Methode

Untersucht wurden neun Patienten (Durchschnittsalter 54,5 Jahre) nach großen rekonstruktiven Eingriffen der Bauchgefäße in thorakaler Katheter-Periduralanaesthesie (sensibler Block Th_4-S_5), die während des Eingriffs durch Intubation sowie Beatmung mit einem N_2O/O_2-Gemisch und Diazepam supplementiert wurde. Zur Periduralanaesthesie verwandten wir 20 bis 30 ml Bupivacain 0,5%. Die Bestimmung der Sauerstoffaufnahme wurde postoperativ mit einem Meßschrank der Fa. Heinemann & Gregori durchgeführt. Dieses Gerät besteht aus einer pneumatischen Einheit, einem Sauerstoffanalysator, einer Recheneinheit und einem 12-Kanal-Punktschreiber. Die Patienten lagen unter einer Haube aus durchsichtiger Folie, aus der kontinuierlich mit der pneumatischen Einheit ein konstantes Luftvolumen abgesaugt wurde. Die Sauerstoffaufnahme des Patienten wird als Produkt des abgesaugten Luftvolumens und der durch den O_2-Analysator bestimmten Sauerstoffgehaltdifferenz zwischen der frei in die Haube eintretenden Raumluft und der abgesaugten Luft errechnet, die gemessenen Werte werden auf STPD-Bedingungen reduziert. Neben der Sauerstoffaufnahme wurden die rektale Temperatur und bei sechs Patienten kontinuierlich die Herzfrequenz und der mittlere arterielle Druck registriert.

Ergebnisse

Die Sauerstoffaufnahme betrug in der ersten Meßperiode, ca. 30 min nach Beendigung des operativen Eingriffs, 5,1 ± 0,5 ml O_2/kg KG x min (n = 7), sie lag damit um 54,5% über dem nach Körpergewicht, Alter und Geschlecht bestimmten Grundumsatzwert [1] (Abb. 1). Die Patienten waren zu diesem Zeitpunkt wach, voll orientiert und analgetisch bis Th_5. Zwei Patienten konnten nicht in die statistische Auswertung einbezogen werden, da ihre Sauerstoffaufnahme

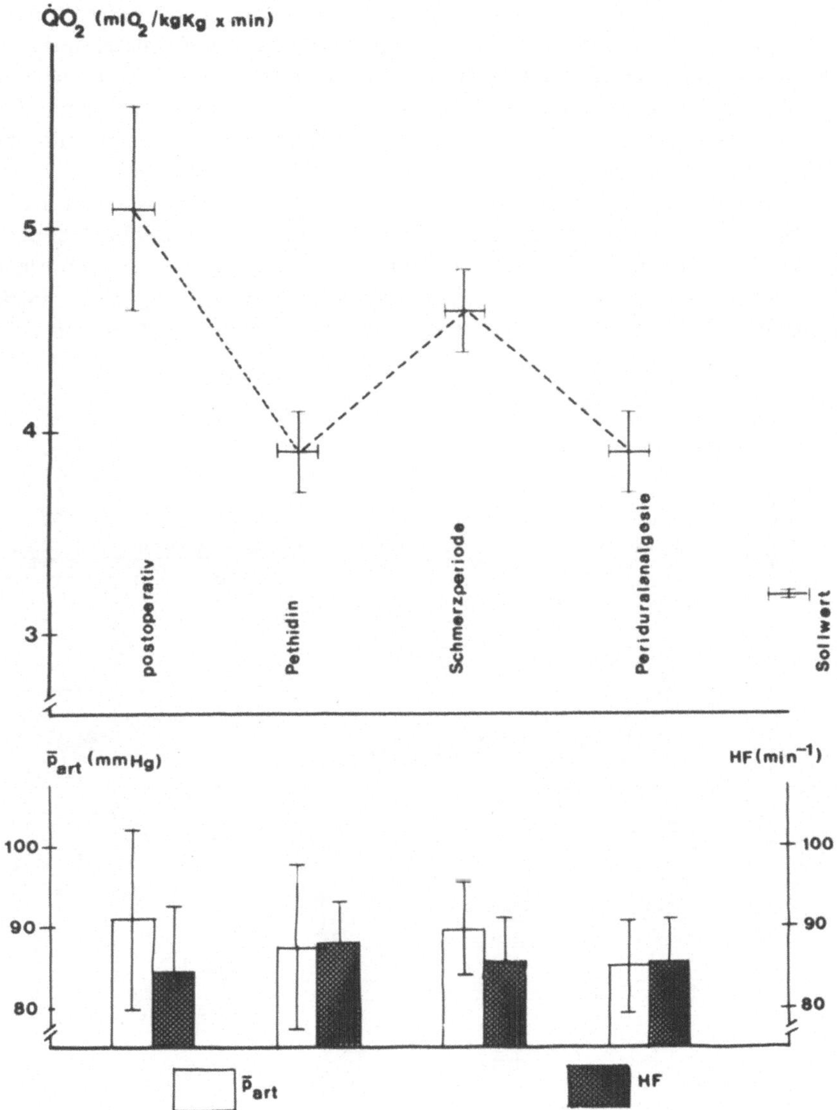

Abb. 1. Verhalten von Sauerstoffaufnahme (QO_2), arteriellem Mitteldruck ($\bar{p}_{art}$) und Herzfrequenz während der einzelnen Meßperioden, Erläuterungen siehe Text

infolge starken Kältezitterns außerhalb des Meßbereiches unseres Analysators (über 600 ml O_2/min) lag. Bei diesen sowie weiteren fünf Patienten des Gesamtkollektivs war das Kältezittern so stark, daß wir Pethidin in einer Dosierung von 0,5 mg/kg KG verabreichten. Dies führte in allen Fällen zur Beseitigung des Kältezitterns und zu einer Abnahme der Sauerstoffaufnahme auf 3,9 ± 0,2 ml O_2/kg KG x min (n = 7), dies entspricht 118,2% des Grundumsatzes.

In der postoperativen Schmerzphase, vom Patienten wurden ziehende und stechende Schmerzen angegeben, stieg die Sauerstoffaufnahme auf 4,6 ± 0,2 ml O_2/kg KG x min (n = 9), sie war damit um 39,4% über dem Grundumsatzwert erhöht. Zu diesem Zeitpunkt injizierten wir Bupivacain 0,5% 5 ml als Bolus in den liegenden Periduralkatheter und starteten gleichzeitig die kontinuierliche Periduralanalgesie mit Bupivacain 0,125% 6 ml/h über einen Perfusor. Diese Maßnahmen führten zu Analgesie und zu einer Abnahme der Sauerstoffaufnahme auf 3,9 ± 0,2 ml O_2/kg KG x min (n = 9), entsprechend 118,2% des Grundumsatzwertes. Die Abnahme der Sauerstoffaufnahme gegenüber der Schmerzperiode um 15,2% ist mit einem $p < 0{,}001$ statistisch signifikant (es wurde der Student t-Test für gepaarte Daten benutzt). Arterieller Mitteldruck und Herzfrequenz zeigten während der einzelnen Meßperioden keine signifikanten Änderungen; die arterielle Gasanalyse postoperativ ergab bei normalem Säuren-Basen-Status ein PO_2 von 80,1 ± 2,7 mmHg, das PCO_2 betrug 38,4 ± 2,7 mmHg (Werte bei Luftatmung). Die Abb. 2 und 3 demonstrieren die für das Gesamtkollektiv dargelegten Daten

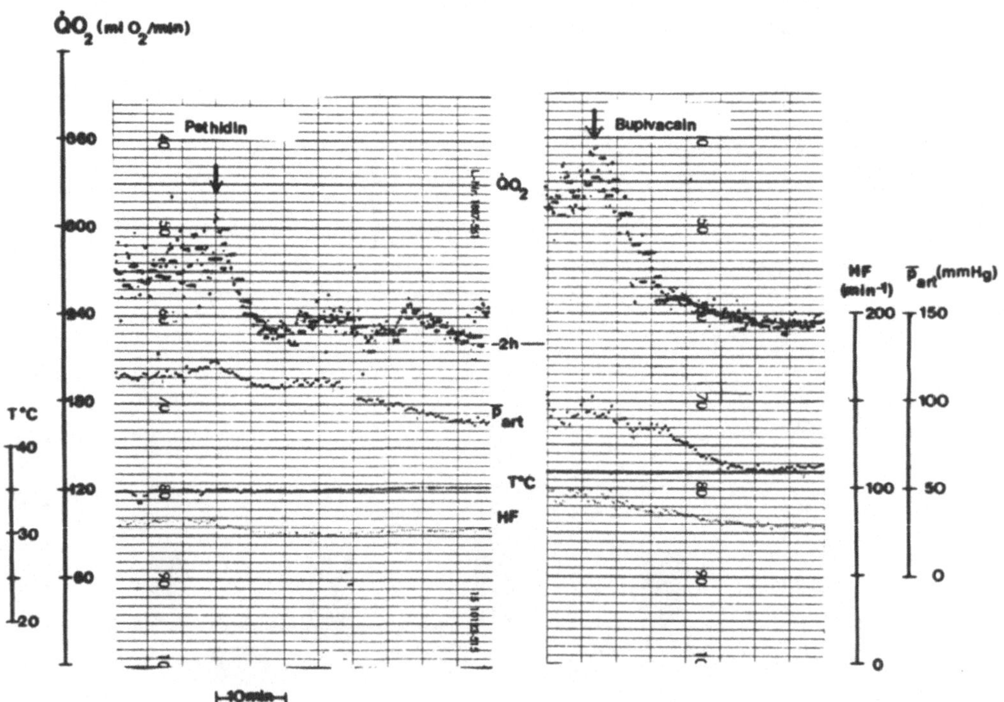

Abb. 2. Ausschnitte aus der Originalregistrierung bei einem Patienten nach aortofemoralem Bypass, linker Teil der Abbildung: Wirkung von Pethidin auf die Sauerstoffaufnahme bei Kältezittern, rechter Teil der Abbildung: Anstieg der Sauerstoffaufnahme in der Schmerzphase und die Kupierung durch Periduralanalgesie mit Bupivacain

anhand von Originalregistrierungen. Unsere Ergebnisse zeigen, daß es in der unmittelbaren postoperativen Phase bei guter Analgesie infolge Kältezitterns zu einer um 54,5% über dem Grundumsatzwert erhöhten Sauerstoffaufnahme kommen kann. Die Gabe von Pethidin reduziert in einer Dosierung von 0,5 mg/kg KG die Sauerstoffaufnahme auf 118,2% des Grundumsatzwertes durch die Beseitigung des Kältezitterns.

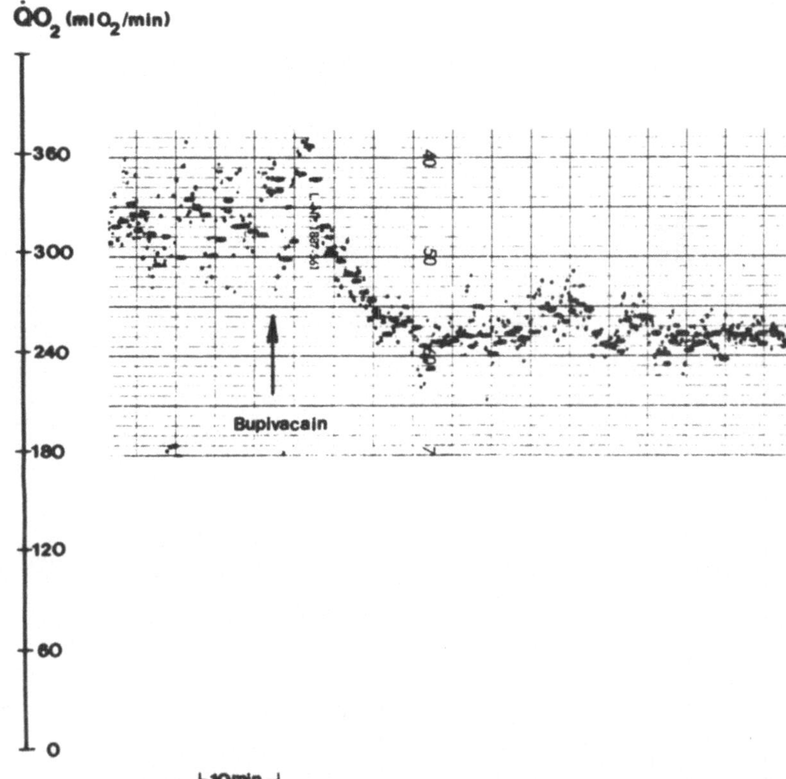

Abb. 3. Abfall der schmerzbedingten Erhöhung der Sauerstoffaufnahme durch Periduralanalgesie mit Bupivacain bei einem Patienten nach aortofemoralem Bypass

Die Sauerstoffaufnahme steigt mit Abklingen der Periduralanaesthesie auf 139,4% des Grundumsatzwertes (Abb. 4). Die postoperative kontinuierliche Periduralanalgesie führt in diesem Stadium zu einer Abnahme der Sauerstoffaufnahme auf 118,2% des Grundumsatzwertes, sie ist damit in der Lage, die schmerzbedingte Erhöhung der Sauerstoffaufnahme vollständig zu blockieren.

Literatur

1. Balke B, Harden KA, Young RC (1971) Ventilation and gas exchange. Fed. Proc. 36:78
2. Muneyuki M, Ueda Y, Urabe N, Takeshita H, Inamoto A (1968) Postoperative pain relief and respiratory function in man. Anesthesiology 29:304
3. Neuhof H, Hey D, Glaser E, Wolf H, Lasch HG (1973) Schocküberwachung durch kontinuierliche Registrierung der Sauerstoffaufnahme und anderer Parameter. Dtsch Med Wochenschr 98:1227
4. Reeves JT, Grover RF, Filley GF, Blount SG Jr (1961) Cardiac output in normal resting man. J Appl Physiol 16:276
5. Sjögren S, Wright B (1972) Circulatory changes during continuous epidural blockade. Acta Anaesthesiol Scand 16:5
6. Spence AA, Smith G (1971) Postoperative analgesia and lung function: A comparison of morphine with extradural block. Br J Anaesth 43:144

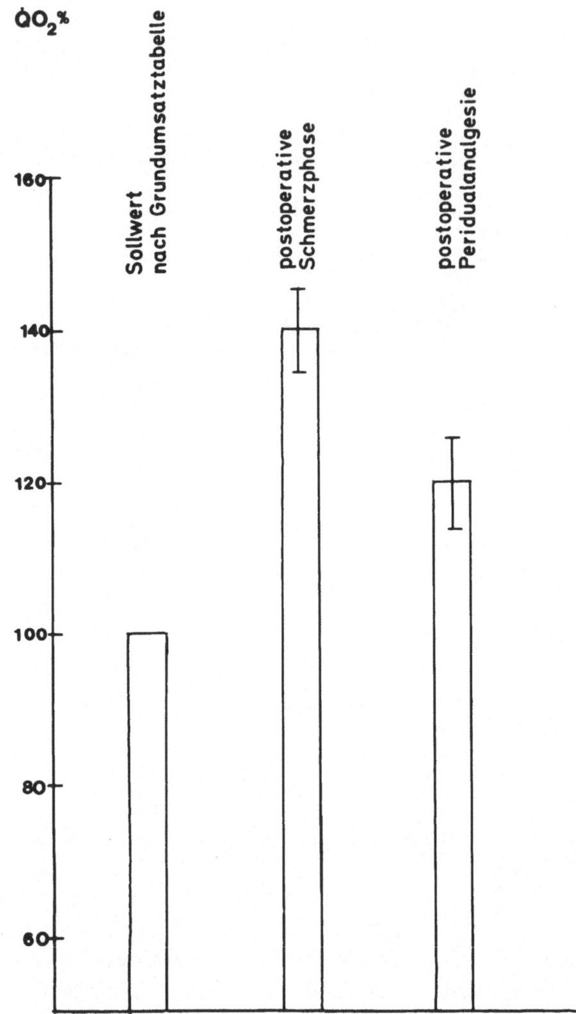

Abb. 4. Verhalten der Sauerstoffaufnahme gegenüber dem Grundumsatzwert in der postoperativen Schmerphase und bei postoperativer Periduralanalgesie mit Bupivacain

Diskussion

Frage: Did you use bupivacain with or without adrenalin?
Fournell: We used bupivacain without adrenalin.
Frage: Haben Sie auch die CO_2-Werte bei den Patienten bestimmt, um etwa über die Ventilation aussagen zu können?
Fournell: Ja, der arterielle PCO_2 betrug 38,4 ± 2,7 mm Hg.
Frage: Haben Sie auch parallel Herzminutenvolumenbestimmungen durchgeführt und konnten Sie sehen, ob die Sauerstoffverbrauchwerte parallel mit der Hämodynamik verlaufen oder geht dies auf Rechnung einer besseren Utilisation?
Fournell: Nein, wir haben bisher keine Bestimmung des Herzzeitvolumens durchgeführt.
Frage: Wie sind nun die Unterschiede zwischen der Pethidinanalgesie und der Periduralanalgesie?
Fournell: Die Gabe von 0,5 mg/kg Körpergewicht Pethidin dient nur zur Beseitigung des Kältezitterns in der postoperativen Phase. Die Patienten waren ja zu diesem Zeitpunkt durch die noch bestehende Periduralanaesthesie des operativen Eingriffes voll analgetisch. Sie hatten nur ein Kältezittern. Die Steigerung des Sauerstoffverbrauches auf 154% des Ausgangswertes – im Extremfall um einige 100% – ist nicht zu erklären

durch mangelnde Analgesie, sondern lediglich durch das Kältezittern, Alleiniger Schmerz ist nicht in der Lage, den Sauerstoffverbrauch so sehr zu steigern. Das zeigt sich auch in den Untersuchungen dadurch, daß die Gabe von Pethidin in der postoperativen Phase den Sauerstoffverbrauch auf exakt den gleichen Wert reduziert wie nachher bei der Reinstitution der Periduralanalgesie. Das war nämlich beides 118,2% des Grundumsatzwertes.

Frage: Ist es richtig, daß Sie eine Blockade von Th_4 abwärts gesetzt haben? Es ist doch anzunehmen, daß Sie dadurch den Sympathikus so gut wie ganz ausgeschaltet hatten. Die Frage wäre: Bei einer gezielten Periduralanaesthesie segmentär, die den wirklich schmerzhaften Bereich betrifft, ist unter diesen Umständen eine Verringerung des Sauerstoffverbrauches anzunehmen. Ich meine, die Sympathikusblockade an sich setzt den Metabolismus herab und könnte dadurch zu einer Verringerung der Sauerstoffaufnahme führen.

Fournell: Ja, wir können jedoch mit unserer Methode nicht differenzieren zwischen dem Effekt einer reinen segmentalen Periduralanaesthesie und den Auswirkungen der Blockierung des Sympathikus auf den Sauerstoffverbrauch. Es ist jedoch bekannt, daß in der postoperativen Phase der Sauerstoffverbrauch unabhängig vom Narkoseverfahren erhöht ist; bei der Periduralanaesthesie ist er jedoch im Verhältnis zu den anderen Narkoseverfahren weniger erhöht. Gleich gute Analgesie in der postoperativen Phase unterstellt, mag dies vielleicht darauf hinweisen, daß nicht nur die Analgesie bei der Periduralanaesthesie ins Gewicht fällt, sondern auch die Sympathikusblockade eine Rolle spielt.

II. Herzkreislauffunktion bei Risikopatienten während Periduralanaesthesie

Vorsitz: J. Lassner, Paris und J.O. Arndt, Düsseldorf

The Influence of Hypovolaemia and Shock on the Haemodynamic Alterations Due to Regional Anaesthesia

M. Stanton-Hicks

Much of the information concerning the influence of hypovolaemia and shock on those circulatory changes consequent upon regional anaesthetic procedures is anecdotal and poorly documented. The first serious attempt to observe such circulatory changes which occur during epidural anaesthesia resulted in what has become a classic paper on the subject: Bonica et al. [3] described the effects of acute blood loss in a group of human volunteers during epidural anaesthesia with either plain lidocaine or adrenaline containing solutions. Although this study relates to one form of regional anaesthesia there are a number of lessons which can be learned. The amount of blood withdrawn was approximately 13% of the patient's blood volume, a not uncommon situation encountered in the operating room and following trauma. In fact, earlier studies performed by cardiologists had determined that losses of 20% of the normal blood volume in healthy subjects were attended by little change in mean arterial pressure, compensation being provided by an appropriate sympathetic endocrine response [8, 9]. When however, an extensive sympathetic block is superimposed upon even this moderate degree of hypovolaemia it is evident that considerable individual variation in the cardiac rate (CR), total peripheral resistance (TPR), and cardiac output (CO) occurs. Fig. 1 compares TPR, CO, and mean arterial pressure during epidural block in several situations. It is reasonable to assume that with somatic

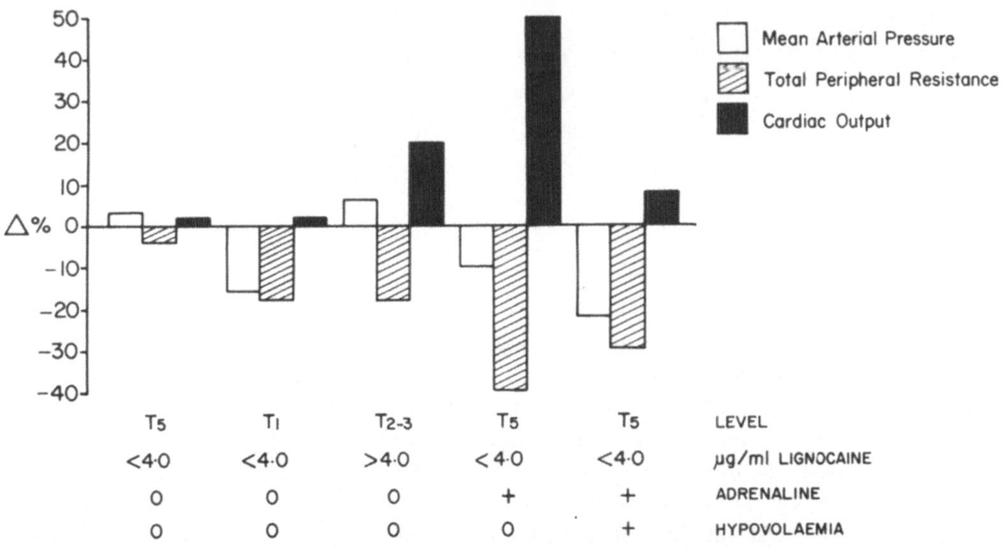

Fig. 1. The cardiovascular effects of epidural anaesthesia under the influence of, (a) different segmental levels, (b) local anaesthetic blood level, (c) presence of adrenaline, (d) hypovolaemia (after Covino and Vassallo [4])

anaesthesia to the fifth thoracic dermatome, as was the case in those studies, the sympathetic block involved at least T_4, and possibly also T_3 – from which spring the lowest cardioaccelerator nerves and therefore most of the sympathetic outflow is affected. The pharmacological adrenalectomy, while conferring other potential advantages on the normovolaemic patient, removes a potent endocrine response from playing its part in the haemodynamic restitution during hypovolaemia. The only mechanism available to effect any degree of compensation is therefore stimulation of the upper cardiac fibres increasing cardiac output and causing vasoconstriction in the upper limbs. When adrenaline was omitted from the local anaesthetic solutions used in the above study such severe hypotension occurred that the study had to be terminated in five of seven subjects and the circulatory collapse required restitution with intravenous ephedrine (Fig. 2). In normovolaemic man, quite the reverse is the case as has already

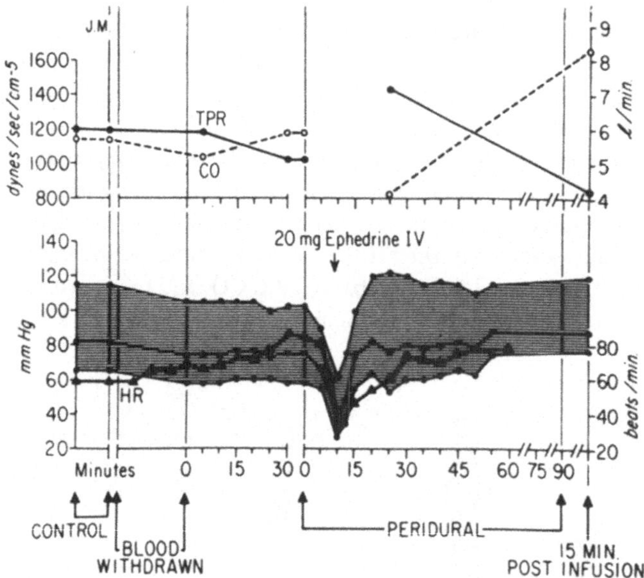

Fig. 2. Alterations in MAP, CR, CO, and TPR in one human subject after acute blood loss and epidural anaesthesia with plain lidocaine 2%, to T_5. (Bonica et al. [3])

been discussed. Here, the widespread β adrenergic effects interfere with the circulatory adjustments in the face of sympathetic block. It is quite clear that the reasons for the greater stability which is seen after epidural block with adrenaline containing solutions are, (1) the α venoconstriction in the great veins, (2) the β stimulation of the heart and (3) the smaller circulating blood levels of local anaesthetic, all of which help to offset the circulatory effects of hypovolaemia (Fig. 3). The degree of hypotension which accompanied the use of adrenaline containing solutions was only about one-third of that which occurred when it was omitted from the local anaesthetic (Fig. 4). In another study, Kennedy et al. [5] observed the haemodynamic effects of subarachnoid block under similar conditions imposed by acute blood loss. The main differences between this and the epidural studies are the greater reduction in MAP and smaller fall in TPR in the epidural group. Lidocaine induced cardiac depression is the most probable ex-

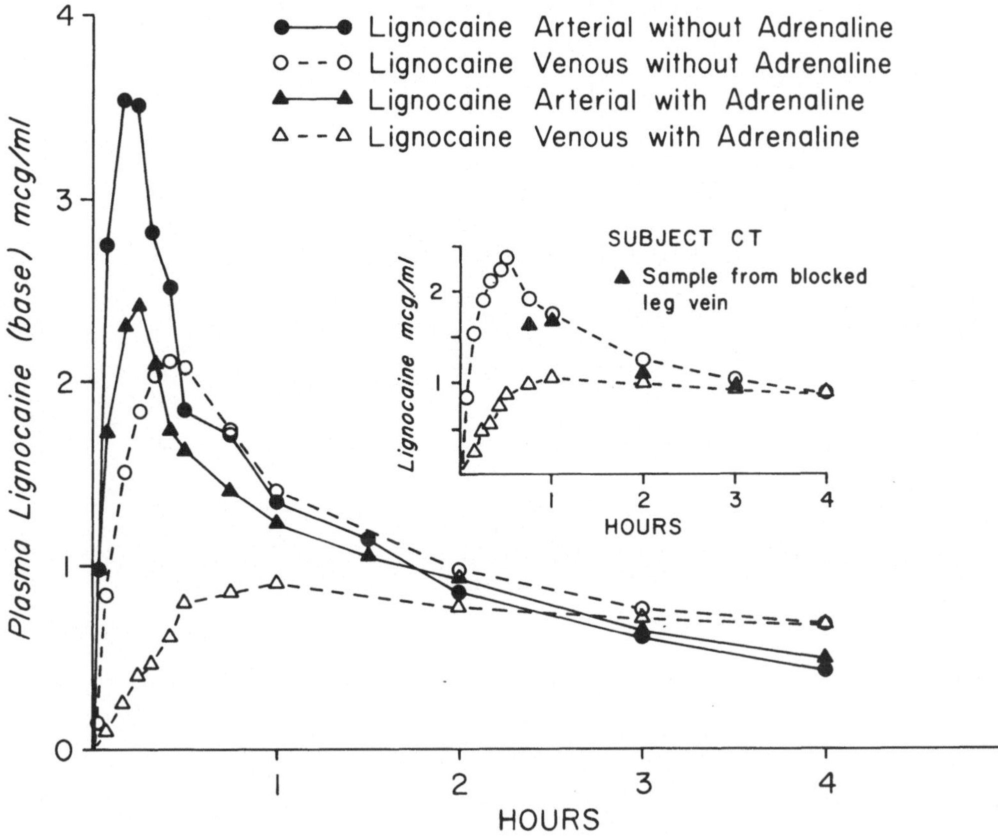

Fig. 3. Profile of local anaesthetic concentrations in the blood after epidural anaesthesia using plain and adrenaline containing solutions

planation for the greater hypotension senn in the epidural study while the differences in TPR may be due to the more rapid onset of sympathetic block in spinal anaesthesia.

The effects of the local anaesthetic both direct and indirect, on the myocardium have been discussed earlier (Fig. 5), and it will suffice to say that Jorfeldt et al. [4], showed that at least mepivacaine and bupivacaine in certain concentrations cause myocardial stimulation. This property is also shared by lidocaine. In the presence of acute blood loss, it can be argued that a relatively higher blood level of lidocaine will be achieved and in addition a relatively higher proportion of the cardiac output is available to the myocardium via the coronary circulation. Carrying this thesis further therefore one would expect a higher total dose of local anaesthetic to be available to the myocardium. In the absence of β adrenergic stimulation, serious myocardial depression could occur. The vasoactivity of local anaesthetics is another factor which must be considered. Since we know that constricted vessels are dilated at certain drug concentrations, (all local anaesthetics relax drug-induced arterial contractions in concentrations greater than 1 x 10^{-5} M), one might consider the effect of these concentrations on those vascular beds which are constricted in response to shock. The normal circulatory response to acute blood loss is, arteriolar constriction in the skin, venoconstriction of the capacitance vessels,

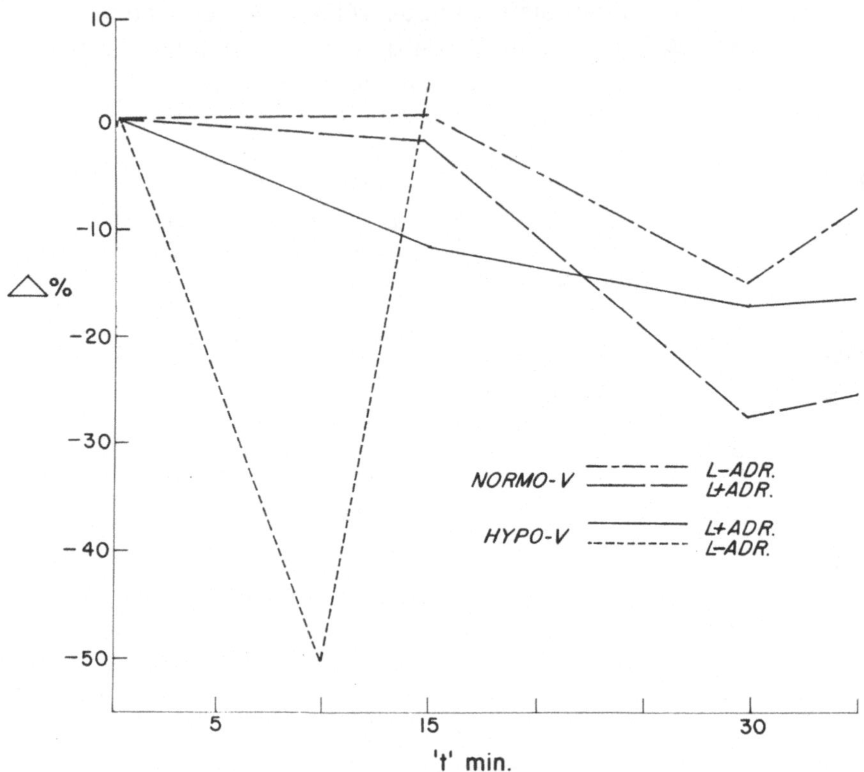

Fig. 4. Changes in MAP after epidural anaesthesia to T_5 using lidocaine 2% with and without adrenaline 5 μg/ml in the presence of (a) normovolaemia and (b) hypovolaemia

redistribution of blood from the splanchnic circulation and tachycardia. Quite apart from the direct effects of local anaesthetics on different vascular beds, the consequences of this situation on the kinetics of drug uptake and disposition are profound. The effect of a reduction in systemic pressure on hepatic and renal function has already been considered. Obviously metabolism and excretion of these drugs will be affected by hypovolaemia and shock, the degree of impairment being a function of the circulatory insufficiency. Under such circumstances one would expect higher blood levels of local anaesthetic, thereby raising the possibility of either cardiac or CNS toxicity precipitating circulatory collapse. However, such a situation, while a theoretical possibility, may in fact not occur as can be seen by the following experimental data. A consideration which would tend to prevent high circulating local anaesthetic levels from developing is the reduction in blood flow in the "depot site", such that its uptake by the systemic circulation is impaired. Experiments in epidural dogs [7] revealed a 30% lower peak blood level and the peak was delayed 40% compared with control, after acute haemorrhage. In spite of this the relatively greater perfusion of the heart may result in a greater extraction of lidocaine by the myocardium. Another aspect relates to the distribution volume which during haemorrhage is reduced and therefore would both elevate the blood level relative to this vol-

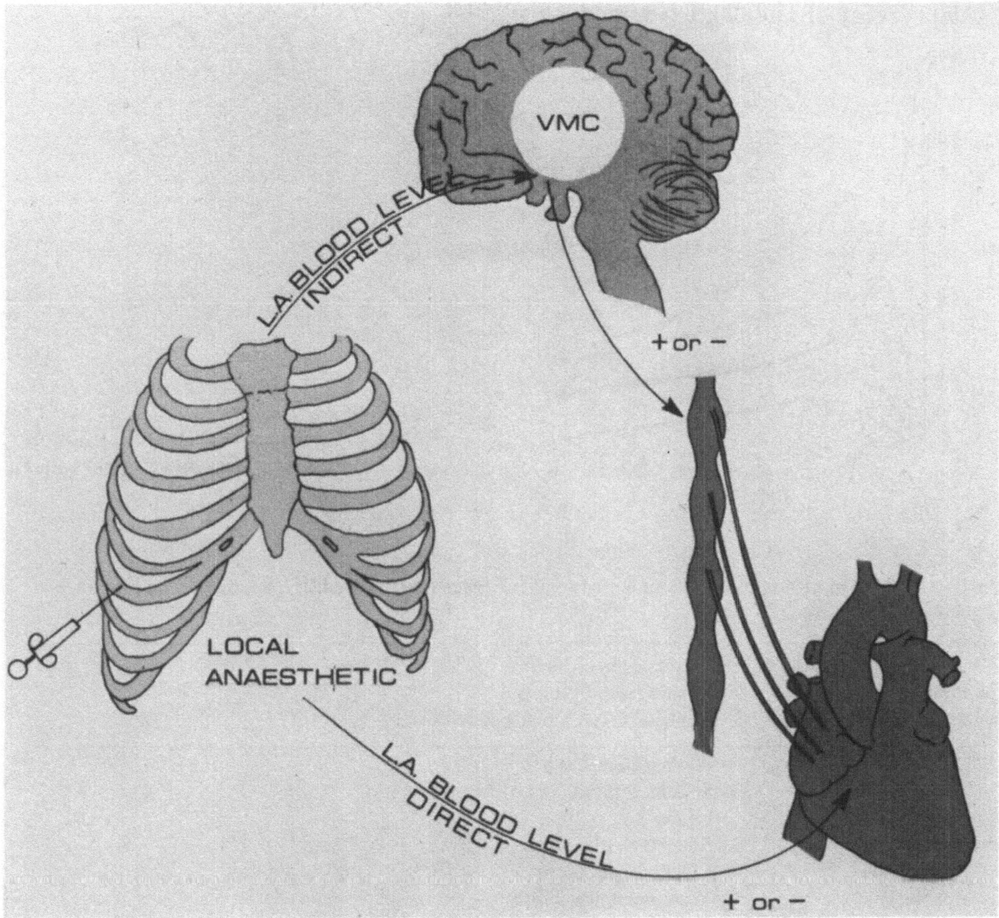

Fig. 5. Schematic drawing showing the two mechanisms by which local anaesthetics exert their influence on the myocardium

ume and also reduce its clearance [1]. Since haemorrhage results in a redistribution of blood from non-essential organs, absorption of local anaesthetic is affected more than is its disposition. Although the liver has a tremendous metabolic reserve and the extraction ratio of lidocaine in man is high, some 60% being removed in a single passage, Benowitz et al. [1, 2], showed in monkeys than when 30% of the blood volume was lost, the hepatic extraction ratio fell from 75% to 43%, so the potential for prolonged circulatory effects of local anaesthetics must be a consideration in hypovolaemia and shock.

Some of the common regional anaesthetic procedures have already been discussed in relation to the blood levels of local anaesthetics which follow equivalent doses of drug. Fig. 6 clearly demonstrates these differences. Table 1 classifies the common techniques in the order of importance relating to the degree with which each can influence the haemodynamic changes in hypovolaemia and shock.

The importance of epidural and spinal anaesthesia in relation to hypovolaemia has been stressed, while the use of coeliac plexus anaesthesia with or without intercostal blocks has not

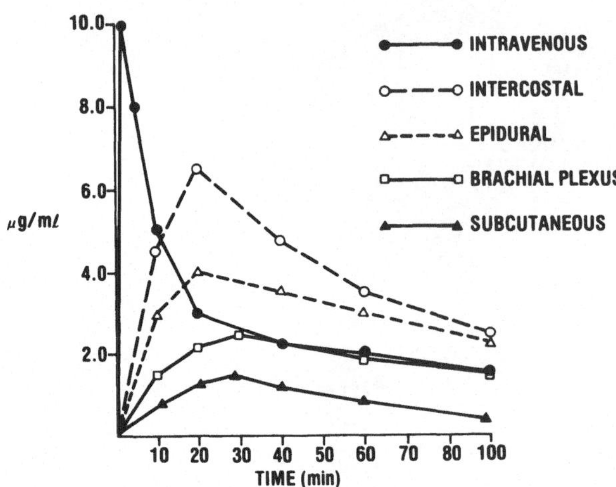

Fig. 6. Comparative peak blood levels of lidocaine after equivalent doses in various anatomical sites

Table 1. Classification of common techniques of regional anaesthesia (Order of haemodynamic influence in hypovolaemia and shock)

Major conduction anaesthesia	1. Epidural anaesthesia 2. Subarachnoid block 3. Coeliac plexus block ± Intercostal blocks
Regional and local anaesthesia	1. Plexus anaesthesia 2. Sciatic, femoral and obturator blocks 3. Bier block 4. Field blocks 5. Terminal nerve blocks

yet been mentioned because of the infrequent use of this technique for abdominal surgery at the present time. Certainly the sympathetic block would be expected to cause the same degree of circulatory embarrassment as would spinal or epidural anaesthesia to the same level. The dose of local anaesthetic which is necessary for adequate analgesia of both the abdominal wall and viscera is much larger than that which is required for epidural anaesthesia of the same number of dermatomes, an aspect which would make this a poor technique in the face of hypovolaemia. Intercostal blocks by themselves are more likely to be used for postoperative analgesia or chest wall trauma. Although it is an axiom of good regional anaesthetic practice to use the smallest dose of local anaesthetic which will achieve satisfactory anaesthesia, the principle is even more important in relation to systemic hypovolaemia.

Except for Bier's block, which is a special case, the remaining regional anaesthetics are associated with only small or moderate drug levels. Interestingly, Mazze and Dunbar [6] found lower quantitites of local anaesthetics after tourniquet release in Bier's block compared with brachial plexus block. However, these results must be interpreted with the realization that after tourniquet release, the peak occurs within a minute and the level will be higher, the shorter the time interval after injection. After 10-20 min most of the local anaesthetic is bound in the tissues, therefore the hazard of high drug blood levels is greatest with short procedures or when inadvertant cuff release occurs prior to tissue binding of the local anaesthetic. in fact half of the total dose is still tissue bound 30 min after tourniquet release [10].

Finally, mention must be made of the physical characteristics of the different regional anaesthetic sites in relation to the local anaesthetic binding properties. Those local anaesthetics such as bupivacaine and etidocaine which are highly fat soluble are rapidly bound to lipid structures and are associated with lower circulating blood levels than their less fat soluble counterparts. However, as has already been shown, the same dose of etidocaine is responsible for much higher blood levels when it is used for intercostal blocks than for epidural anaesthesia. The reason is that multiple injections in the intercostal spaces exposes a larger vascular surface area and therefore more drug is absorbed into the circulation. Although prilocaine has about the same degree of lipid solubility as lidocaine, it has less vasodilator action when used in the same concentration and it is respinsible for much lower blood levels as a consequence.

In summary then, major conduction anaesthesia when used in conjunction with hypovolaemia can be associated with serious circulatory depression. It should not be used in shocked patients until the circulatory status has first been restored. The smallest dose of local anaesthetic agent which will produce the desired effect should be used and a vasoconstrictor having both α and β stimulatory effects should always accompany these blocks. Other regional anaesthetic procedures are safe to use in the presence of hypovolaemia and shock, but intercostal blocks should only be performed with agents having a high lipid affinity like bupivacaine and etidocaine. Bier blocks are excellent but care must be taken to ensure that no release of the tourniquet occurs within 20 min and because of the lower cardiotoxicity on a w/w basis, prilocaine is probably the agent of choice. A double tourniquet should always be used.

References

1. Benowitz N, Forsyth RP, Melmon KL, Rowland M (1974) Lidocaine disposition kinetics in monkey and man II. Effects of hermorrhage and sympathomimetic drug administration. Clin Pharmacol Ther 16:99
2. Benowitz N, Forsyth RP, Melmon KL, Rowland M (1974) Lidocaine disposition kinetics in monkey and man I. Prediction by a perfusion model. Clin Pharmacol Ther 16:87
3. Bonica JJ, Kennedy WF Jr, Akamatsu TJ, Gerbershagen HJ (1972) Circulatory effects of peridural block III. Effects of acute blood loss. Anesthesiology 36:219
4. Jorfeldt L, Löfstrom B, Pernow B, Wahren J (1970) The effect of mepivacaine and lidocaine on forearm resistance and capacitance vessels in man. Acta Anaesthesiol Scand 14:183
5. Kennedy WF, Bonica JJ, Akamatsu TJ, Ward RJ, Martin WE, Grinstein A (1968) Cardiovascular and respiratory effects of subarachnoid block in the presence of acute blood loss. Anesthesiology 29:29
6. Mazze RI, Dunbar RW (1966) Plasma lidocaine concentrations after caudal, lumbar, epidural, axillary block and intravenous regional anesthesia. Anesthesiology 27:574
7. Morikawa KI, Bonica JJ, Tucker GT, Murphy TM (1974) Effect of acute hypovolaemia on lignocaine absorption and cardiovascular response following epidural block in dogs. Br J Anaesth 46:631
8. Ralston LA, Cobb LA, Bruce RA (1961) Acute circulatory effects of arterial bleeding as determined by indicator-dilution curves in normal human subjects. Am Heart J 61:770
9. Rothe CF (1970) Heart failure and fluid loss in hemorrhagic shock. Fed Proc 29:1854
10. Tucker GT, Boas RA (1971) Pharmacokinetic aspects of intravenous regional anesthesia. Anesthesiology 34:538

Diskussion

Question: Dr. Stanton-Hicks, may I ask you to comment on your contention that the advantage of the adrenaline containing anaesthetic solution in the case of hypovolaemia would be connected with a lower blood level of the anaesthetic?

Stanton-Hicks: There are data available in dogs which are bled by 30% of their blood volume showing far lower blood levels of the local anaesthetics when adrenaline containing solution was used, compared to a plain solution. In Hypovolaemic and shock states there is a redistribution of blood from non-essential to essential organs and by this reduced perfusion the uptake of the local anaesthetic into the blood from the site of the injection is also reduced. Thus the uptake of the local anaesthetic from the site of injection is reduced either by adrenaline or by the reduced perfusion in the hypovolaemic state. Bonica's results seem complicated to me because his experiments were dual experiments. In his series, an adrenaline containing solution was always given before the plain solution on the same day. It may well be that this was an additional factor in that some of the local anaesthetic from the first study was still bound in the myocardium when the plain solution in the second study was injected, increasing the amount of the local anaesthetics in the myocardium and thus causing the facts in the second series.

Haemodynamic Adaptation During Peridural Analgesia in Elderly Patients

G. Engberg and L. Wiklund

It has been known for a relatively long time that the circulatory disturbances that occur during epidural or spinal analgesia increase both with the age of the patient and with the extent of the analgesia. Through the many excellent studies reported from Seattle, Washington, it has in fact been established that these disturbances – arterial hypotension and a decreased cardiac output – are of a different order of magnitude and of greater clinical significance in older patients [2]. Further, attention has been drawn to the difference in circulatory adaptation between healthy volunteers not undergoing surgery and elderly patients with a poor circulation [2, 3, 4] of whom we meet so many nowadays in our daily clinical work. Especially when the blockades have reached the upper thoracic segments, the circulatory adaptation of the older patients has been found to be more difficult to control. From the findings of Otton and Wilson [14], among others, this would seem to be attributable to a blockade of the sympathetic cardiac nerves, i.e. the nerves that increase the power of contraction of the heart and the heart rate. The elimination of this sympathetic stimulation of the heart [13] generally has the effect that the heart cannot compensate for the lower degree of ventricular filling following peripheral vasodilatation. Furthermore, in clinical practice two other drugs are used in conjunction with these forms of analgesia. These are atropine, which eliminates vagal influence of the heart [14], and adrenaline in the local anaesthetic solution, which apart from its increasing effect on the heart rate decreases the total peripheral resistance and somewhat increases cardiac output [4, 11].

During the initial trial of etidocaine about 8 years ago, we came up against the problem of a rapid fall in blood pressure after induction of epidural analgesia with this drug [7, 11]. Two such examples of cardiovascular collapse then occurred during a trial series in which epidural blockades up to between C_8 and T_3 were generally attained in elderly patients [8, 9]. The patients were premedicated with morphine and scopolamine and also received 300 ml fluid i.v. immediately before the blockade. Fig. 1 shows the rapidly decreasing arterial blood pressure, the decrease in pulmonary arterial pressure so that it became slightly negative during di-

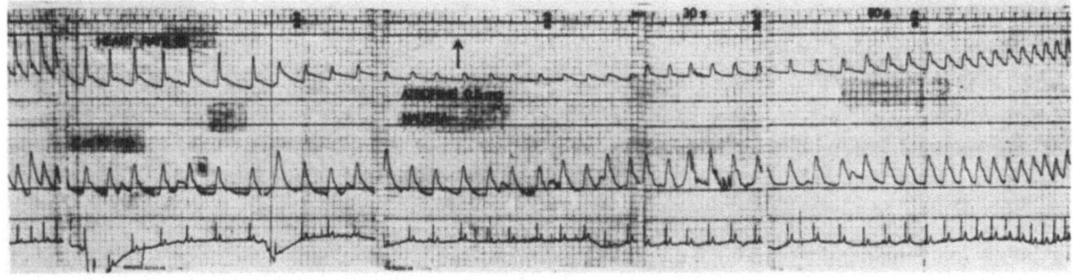

Fig. 1. Recordings of arterial blood pressure (upper tracing, 0-100 mm Hg), pulmonary arterial blood pressure (middle tracing, 0-40 mm Hg) and ECG (lower tracing) in one patient before and during a sudden decrease in these blood pressures and heart rate. Etidocaine adrenaline was used without ephedrine premedication. Above the upper tracing, time is marked in seconds

astole, and the rapid fall in heart rate to 28 beats/min. After i.v. administration of atropine the circulation was restored within 60 s to the values recorded before the collapse. Another example of a similar collapse is shown in Fig. 2; about 20 min before this recording was made the elderly patient had had an injection of 20 ml 1% etidocaine (plain) through an epidural catheter.

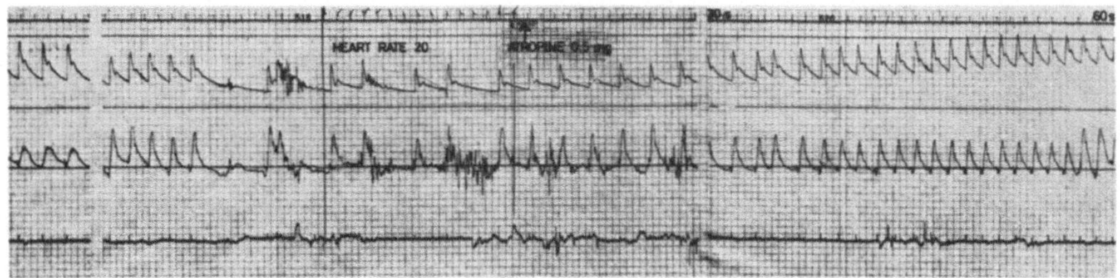

Fig. 2. Recordings of arterial blood pressure (upper tracing, 0-100 mm Hg), pulmonary arterial blood pressure (middle tracing, 0-40 mm Hg) and ECG (lower tracing) before and during a sudden decrease in these blood pressures and heart rate. Etidocaine plain was used without ephedrine premedication. Above the upper tracing, time is marked in seconds

Fortunately the majority of our elderly patients do not react so dramatically to administration of a high level epidural blockade. Almost invariably, however, there is a considerable fall in blood pressure, which occurs most rapidly after administration of etidocaine, but the magnitude of the fall is the same for both etidocaine and bupivacaine (Figs. 3 a and b). The rapid

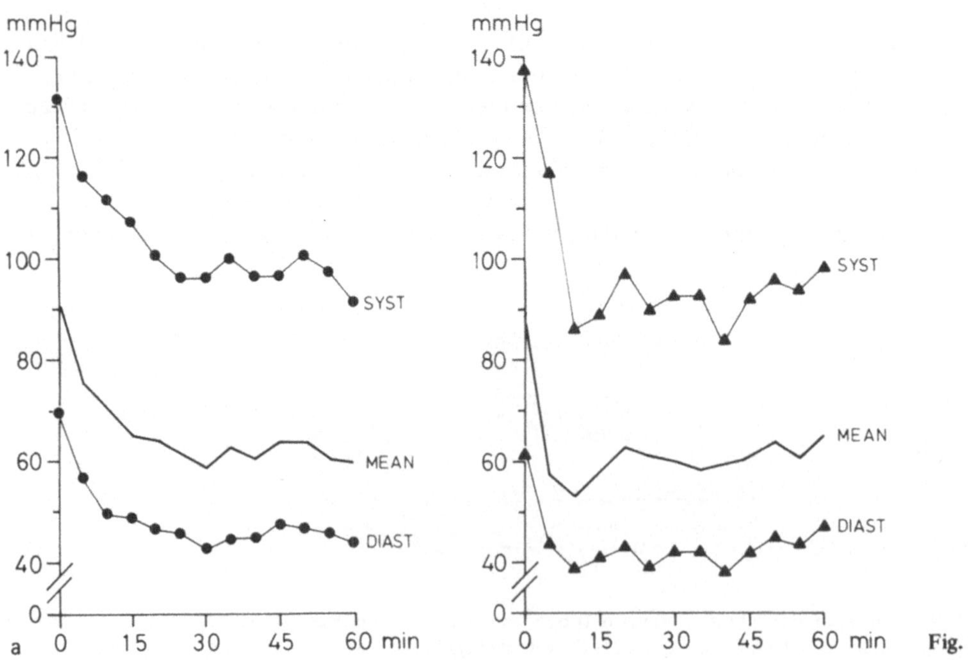

Fig. 3a

blood pressure decrease, especially, often causes nausea, pallor and cold sweating, and sometimes even isolated aberrant ECG complexes. As seen in Fig. 4, however, this blood pressure reaction is not generally accompanied by bradycardia and the cardiac output remains at the same level. The only noteworthy event that normally takes place is that the total peripheral resistance decreases and so do the pressures in the pulmonary artery. One may ask what it is that makes the patient feel ill when the blood pressure falls rapidly. Although we have no measurement results in this respect from this series, the cause may be stated with certainty to lie in a diminished cerebral blood flow and sometimes deterioration of coronary perfusion. It should be kept in mind that these vascular areas in particular are more pressure dependent in older people, who often have a slight or even manifest hypertension [5, 6, 12].

We solved the problem of this rapid fall in blood pressure on induction of high epidural blockades with etidocaine and bupivacaine in elderly patients by starting to use the old well-known drug ephedrine, which has both an ionotropic effect on the heart and a constrictive effect on the peripheral vessels [1, 15]. We gave 50 mg ephedrine subcutaneously or intramuscularly into the patient's back at the same time as the epidural catheter was inserted. The same dose of local anaesthetic then had no significant effect on the pulmonary arterial pressures

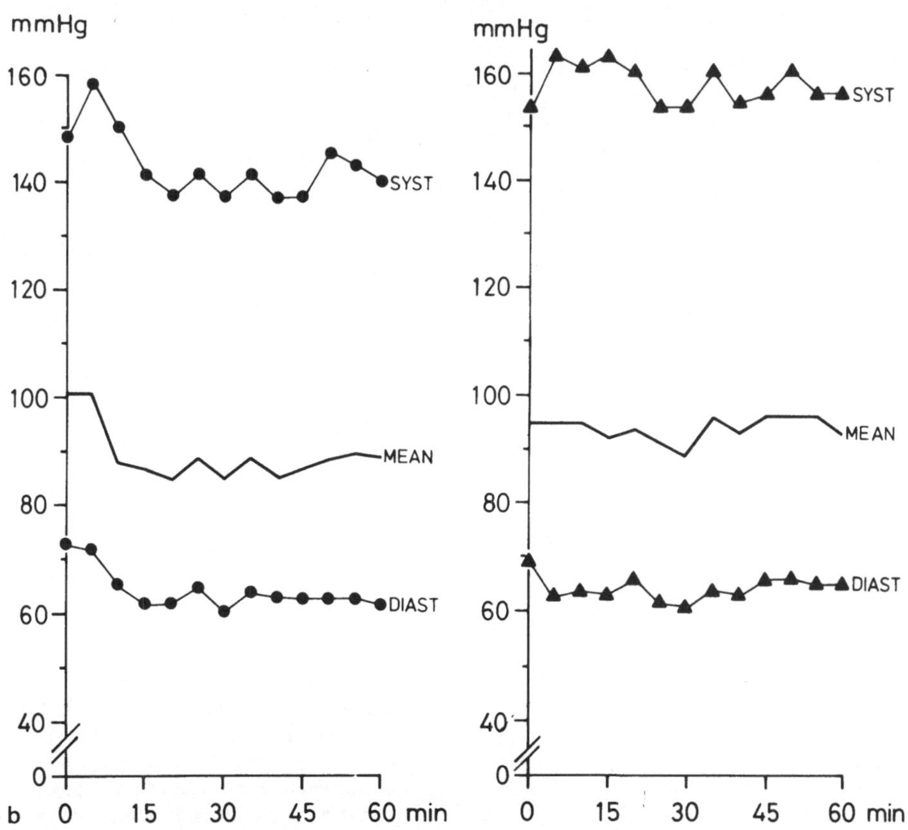

Fig. 3a and b. Systolic, mean and diastolic arterial blood pressure (mean values) before and during epidural blockade with bupivacaine adrenaline (● ○) and etidocaine adrenaline (▲ △) without *(3a)* and with *(3b)* ephedrine premedication

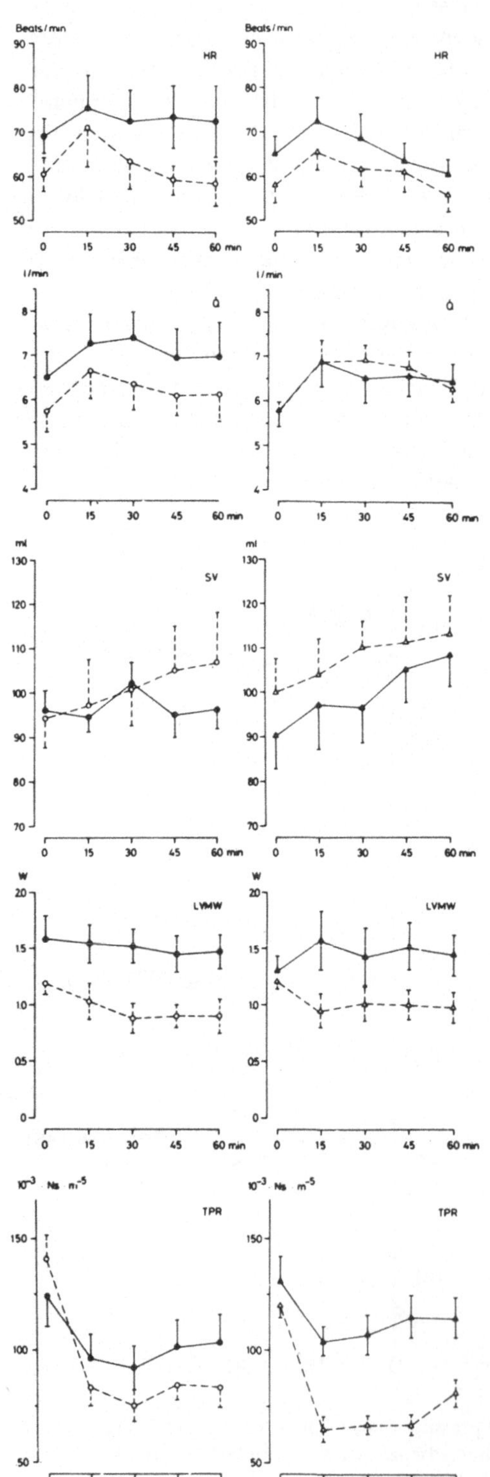

Fig. 4. Heart rate, cardiac output (Q̇), stroke volume (SV), left ventricular minute work (LVMW) and total peripheral resistance (TPR) before and during epidural blockade with bupivacaine adrenaline (left) and etidocaine adrenaline (right). Dashed lines and open symbols represent groups without, and solid lines and filled symbols represent groups with ephedrine premedication. The values are presented as means ± standard error

(Fig. 5), and the arterial blood pressure remained stable. We noted, moreover, that these effects were attained without any increase in heart rate or heart work (see Fig. 4). The total peripheral vascular resistance increased somewhat as a result of the ephedrine injection, but even then it remained significantly below the pre-anaesthesia level (see Fig. 4).

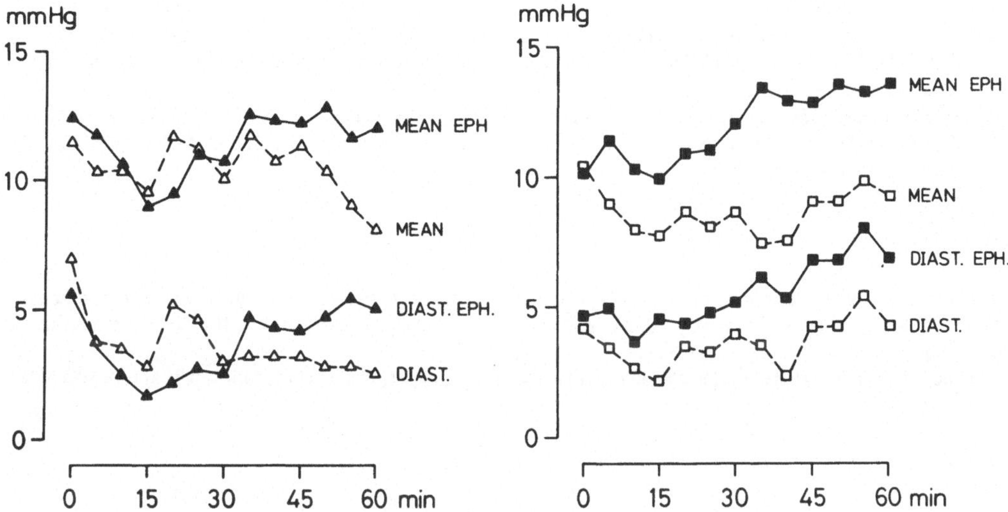

Fig. 5. Mean and diastolic pulmonary arterial blood pressure before and during epidural blockade with etidocaine adrenaline (left) and etidocaine plain (right), with and without ephedrine premedication

In summary, it should be borne in mind that the circulation of the central nervous system and the coronary blood flow are more sensitive to blood pressure decreases in elderly patients than in young ones. We have eliminated the difficulty in blood pressure regulation which is often encountered in older patients after induction of a high epidural blockade, by premedication with ephedrine. With the use of this drug we have maintained a stable blood pressure without any increase in the work of the heart, and as a result the patients have felt much better.

References

1. Aviado DM (1970) Sympathomimetic drugs. Springfield, pp 95-156
2. Bonica JJ, Backup PH, Anderson CE, Hadfield D, Crepps WF, Monk BF (1957) Peridural block: Analysis of 3.637 cases and a review. Anesthesiology 18:723
3. Bonica JJ, Berges PU, Morikawa K (1970) Circulatory effects of peridural block: I. Effects of level of analgesia and dose of lidocaine. Anesthesiology 33:619
4. Bonica JJ, Akamatsu TJ, Berges PU, Morikawa K, Kennedy WF Jr (1971) Circulatory effects of peridural block: II. Effects of epinephrine. Anesthesiology 35:514
5. Duke PC, Wade JG, Hickey RF, Larson CP (1976) The effect of age on baroreceptor reflex function in man. Can Anaesth Soc J 23:111
6. Eckenhoff JE, Hafkenschiel JH, Foltz EL, Driver RL (1948) Influence of hypotension on coronary blood flow, cardiac work, and cardiac efficiency. Am J Physiol 152:545
7. Engberg G (1977) The use of ephedrine in epidural analgesia. Ups J Med Sci 82:183
8. Engberg G, Wiklund L (1978) The use of ephedrine for prevention of arterial hypotension during epidural Blockade. Acta Anaesthesiol Scand [Suppl] 66:1

9. Engberg G, Wiklund L (1978) The circulatory effects of intravenously administered ephedrine during epidural blockade. Acta Anaesthesiol Scand [Suppl] 66:27
10. Engberg G, Holmdahl MH Jr, Edström HH (1974) A comparison of the local anaesthetic properties of bupivacaine and two new longacting agents, HS 37 and etidocaine, in epidural analgesia. Acta Anaesthesiol Scand 18:277
11. Kennedy WF Jr, Bonica JJ, Ward RJ, Tolas AG, Martin WE, Grinstein A (1966) Cardiorespiratory effects of epinephrine when used in regional anesthesia. Acta Anaesthesiol Scand 23:320
12. Lassen NA, Christensen MS (1976) Physiology of cerebral blood flow. Br J Anaesth 48:719
13. Levy MN (1971) Sympathetic – parasympathetic interactions on the heart. Circ Res 19:437
14. Otton PE, Wilson EJ (1966) The cardiocirculatory effects of upper thoracic epidural analgesia. Can Anaesth Soc J 13:541
15. Ward RJ, Kennedy WF, Bonica JJ, Martin WE, Tolas AG, Akamatsu T (1966) Experimental evaluation of atropine and vasopressors for the treatment of hypotension of high subarachnoidal anesthesia. Anesth Analg 45:621

Discussion

Question: How much fluid do you routinely administer to the patients before induction of epidural anesthesia, especially in those cases with a high epidural; do you have any regimen or is it different from patient to patient?

Wiklund: It is different from anaesthesiologist to anaesthesiologist, but I should think it is about 300-500 ml normally.

Änderung der Hämodynamik während Regionalanaesthesie beim Hypertoniker

H.J. Wüst, W. Sandmann, G. Florack und O. Richter

Die praeoperative Herzkreislauffunktion beim Hypertoniker wird in der Regel von einem erniedrigten Schlag- und Herzzeitvolumen bei erhöhtem totalen peripheren Widerstand gekennzeichnet [1]. Dabei ist das zirkulierende Blutvolumen reduziert [1, 3]. Durch die Wirkungen der Anaesthetika auf den Herzmuskel und die Gefäßmuskulatur kann es bei Narkoseeinleitung in dieser Ausgangssituation zu unkontrollierten Blutdruckabfällen kommen [4]. Auf der anderen Seite droht bei hypertensiven Krisen das Linksherzversagen [2], so daß druck- und widerstandsentlastende Maßnahmen notwendig werden. Die kontinuierliche Epiduralanaesthesie stellt durch die begleitende Sympathikolyse ein solches Verfahren dar. Über die Kreislaufveränderungen während thorakaler Epiduralanaesthesie liegen jedoch bisher keine detaillierten Ergebnisse vor.

Methodik

Es wurden die initialen Einflüsse einer ausgedehnten thorakalen Epiduralanaesthesie (sensibler Block T_5-S_5, 18 Dermatome) auf die Drucke im großen und kleinen Kreislauf sowie auf das Herzzeitvolumen bei 13 Normo- und 19 Hypertonikern verglichen. Zur thorakalen Epiduralanaesthesie erhielten die Patienten 20 ml (davon 5 ml Testdosis) der 0,5%igen Bupivacainlösung ohne Adrenalinzusatz über den bei $T_{8/9}$ eingeführten Epiduralkatheter. Es wurden 1500 ml Elektrolytlösung in dieser Phase infundiert.

Ergebnisse

Herzfrequenz, arterieller Mitteldruck und totaler peripherer Widerstand (Abb. 1)

Die Herzfrequenz, der arterielle Mitteldruck sowie der totale periphere Widerstand zeigen in der Einleitungsphase der hohen thorakalen Epiduralanaesthesie in der hypertensiven Gruppe eine deutliche Reduktion. Beim normotonen Patienten dagegen nimmt der arterille Mitteldruck ab, ohne daß sich der Widerstand ändert und bei den vier Patienten mit einer Nierenarterienstenose ändern sich weder der arterielle Mitteldruck noch der totale periphere Widerstand. Der praeoperativ deutlich höhere Blutdruck und periphere Widerstand in der hypertensiven Gruppe wird dadurch den Werten der normotensiven Gruppe angeglichen.

Herz und Schlagindex (Abb. 2)

In der normotensiven Gruppe führt die Abnahme des Herz- und Schlagindexes zur Senkung des arteriellen Mitteldruckes. Nach Infusion von weiteren 750 ml Elektrolytlösung steigen Herz- und Schlagindex wieder leicht an. Bei unverändertem Schlagindex nimmt der Herzindex beim Hypertoniker frequenzbedingt leicht ab.

Bei den 4 Patienten mit einer Nierenarterienstenose nimmt der Herz- und Schlagindex bis 30 Minuten nach Bupivacaininjektion ab, steigt dann aber ohne Volumengabe auf den Ausgangswert an.

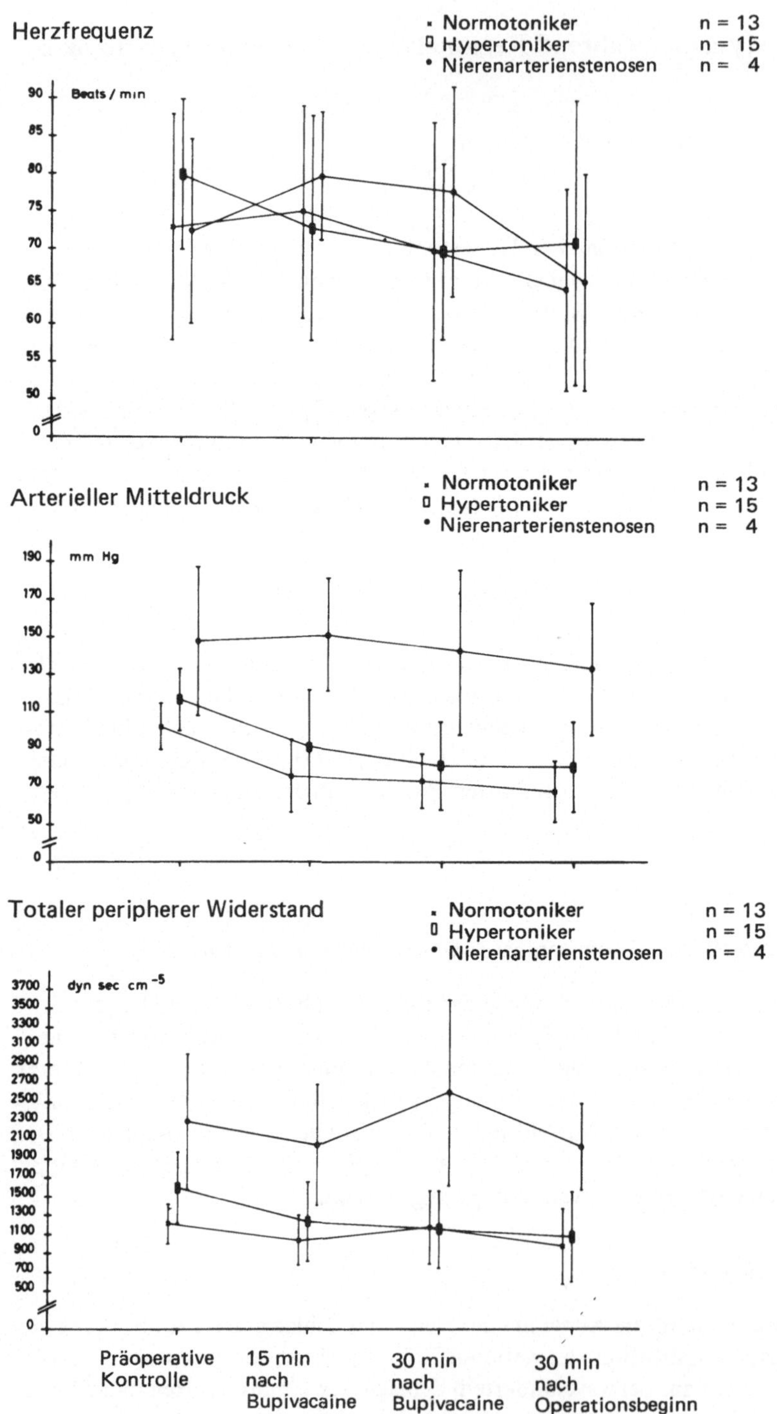

Abb. 1. Verhalten der Herzfrequenz, des arteriellen Mitteldruckes und des totalen peripheren Widerstandes beim normotensiven, hypertensiven Patienten und vier Patienten mit einer renovasculären Hypertonie während der Einleitungsphase einer hohen thorakalen Epiduralanaesthesie

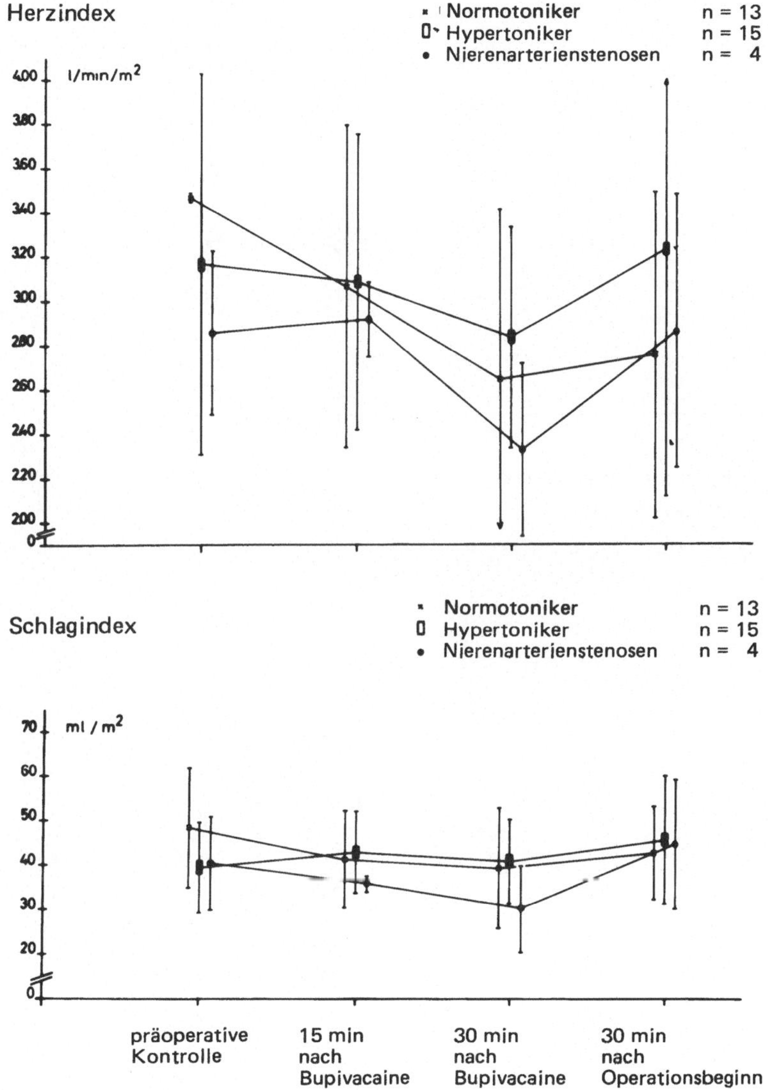

Abb. 2. Verhalten des Schlag- und Herzindexes in der Einleitungsphase der hohen thorakalen Epiduralanaesthesie

Drucke im rechten Vorhof, in der Arteria pulmonalis und in den Lungenkapillaren (Abb. 3)

Entsprechend der Infusionstherapie ändern sich die Drucke im rechten Vorhof, in der Arteria pulmonalis und den Lungenkapillaren nicht wesentlich.

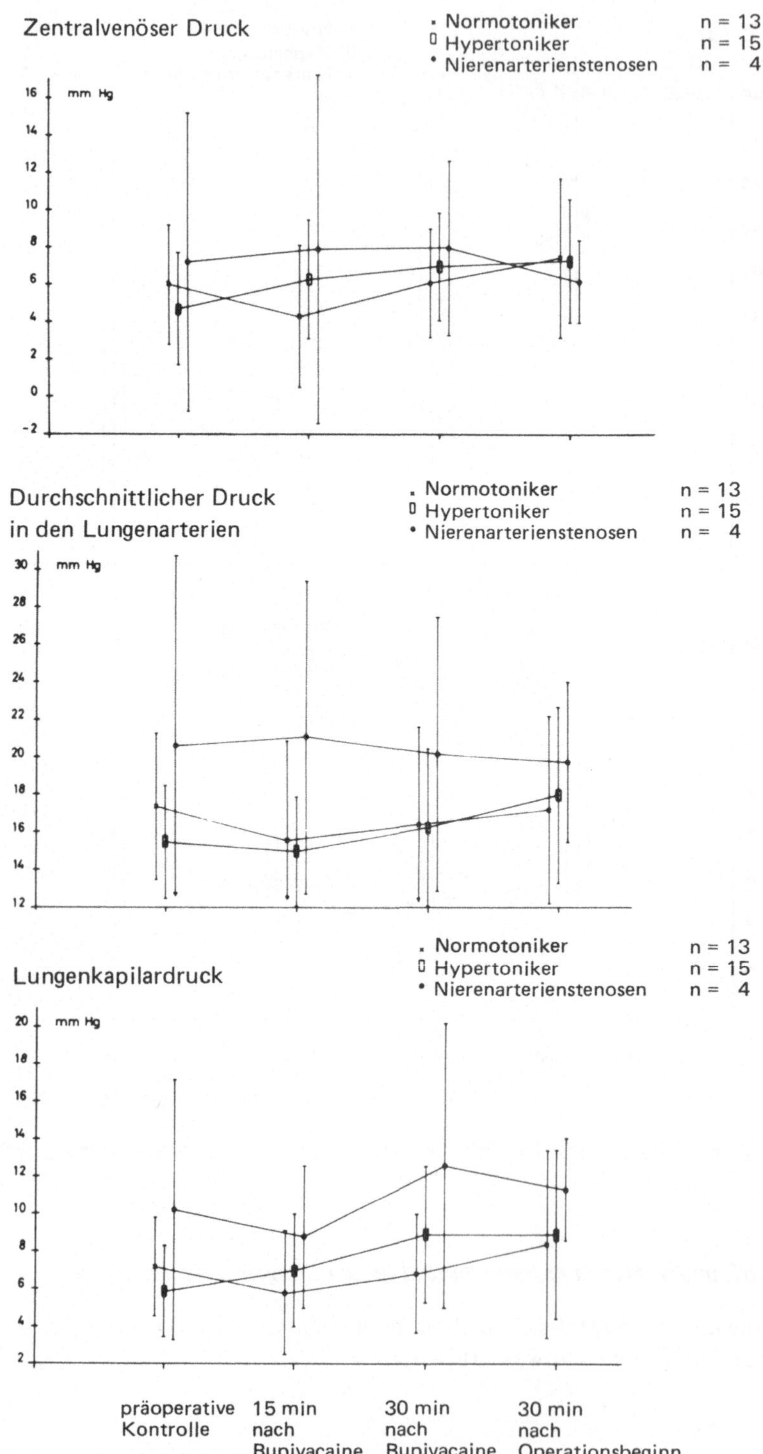

Abb. 3. Verhalten der rechtskardialen Drucke

Zusammenfassung

Die Einleitung der thorakalen Epiduralanaesthesie normalisierte die Druck- und Widerstandsbelastung beim Hypertoniker. Dabei nahm das Herzzeitvolumen frequenzbedingt ab. Für die Aufrechterhaltung eines ausreichenden Schlag- und Herzzeitvolumens erwies sich die ausreichende Volumensubstitution als eine unbedingte Notwendigkeit, da bei diesen Patienten bereits praeoperativ eine Hypovolämie bestand.

Literatur

1. Brismar B, Borgenwald L, Cronenstrand R, Jorfeldt L, Jublin-Dannfelt A (1977) The cardiovascular effects of neuroleptanaesthesia. Acta Anaesthesiol Scand 21:100
2. Gal TJ, Cooperman LH (1975) Hypertension in the immediate postoperative period. Br J Anaesth 47:70
3. Guyton AC, Young DB, Olue JW de, Ferguson JD, Mc Laa RE, Cevese A, Trippodo NC, Hali JE (1975) The role of the kidney in hypertension. In: Berglund G, Hanssen L, Werkö L (eds) Pathophysiology and management of arterial hypertension. Lindgren and Söner, Mölndal
4. Prys-Roberts C, Meloche R, Foex P (1971) Studies of anaesthesia in relation to hypertension I. Cardiovascular responses of treated and untreated patients. Br J Anaesth 43:122

Diskussion

Frage: Können die empfohlenen 1500 ml beim Hypertoniker nach dem Abklingen des Anaesthesieeffektes nicht eventuell unangenehme Folgen haben?

Wüst: Das ist möglich, wenn Sie die Volumensubstitution mit lang wirksamen Mitteln wie Macrodex und auch Humanalbumin betreiben. Dann kann es, nicht so sehr auf der arteriellen Seite, aber im kleinen Kreislauf, zu erheblichen Reaktionen kommen. Die rechtskardialen Drucke steigen in Extremfällen sehr stark an. So haben wir Steigerungen des Druckes in der Arteria pulmonalis um 20 und mehr mm Hg gesehen. Diese Drucksteigerungen wurden aber nur beobachtet, wenn keine Analgesie mehr bestand.

Es ist deshalb die Frage, ob man einem Hypertoniker eine derartig große Menge Flüssigkeit anbieten soll. Erhielte aber der Patient keine Periduralanaesthesie, würde man derartige große Mengen nicht geben, das ist potentiell gefährlich. Es ist notwendig, beim gefäßchirurgischen Patienten, unabhängig von der Narkoseart, reichlich Volumen in der Anfangsphase der Narkose zu geben, weil das zirkulierende Blutvolumen, wie bereits Guyton 1965 und Brismar 1977 gezeigt haben, im Vergleich zu gleichaltrigen gesunden Patienten reduziert ist. Hierfür dürfte die deutliche Reduktion des Herzminutenvolumens und des arteriellen Mitteldruckes bei den 23 Patienten unter Neuroleptanaesthesie ein Anzeichen sein. Die Gabe von 1500 ml Elektrolytlösung bei diesen Patienten verhinderte, wie gezeigt, den Abfall des Blutdruckes und des Herzindex nicht.

Erst nach Beginn der Operation normalisiert sich der Druck und der Herzindex wieder. Unter dem Einfluß der Epiduralanaesthesie dagegen werden diese extremen Kreislaufeffekte, die in der Regel etwa eine halbe Stunde anhalten, abgeschwächt werden. Bei einer drei- bis fünfstündigen Operationsdauer besteht dann, wenn Sie Elektrolytlösung gegeben haben, genügend Zeit zur Entlastung durch Ausscheiden über die Nieren.

Frage: Sie würden sich grundsätzlich dafür aussprechen, eine größere Menge an Flüssigkeit anzubieten, bevor Sie zu einem Vasokonstriktor greifen?

Wüst: Ja, ich würde eher Volumen geben, da diese Patienten, wie bereits gesagt, hypovolämisch sind und zur Aufrechterhaltung einer ausreichenden Nierenfunktion in der postoperativen Phase ein ausreichendes Volumenangebot benötigen.

Frage: In der Geburtshilfe werden immer häufiger betastimulierende Agentien verwendet. Kann jemand über die Zusammenwirkung oder den Effekt der Betastimulationen unter Periduralanaesthesie etwas aussagen?

Antwort: Wenn wir Patientinnen mit einer Periduralanaesthesie Betastimulatoren zur Wehenausschaltung geben, haben wir keine wesentlichen Veränderungen am Kreislauf gesehen. Das sind die Ergebnisse der Untersuchungen von mehreren hundert Patientinnen.

Bemerkung aus dem Auditorium: Wir haben häufiger nach Gabe der Hauptdosis von 8 ml Bupivacain 0,25%ig unter der Geburt eine Zunahme der Wehentätigkeit beobachtet. Sie machte manchmal den notfallmäßigen Einsatz von betastimulierenden Substanzen notwendig. Von seiten der Mutter haben wir hier keine Komplikationen gesehen.

Der Einfluß der thorakalen Periduralanalgesie auf den Schweregrad einer akuten Myokardischämie beim Hund mit offenem Thorax

H. Vik-Mo, S. Ottesen und H. Renck

Eine wachsende Anzahl von Patienten mit koronarer Herzkrankheit sind chirurgische Operationskandidaten. Chirurgische Eingriffe bedeuten in dieser Patientengruppe eine größere Gefahr für Herzinfarkt [15]. Der Einfluß der Anästhesie auf die Entstehung einer Myokardischämie sollte deswegen sorgfältig geschätzt werden. Die thorakale Periduralanalgesie (TPA) hat sich als eine sehr gute Alternative für sowohl intraoperative [4, 7] als auch postoperative Analgesie [6, 8, 11, 12] gezeigt.

Die vorliegende Untersuchung wurde vorgenommen, um den Einfluß der TPA auf die hämodynamischen [14] und metabolischen [3] Determinanten des myokardialen Sauerstoffverbrauchs ($M\dot{V}O_2$) zu studieren. Da außerdem die Größe eines akuten Herzinfarktes hauptsächlich vom lokalen Verhältnis von Sauerstoffangebot und -verbrauch des Herzmuskels abhängt, wurde auch der Einfluß der TPA auf den Schweregrad einer akuten Myokardischämie studiert.

Methode

8 Bastardhunde wurden in Vollnarkose mit Pentobarbital-Natrium untersucht. Das Herz wurde durch eine Thorakotomie freigelegt.

Ein Zweig der linken anterioren Arteria descendens wurde freigelegt in der Absicht, ihn später zu verschließen (Abb. 1).

Das Verhalten der Herzfrequenz (HR), des systolischen linken Ventrikeldrucks (LVSP) als ein Maß der Herzmuskelspannung, und die maximale Steigerungsgeschwindigkeit des linken Ventrikeldrucks (LV dP/dt max) als ein Maß der Herzmuskelkontraktilität wurden als Ausdruck der hämodynamischen Determinanten für den $M\dot{V}O_2$ gemessen.

Als metabolische Determinanten wurden freie Fettsäuren (FFA), Glukose und Laktat im arteriellen Blut und ihre Aufnahme im Herzmuskel bestimmt.

Die Koronardurchblutung (MBF) wurde mittels Wasserstoffdesaturationstechnik [1] gemessen. Der MVO_2 konnte nach Bestimmung der Sauerstoffspannung und -sättigung im arteriellen und Sinus Coronarius-Blut berechnet werden.

Um den Schweregrad der Myokardischämie einzuschätzen, wurden ST-Segmentstudien im epikardialen EKG an 10-15 Stellen des linken Ventrikels vorgenommen [10]. Diese Stellen waren sowohl inner- als auch außerhalb des Versorgungsgebietes der zu verschließenden Koronararterie lokalisiert, als auch fern vom Verschluß. Die Summe der ST-Segmenthebungen in 10-15 EKG-Registrierungen, 10 Min nach dem Verschluß der Koronararterie, wurde als Index des Schweregrads der Ischämie benutzt, während die Anzahl von ST-Segmenthebungen, größer als 2 mV, als Index der Ischämieausbreitung verwendet wurde [10, 13].

Folgende experimentelle Situationen wurden untersucht (Abb. 2): **(1.)** Zuerst wurden Registrierungen in einem Leerversuch durchgeführt, begleitet von **(2.)** einem Verschluß der Koronararterie unter Kontrollbedingungen und Registrierung 10 Min danach. **(3.)** Der Leerversuch wurde 30 Min nach Wiederöffnen der Koronararterie wiederholt. **(4.)** Jetzt erfolgte die Induktion der TPA mit 2,5 ml 0,5% Bupivacain, begleitet von Registrierung nach 30 Min, und

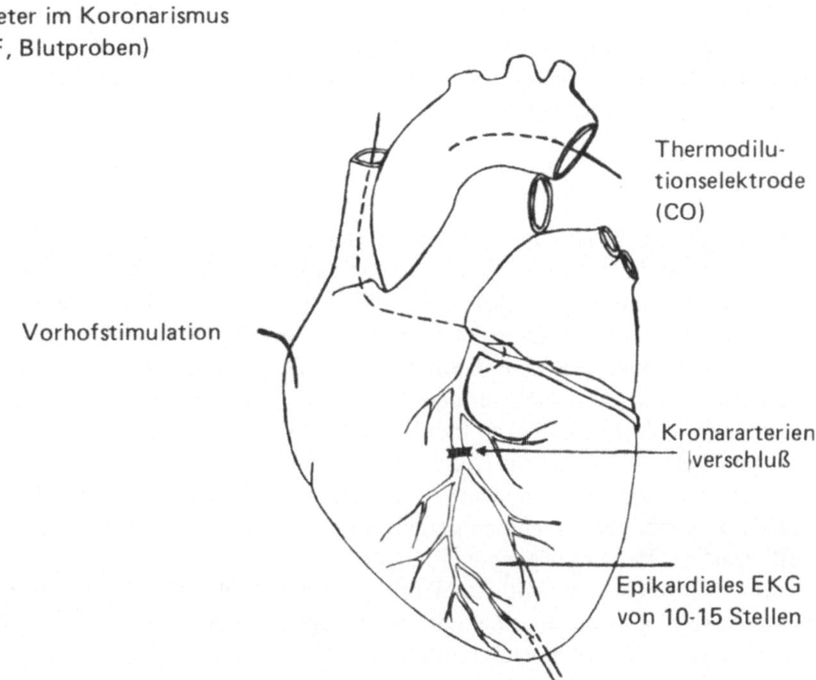

Abb. 1. Experimentelle Herzpräparation

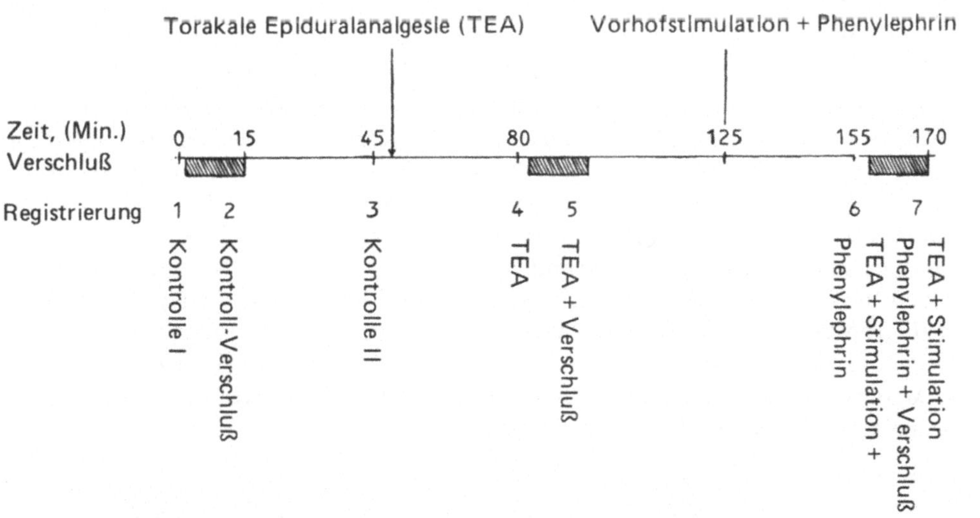

Abb. 2. Experimentelle Situation und Zeitverlauf der Untersuchung. 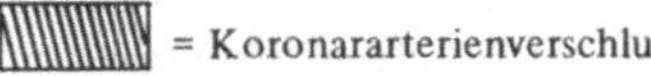 = Koronararterienverschluß

(5.) Verschluß der Koronararterie wie im Leerversuch. (6.) 30 Min nach Wiederöffnen der Arterie erfolgte eine Infusion von Phenylephrin und Vorhofstimulation, bis die HR und der arterielle Blutdruck auf Leerversuchswerte resituiert waren. (7.) Zuletzt wurde die Koronararterie noch einmal verschlossen.

Ergebnisse

Abb. 3 zeigt, daß die hämodynamischen Determinanten des $M\dot{V}O_2$ ihre Minimalwerte 15 Min. nach Induktion der TPA erreicht hatten und danach stabil blieben. Dies entspricht einer Abnahme der HR von ungefähr 20%, des LVSP von 30% und des LV dP/dt max von etwa 40%.

Die metabolische Wirkung der TPA (Abb. 4) ergab eine ungefähr 30%-Abnahme von sowohl $M\dot{V}O_2$ als auch von MBF. Obwohl die Konzentrationen von FFA, Glukose und Laktat im Arterienblut im Vergleich mit dem Leerversuch unverändert blieben, nahmen ihre Nettoaufnahmen im Herzmuskel nach Induktion der TPA signifikant ab. Dieser Abfall war für FFA 70%, für Glukose 40% und für Laktat 45%.

Nachdem die Leerversuchwerte des arteriellen Blutdrucks und der HR mit Phenylephrin und Vorhofstimulation wiederhergestellt waren, stiegen auch Substrataufnahme und Sauerstoffbedarf des Herzens wieder an.

Die TPA zeigte eine deutliche Wirkung auf die Myokardischämie. Als Summe der ST-Segmenthebungen ausgedrückt, nahm der Schweregrad des Herzinfarktes im Vergleich mit dem Verschluß im Leerversuch nach Induktion der TPA signifikant ab. Die Ischämieausbreitung blieb dagegen im wesentlichen unverändert.

Nach Wiederherstellung des arteriellen Blutdrucks und der HR auf Leerversuchswerte nahmen $M\dot{V}O_2$ und Schweregrad des Herzinfarktes wieder zu.

In dieser Weise stimmten die Veränderungen der Myokardischämie in dieser Untersuchung gut mit den gemessenen Veränderungen der hämodynamischen Determinanten des Herzmuskelstoffwechsels überein.

Diskussion

Nach Angaben der Literatur ist die Durchblutung im Endokard bei einer Myokardischämie noch mehr beeinträchtigt als die im Epikard [2]. Auch bei Stimulation des Ganglion stellatum beim Hund nimmt die Durchblutung im Endokard auf Kosten des Epikards ab [16], während die erstere bei einer Sympathikusblockade wie bei der TPA zunimmt [5]. Vielleicht hat dieser Mechanismus eine Rolle bei der Reduktion der Myokardischämie bei der TPA gespielt. Eine Hemmung der stimulierten Lipolyse, die normalerweise im ischämischen Myokard vorkommt, könnte außerdem auch günstig auf den Schweregrad des Herzinfarktes eingewirkt haben [9].

Die Ergebnisse dieser Untersuchung lassen vermuten, daß der Sauerstoffgehalt eines ischämischen Myokards durch die TPA verbessert wird. Die Konklusion ist, daß die TPA die Schwere einer Myokardischämie hauptsächlich durch eine Reduktion der mechanischen Aktivität und damit des Stoffwechsels des Herzens reduziert.

Literatur

1. Aukland K, Bower BF, Berliner RW (1954) Measurement of local blood flow with hydrogen gas. Circ Res 14:164
2. Becker LC, Fortuin NJ, Pitt B (1971) Effect of ischemia and antianginal drugs on the distribution of radioactive microspheres in the canine left ventricle. Circ Res 28:263

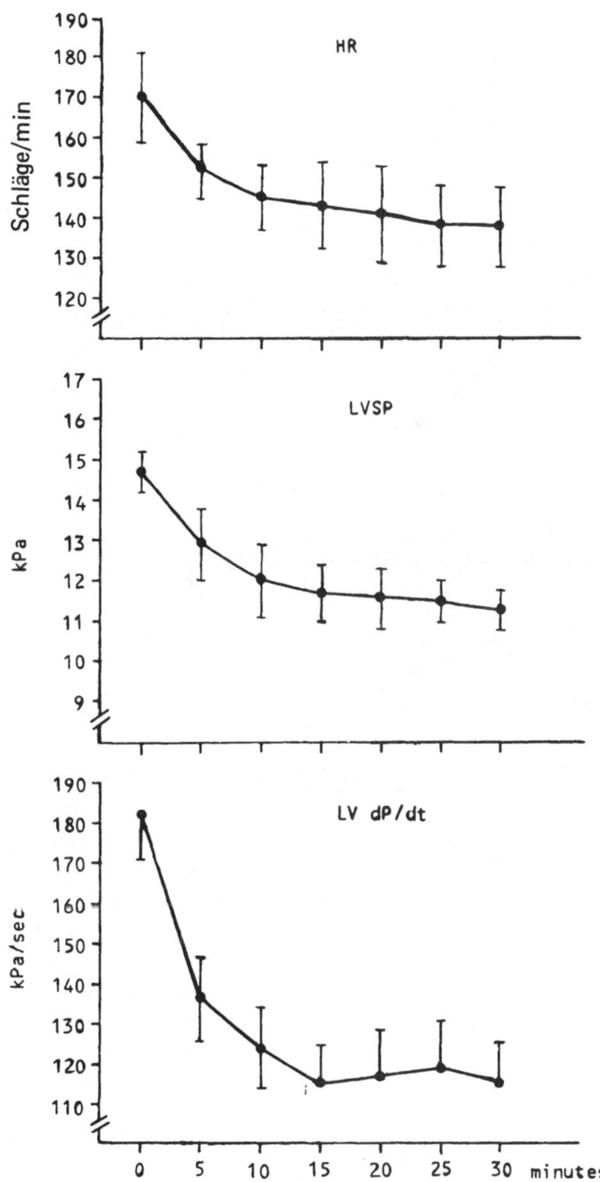

Abb. 3. Akute Wirkung der thorakalen periduralanalgesie auf HR, LVSP und LV dP/dt max

3. Bing RJ (1965) Cardiac metabolism. Physiol Rev 45:171
4. Bonica JJ, Backup PH, Anderson CE, Hadfield D, Crepps WF, Monk BF (1957) Peridural block: Analysis of 3637 cases and a review. Anesthesiology 18:723
5. Bramwell RS, Zborowska-Sluis DT, Bromage PR, Klassen GA (1977) The effect of epidural blockade on the canine coronary circulation. Meeting Amer. Soc. Anesth., New Orleans, Abstracts p 769
6. Bromage PR (1967) Extradural analgesia for pain relief. Br J Anaesth 39:721
7. Dawkins CJ, Steel GC (1971) Thoracic extradural (epidural) block for upper abdominal surgery. Anaesthesia 26:41

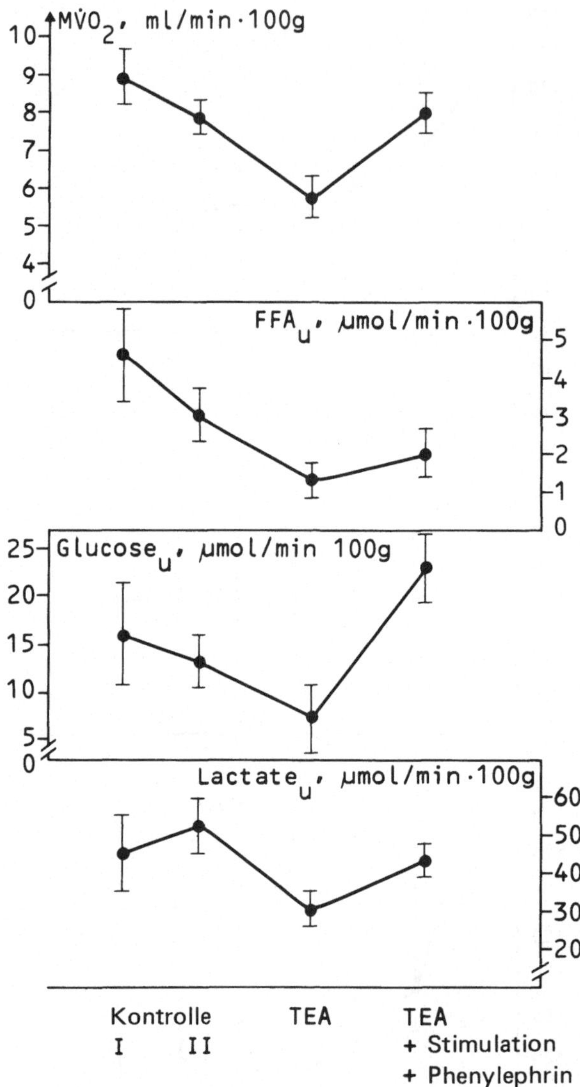

Abb. 4. Akute Wirkung der thorakalen Periduralanalgesie auf $M\dot{V}O_2$, FFA, Glukose und Laktat

8. Hollmen A, Saukonen J (1972) The effects of postoperative epidural analgesia versus centrally acting opiates on physiological shunt after upper abdominal operations. Acta Anaesthesiol Scand 16:147
9. Hough RS, Gevers W (1975) Catecholamine release as mediator of intracellular enzyme activation in ischemic perfused rat heart. S Afr Med J 49:538
10. Maroko PR, Kjekshus JK, Sobel BE, Watanabe T, Covell JW, Ross J, Braunwald E (1971) Factors influencing infarct size following experimental coronary artery occlusion. Circulation 43:67
11. Renck H, Edström H, Kinnberger B, Brandt G (1976) Thoracic epidural analgesia – II: Prolongation in the early postoperative period by continuous injection of 1.0% bupivacaine. Acta Anaesthesiol Scand 20:47
12. Saady A (1974) Pulmonary consequences of upper abdominal surgery – therapeutic considerations. Anaesth Intensive Care 2:221

13. Sayen JJ, Sheldon WF, Pierce G, Kuo PT (1958) Polarografic oxygen, the epicardial electrocardiogram and muscle contraction in experimental acute regional ischemia of the left ventricle. Circ Res 6:779
14. Sonnenblick EH, Ross J Jr, Braunwald E (1968) Oxygen consumption of the heart. Newer concepts of its multifactorial determination. Am J Cardiol 22:328
15. Tarhan S, Moffitt EA, Taylor WF, Giuliani ET (1972) Myocardial infarction after general anesthesis. JAMA 220:1451
16. Uchida Y, Ueda H (1972) Non-uniform blood flow through the ischemic myocardium induced by stellate ganglion stimulation. Jpn Circ J 36:673

Diskussion

Frage: Ich wollte nur wissen, ob das eine Methode ist, einen Herzinfarkt zu behandeln?
Ottesen: Ja, und zwar in Angleichung an die Theorie der Propranolol-Wirkung beim akuten Herzinfarkt, die besagt, daß Propranolol die Infarktgröße reduziert. Obwohl Propranolol direkt auf den Rezeptor wirkt, die thorakale Periduralanalgesie jedoch praeganglionär wirkt, könnte man die Wirkung der beiden auf das Herz vergleichen. Es hat sich außerdem gezeigt, daß die thorakale Periduralanalgesie durch die begleitende Sympathikusblockade antiarrhythmisch wirkt. Die gleiche Wirkung wird bei der direkten Blockade der Betarezeptoren mit Propranolol beobachtet. Gleichzeitig verhindert sie den Angina pectoris Schmerz, wie Untersuchungen bei Patienten nach einer Herztransplantation gezeigt haben, die keine sympathische Innervation des Herzens besitzen. Den gleichen Effekt hat eine Stellatum-Blockade.

Ich selbst habe es in der Praxis noch nie versucht. Es gibt aber einige Einzelbeobachtungen von Gellmann und Bromage, die eine günstige Wirkung der thorakalen Epiduralanalgesie bei Herzinfarktpatienten beobachtet haben. Es liegen aber bisher keine Ergebnisse einer systematischen Untersuchung vor.
Lennartz: Sie haben wohl heute morgen wie auch heute nachmittag mehrfach LV dP/dt max als Maß der Kontraktilität bezeichnet. Wie können Sie in Ihren Untersuchungen ausschließen, daß die Veränderungen von dP/dt max nicht nur Veränderungen der preload und der afterload sind?
Ottesen: Das kann ich nicht ausschließen. Bekanntlich sind bei der Periduralanalgesie Veränderungen der afterload und der preload sehr groß.
Lennartz: Dann kann man dP/dt max auch nicht als Maß der Kontraktilität bezeichnen.
Ottesen: Wir haben auch dP/dt max durch entwickelten Ventrikeldruck gemessen und er hat sich nicht geändert. Aber im Prinzip darf man Ihnen wohl zustimmen, wenn man den Sympathikustonus ausschaltet, dann nimmt wahrscheinlich die Kontraktilität ab.
Frage: Bei Sofortmaßnahmen bei Myokardpatienten sind die Pulmonalkapillardrucke und das Herzminutenvolumen von entscheidender Bedeutung. Deshalb hätte mich interessiert, wie sich die Pulmonalkapillardruckwerte in dieser Untersuchungsserie unter thorakaler Epiduralanaesthesie verhielten.
Ottesen: Wir haben die pulmonalen Verschlußdrucke oder den linksventrikulären enddiastolischen Druck nicht gemessen. Das war wegen technischer Schwierigkeiten nicht möglich. Aber ich stimme mit Ihnen überein, daß die Messung notwendig gewesen wäre.
Frage: Sie haben Vorteile für die hohe Periduralanaesthesie beim Bestehen oder künstlich herbeigeführten Herzinfarkt dargelegt. Wir sind klinisch häufiger in der differenten Situation, wo nämlich der Herzinfarkt befürchtet wird. Selten ist dabei eine hohe Epiduralanaesthesie notwendig, aber gelegentlich kann ein Patient, der vom Herzinfarkt bedroht ist, eine Periduralanaesthesie in der Lumbalgegend gebrauchen können. Würden Sie in dem Falle anraten, die lumbale Epiduralanaesthesie bis in die Thorakalhöhe auszudehnen, um einen Schutz herbeizuführen, obgleich man ja weiß, daß diese Ausdehnung auch mit einem stärkeren Blutdruckabfall einhergeht.
Ottesen: Ich meine, wenn man eine thorakale Periduralanaesthesie so einfach applizieren kann, würde ich das vorziehen. Wenn man die Periduralanalgesie lumbal anlegt, dann muß man ja auch größere Dosen verwenden, um die Ausbreitung hochzubringen.
Arndt: Ich stimme also mit Ihren Befunden durchaus überein. Das ist alles plausibel und kommt eigentlich auch so heraus, wie man es theoretisch erwartet.

Ich bin aber sehr skeptisch, wenn Sie daraus ableiten wollen, daß diese Periduralanaesthesie möglicherweise günstige Effekte haben könne bei Myokardischämie. Ich will Ihnen sagen, warum: Bei diesem experimentellen Präparat fallen Sie auf ein Problem herein: Ihre Tiere haben einen hohen Sympathikotonus, sie haben Herzfrequenzen von 180 und genau da sehen Sie solche Effekte. Sie sehen sie natürlich nicht, wenn diese Tiere 60 Schläge/min hätten, d.h. vorwiegend einen Vagotonus aufweisen, was übrigens auch bei Leuten mit einem Herzinfarkt häufig in der Frühphase nachzuweisen ist. Ich wäre sehr skeptisch, diese Dinge einfach zu übertragen. Ich würde dann erst einmal sehen, wie sieht das unter ganz anderen Bedingungen aus.

Ottesen: Auch ich bin Ihrer Meinung, daß diese Befunde nicht direkt klinisch übertragbar sind. Das war auch nicht unsere Absicht.

Hämodynamische Veränderungen durch Schmerzphasen infolge Tachyphylaxie bei postoperativer Epiduralanaesthesie

H.J. Wüst, W. Sandmann und O. Richter

Durch die kontinuierliche Infusion von Lokalanaesthetika lassen sich die schmerzfreien Intervalle im Verlauf der postoperativen Epiduralanalgesie von durchschnittlich 2 Stunden auf 15 Stunden verlängern. Die Entwicklung einer Toleranz bedingt jedoch immer wieder Schmerzphasen. Bei Patienten unter Epiduralanalgesie können sich aus der sympathikotonen Stimulation durch den Schmerz und der zur Aufrechterhaltung der Herzkreislauffunktion notwendigen Volumensubstitution kardiorespiratorische Probleme entwickeln. Deshalb untersuchten wir den Einfluß einer kontrollierten Schmerzphase auf die Herzkreislauffunktion im kleinen und großen Kreislauf.

Methodik

Bei insgesamt 75 gefäßchirurgischen Patienten nach aortofemoralem Bypass (AFB) wurde der Einfluß einer geplanten Schmerzphase am ersten postoperativen Tag auf die Parameter im großen und kleinen Kreislauf untersucht, und zwar:

1. Orientierend bei 10 Patienten in Hinblick auf Art und Häufigkeit der Kreislaufveränderung.
2. Der Einfluß einer bestehenden Hypertonie auf schmerzbedingte Kreislaufreaktionen (16 Patienten).
3. Der Einfluß der Narkosetechnik (NLA, Halothan, thorakale Epiduralanaesthesie) auf die durch Schmerz induzierten Kreislaufveränderungen (49 Patienten).

Ergebnisse

Die Veränderungen von Herzfrequenz, arteriellem Mitteldruck, Herzindex und TPR während einer Schmerzphase am 1. postoperativen Tag sind in Abb. 1 dargestellt. Nach intraoperativer Epiduralanaesthesie waren die beobachteten Veränderungen nur geringfügig.

Dagegen stiegen die rechtskardialen Drucke deutlich an (Abb. 2), d.h., es kam zu einer Volumenverschiebung aus der Peripherie nach zentral. Möglicherweise wurde eine katecholaminbedingte Vasokonstriktion im kleinen Kreislauf wirksam. Die schmerzbedingten Drucksteigerungen bildeten sich nach Beginn der Analgesie weitgehend zurück.

Ein praeexistenter Hypertonus bedingte eine überschießende sympathikotone Reaktion. Dies zeigen die Parameter des großen und kleinen Kreislaufs.

Die Schmerzausschaltung mit 1 mg/kg Pethidin verbesserte die Kreislaufsituation bis 30 Minuten nach Injektion nicht. Sie führte im Gegenteil bei den Hypertonikern zu einem weiteren Anstieg des Mitteldruckes in der Arteria pulmonalis. Erst der Wiederbeginn der Epiduralanalgesie normalisierte die Kreislaufsituation wieder (Abb. 3).

Einfluß der Narkosetechnik

Auf Grund dieser Ergebnisse erhob sich die Frage nach dem Einfluß der Narkosetechnik auf die schmerzbedingten Kreislaufreaktionen. Bei der Anwendung von gasförmigen wie intravenö-

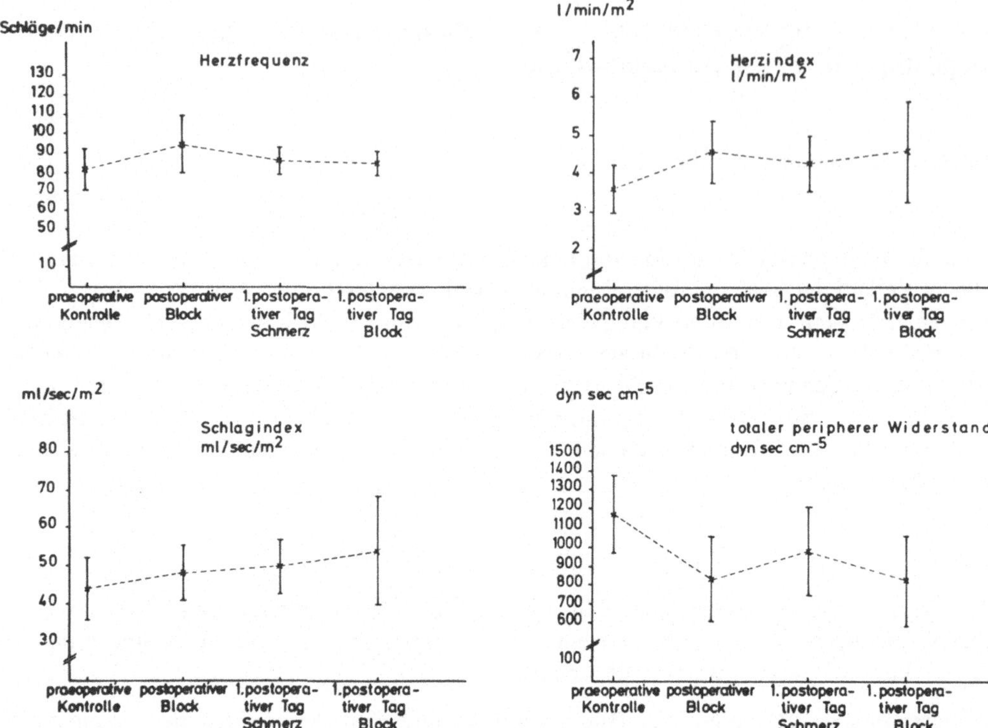

Abb. 1. Mittelwerte und Standardabweichung der Herzfrequenz, des Herz- und Schlagindex sowie des totalen peripheren Widerstandes bei 10 Patienten. Die dargestellten Parameter zeigen während und nach Schmerzphase am 1. postoperativen Tag keine wesentlichen Veränderungen

sen Anaesthetika sind am 1. postoperativen Tag noch relevante Blutspiegel nachweisbar. So betrug die Halbwertszeit von Valium 70 Stunden, die von Fentanyl 1-4 Tage [3]. Eine modifizierende Wirkung des Faktors Narkosemittel war deshalb, wie bereits bei der intraoperativen Herzkreislauffunktion gezeigt, auch bei der Schmerzreaktion in der postoperativen Phase zu erwarten.

In Abb. 4 sind die Kreislaufreaktionen auf den Schmerz in der unmittelbaren postoperativen Phase den Reaktionen auf den Schmerz bei Ausklingen der Epiduralanaesthesie am Morgen des 1. postoperativen Tages gegenübergestellt. Die Abbildung zeigt die Reaktion von HF, MAP, TPR und Herzindex nach NLA, Halothannarkose und Epiduralanaesthesie.

4-6 Stunden nach Operations- und Narkoseende zeigten sich in den drei Narkosegruppen deutliche Unterschiede in der Reaktion auf den Schmerz. Auf den Stimulus stiegen unter Halothan und Epiduralanaesthesie Herzfrequenz, Blutdruck, Herzindex und TPR an. Nach NLA zeigten die Herzfrequenz, der Blutdruck und der TPR die gleiche Reaktion, der Herzindex fiel dagegen signifikant ab.

Erst der Beginn der kontinuierlichen Epiduralanaesthesie glich die Unterschiede in den Parametern in den Narkosegruppen aus. Am Morgen des ersten postoperativen Tages zeigte sich in allen drei Gruppen eine abgeschwächte Reaktion in den Parametern der arteriellen Seite auf den Schmerz.

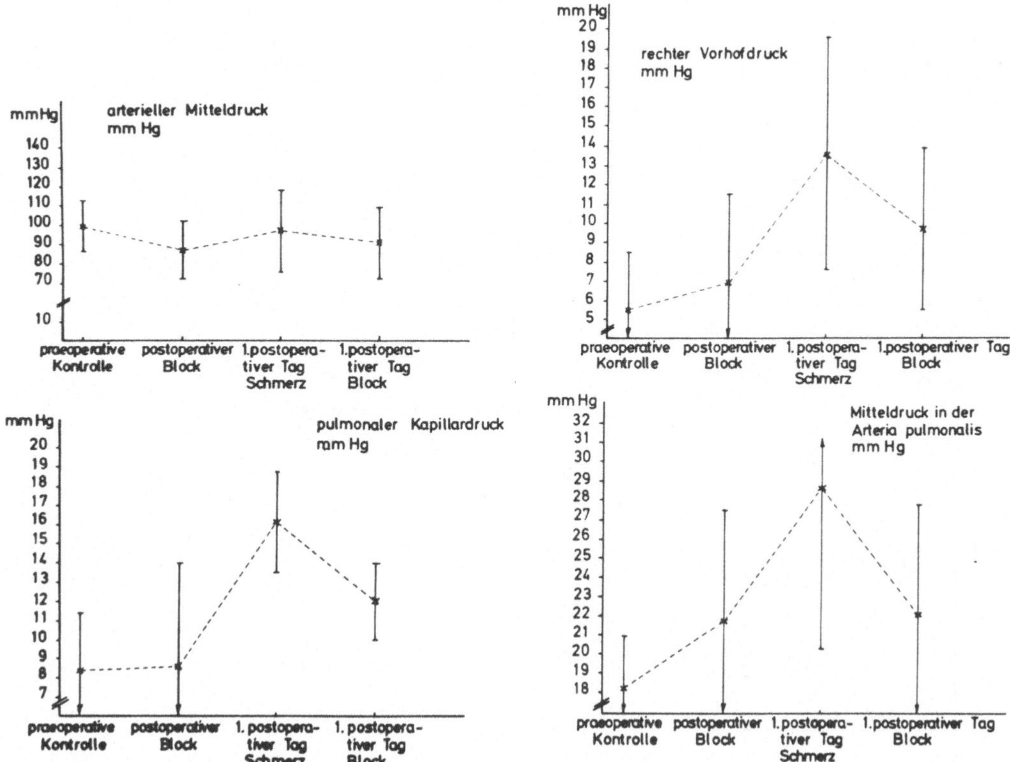

Abb. 2. Mittelwerte und Standardabweichung des arteriellen Mitteldruckes und der rechts-kardialen Drucke bei den gleichen Patienten wie Abb. 1. Im Gegensatz zu der geringen Änderung des arteriellen Mitteldruckes während und nach einer Schmerzphase ergibt sich für die rechtskardialen Drucke eine sehr deutliche Reaktion auf den Schmerz, die sich nach Wiederherstellung der Epiduralanaesthesie zurückbildet

Im kleinen Kreislauf zeigte sich am Beispiel des Mitteldruckes in der Arteria pulmonalis eine unterschiedliche Antwort auf den Schmerzstimulus (Abb. 5). Die Patienten, die nur mit der Epiduralanaesthesie behandelt worden waren, reagierten mit einem minimalen Druckanstieg. Die Reaktion nach Halothannarkose und NLA war dagegen ausgeprägter.

Zusammenfassung

Während Schmerzphasen unter kontinuierlicher Epiduralanaesthesie können die Drucke im kleinen Kreislauf bedrohlich ansteigen. Dabei kann es auch ohne Linksherzversagen zu einem interstitiellen Lungenödem kommen, da der intravasale Druck den onkotischen Druck übersteigen kann. Als Folge wird Flüssigkeit in die Gewebe abgepreßt. Besonders gefährdet sind Hypertoniker, da bei ihnen zusätzlich ein Versagen des linken Herzens durch akute Widerstandsbelastung droht [1, 2]. Die alleinige Behandlung mit Schmerzmitteln konnte die Kreislaufveränderungen nicht mildern. Erst der Wiederbeginn der Epiduralanaesthesie führte zu einer Senkung der Drucke.

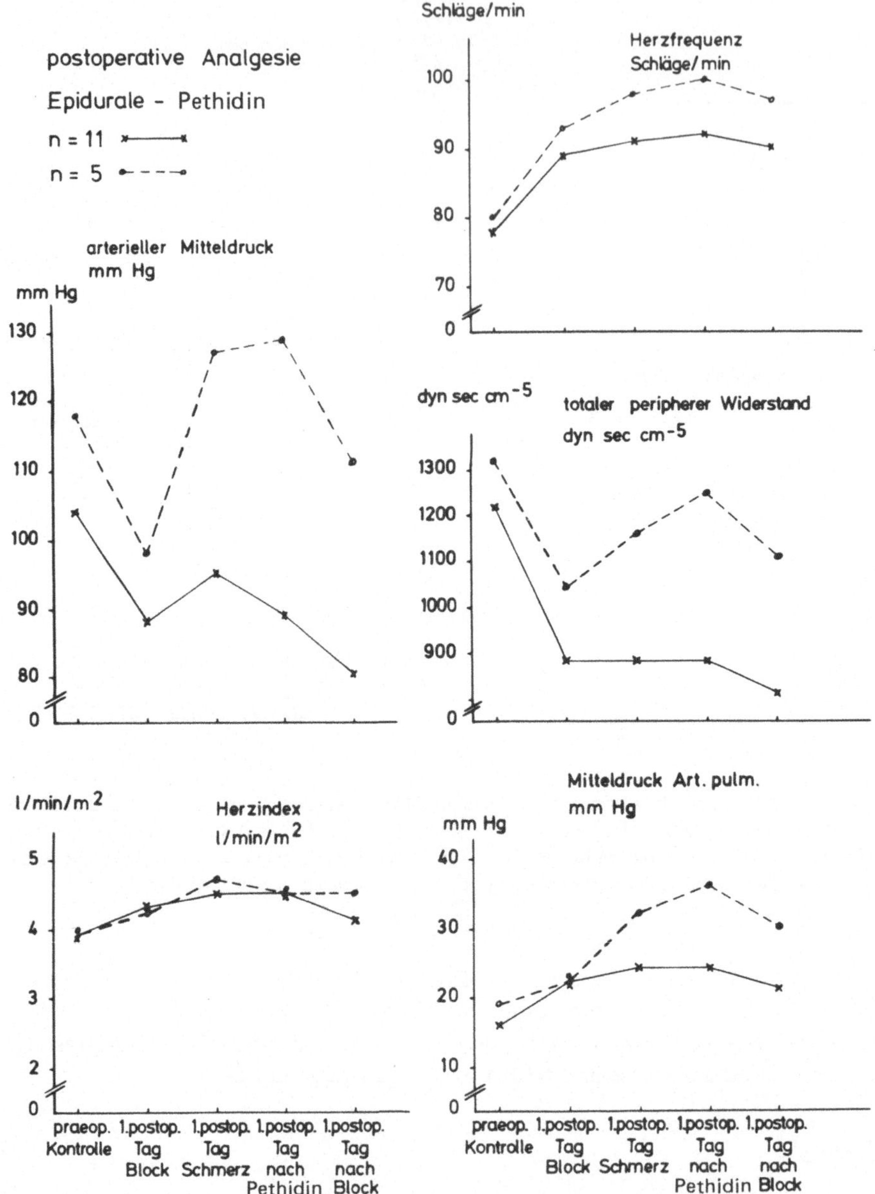

Abb. 3. Darstellung der Kreislaufreaktion beim Normo- (x—x, n = 11) und Hypertoniker (•- - -•, n = 5) auf eine Schmerzphase und die Gabe von 1 mg/kg Dolantin. Schmerzbedingt stieg der arterielle Mitteldruck, der totale periphere Widerstand sowie der Druck in der Arteria pulmonalis beim Hypertoniker deutlicher an als beim Normotoniker. Während 1 mg/kg Dolantin die Kreislaufparameter nicht wesentlich beeinflußt, wird dadurch beim Hypertoniker die hypertensive Reaktion verstärkt. Erst nach Wiederherstellung der Epiduralanaesthesie zeigt sich die Tendenz zur Rückbildung

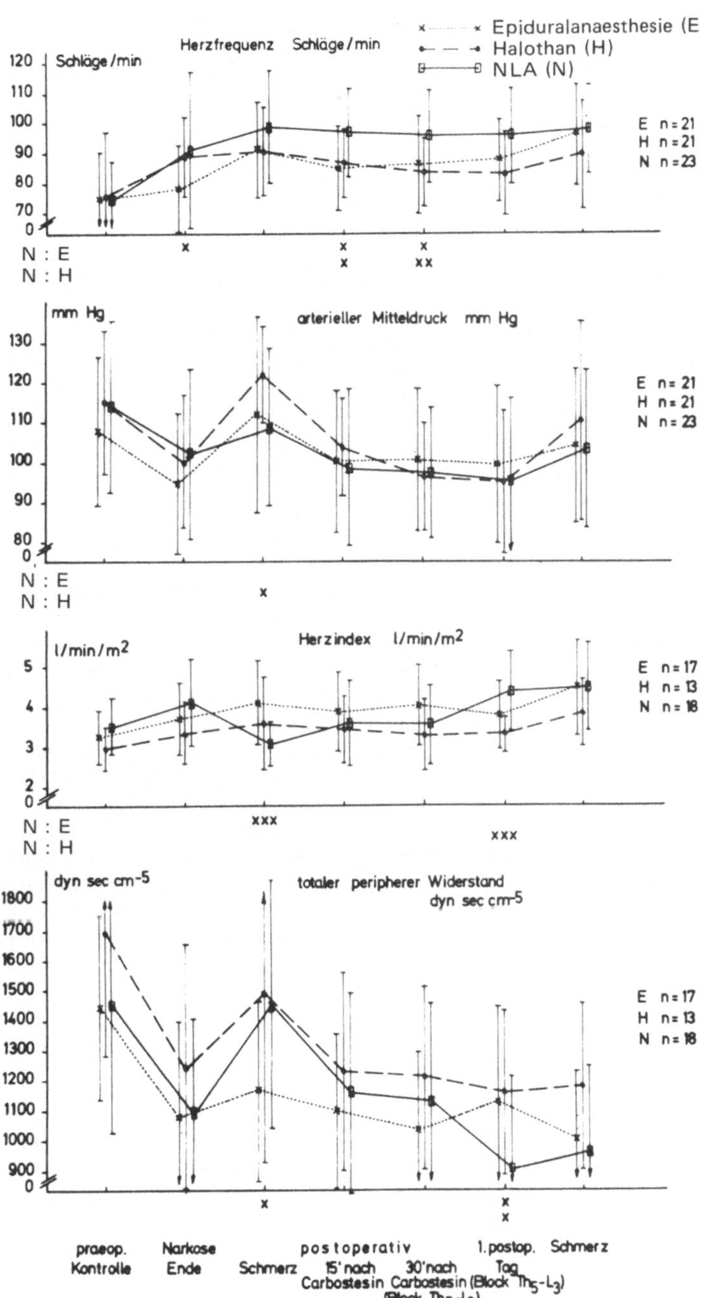

Abb. 4. Gegenüberstellung der Schmerzreaktionen 4-6 Stunden nach Narkoseende und nach Unterbrechung der kontinuierlichen Epiduralanaesthesie am Morgen des 1. postoperativen Tages bei drei Narkoseverfahren. Deutliche sympathikotone Reaktion von Druck und Widerstand in den 3 Narkosegruppen 4-6 Stunden nach Narkoseende. Dabei ist der Herzindex in der Neurolept-Gruppe deutlich abgefallen. Bis 30 Minuten nach Beginn der Epiduralanaesthesie haben sich die Kreislaufparameter in den 3 Narkosegruppen angeglichen. Nach einer kontrollierten Schmerzphase am 1. postoperativen Tag ergibt sich jedoch in den drei Narkosegruppen ein nahezu gleichgerichteter Trend im Verhalten der Kreislaufparameter

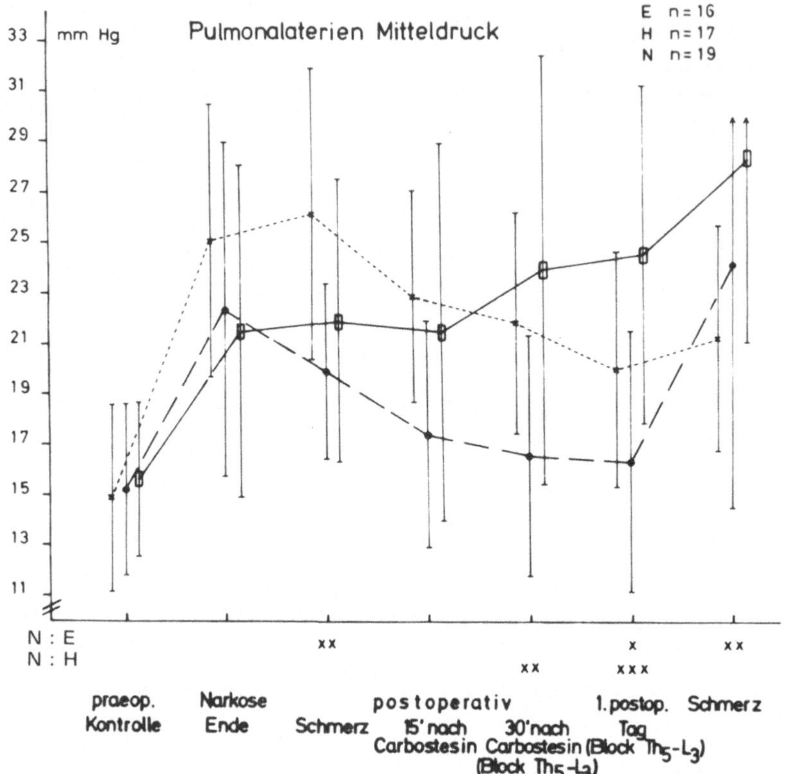

Abb. 5. Gegenüberstellung der Schmerzreaktionen 4-6 Stunden nach Narkoseende und nach Unterbrechung der kontinuierlichen Epiduralanaesthesie am Morgen des 1. postoperativen Tages am Verhalten des Mitteldruckes in der Arteria pulmonalis. Während der Druck in der Arteria pulmonalis in der Schmerzphase 4-6 Stunden nach Narkoseende nicht wesentlich ansteigt, zeigt sich am 1. postoperativen Tag nach Halothan und NLA eine ausgeprägtere Reaktion als in der Epiduralgruppe

Literatur

1. Freis ED (1969) Hypertensive crisis. JAMA 208:338
2. Gal TJ, Cooperman LH (1975) Hypertension in the immediate postoperative period. Br J Anaesth 47:70
3. Wijngaarden V, Soudijn W (1968) The metabolism and excretion of the analgesic fentanyl by wistar rats. Life Sci 7:1239

Diskussion

Frage: Wenn ich Sie richtig verstanden habe, haben Sie gesagt, daß Sie nach Neuroleptnarkose einen geringeren Sauerstoffverbrauch haben als nach der Halothan- und Epiduralnarkose.

Wüst: Nur unter Schmerzbedingungen in der postoperativen Phase war die Sauerstoffaufnahme nach Halothan- und Epiduralnarkose deutlich höher als bei den Patienten, die eine Neuroleptanaesthesie erhalten hatten. Unter diesen Bedingungen zeigen die Patienten der Neuroleptgruppe ebenso wie die Patienten der beiden anderen Gruppe am Verhalten des arteriellen Blutdruckes, der Herzfrequenz und des totalen peripheren Widerstandes eine deutlich sympathikotone Reaktionslage. Während der Herzindex nach Halothan- und Epiduralanaesthesie bei Schmerzen ansteigt, fällt er nach der Neuroleptanaesthesie deutlich ab, d.h. die in der

Zeiteinheit zu den Geweben transportierte Sauerstoffmenge wird reduziert bei unveränderter Aufnahme von Sauerstoff in die Gewebe.

Dabei ist m.E. jedoch die Sauerstoffaufnahme nicht das entscheidende Kriterium, sondern es geht darum: Besteht zwischen der Aufnahme und dem Bedarf ein Gleichgewicht. Hierfür ist die Entwicklung einer metabolischen Azidose ein Kriterium. Der pH-Wert von 7,31 4-6 Stunden nach der Neuroleptanaesthesie deutet aber auf ein Mißverhältnis zwischen Angebot und Bedarf hin, während in der Halothan- und Epiduralgruppe unter Schmerzbedingungen der Sauerstoffbedarf durch das Angebot gedeckt werden kann. Hierfür spricht der normale pH-Wert bei den Patienten dieser beiden Gruppen.

Frage: Nun wollte ich ganz spezifisch wissen, ob Sie die Neuroleptnarkose zur nachklingenden Schmerzbekämpfung erhalten haben, oder ob Sie prinzipiell mit Naloxon antagonisiert haben.

Wüst: Wir haben diesen analgetischen Effekt weitgehend beibehalten. Nur wenn der PCO_2 im arteriellen Blut deutlich über 50 Torr angestiegen und die Atemfrequenz deutlich auf 6-9 Züge/min abgefallen war, griffen wir mit Naloxon ein, da wir die Patienten nicht bis zum Abklingen der atemdepressorischen Wirkung des Fentanyls beatmen wollten.

III. Streß und Endokrinium während Narkose und Operation

Vorsitz: T. Tammisto, Helsinki und H. Lennartz, Marburg

Pathophysiologie des intra- und postoperativen Streß

T. Tammisto

Unter dem Streß-Syndrom versteht man die Veränderungen in der Funktion des Organismus, die durch verschiedene Belastungen wie Angst, Schmerz, Verletzungen, Infektionen u.s.w. hervorgerufen werden. Unabhängig von der Art der auslösenden Belastung gestaltet sich das Syndrom im großen und ganzen gleich, wobei die Aktivierung des neuroendokrinen Systems eine entscheidende Rolle spielt. Diese Aktivierung kann mit einer Lähmungsphase eingeleitet werden und wird dann, falls der Organismus überlebt, in eine anabolische Restitutionsphase umgewandelt. Obwohl der genaue Ablauf und die Bedeutung der einzelnen Funktionsveränderungen und deren komplexen Verflechtungen im Gesamtgeschehen noch nicht aufgeklärt worden sind, bedeutet die Entfaltung dieses Streß-Syndroms eine Sammlung der Abwehrkräfte des Organismus und dient somit dem Überleben des Organismus. Dies braucht aber nicht zu bedeuten, daß alle einzelnen Funktionsveränderungen, ungeachtet des Ausmaßes, des Zeitpunktes und der Zusammenwirkung der Veränderungen, für die Abwehrreaktion immer vorteilhaft sein müssen. Im Gegenteil scheint z.B. eine übertriebene und anhaltende Aktivierung des sympathischen Nervensystems in manchen Situationen eher verhängnisvoll zu werden. Es ist auch denkbar, daß eine an und für sich sinnvolle Abwehrreaktion, die nicht ausreicht, um die Homeostase zu garantieren, sinnlos und sogar schädlich sein kann und – wenn die Homeostase künstlich aufrechterhalten werden muß – Therapieversuchen letzten Endes entgegenwirkt. Die Dämpfung dieser nachteiligen Reaktionen ist deswegen eine wichtige Aufgabe in der Homeostasebehandlung. Leider sind unsere Kenntnisse und pharmakologischen Möglichkeiten zu einer gezielten Therapie vorläufig noch relativ beschränkt, was die Wichtigkeit jeder neuen Information auf diesem Gebiet sehr unterstreicht. Da das Streß-Syndrom eine äußerst bunte Palette der verschiedensten Funktions- und sogar Strukturveränderungen des Organismus anbietet, können wir im Rahmen dieser Ausführungen nur einen flüchtigen Blick darauf werfen.

In der Entstehung des Streß-Syndroms scheinen afferente Reize von der Peripherie zum Hypothalamus eine entscheidende Rolle zu spielen, da deren Unterbrechung die Entfaltung des Streß-Syndroms verhindert. Diese afferenten Reize können direkt am Verletzungsort ausgelöst werden oder sie können durch Folgeerscheinungen der Verletzung wie Blutverlust, Dehydration und pH-Veränderungen entstehen. Es scheint auch wahrscheinlich, daß verschiedene Spaltprodukte des traumatisierten und infizierten Gewebes die Entfaltung des Streß-Syndroms humoral beeinflussen. Es besteht z.B. die Möglichkeit, daß durch Degradierung der Proteine Peptide und Aminosäuren entstehen, Fettsäuren am Verletzungsort in Prostaglandine umgebaut werden und stimulierte Phagozyten pyrogene Proteine produzieren. Durch diese verschiedenen afferenten und humoralen Reize wird der Homeo- und Thermostat des Körperhaushalts, der Hypothalamus, „höher" eingestellt, der Hypothalamus wird also stimuliert. Dies äußert sich erstens als vermehrte Funktion der hypothalamischen Kerne, die die Funktion des autonomen Nervensystems regulieren. Dabei überwiegt die Stimulation der sympathischen ventro- und dorsomedialen Kerne über die der parasympathischen Kerne. Die sympathische Stimulation wird über die thorakolumbale intermediolaterale Säule und von da über den Grenzstrang und über die prävertebralen Ganglien auf die Endorgane übertragen, wodurch die bekannten Symptome des Sympathikotonus zustande kommen. Es entsteht also die von Cannon [1] beschriebene klassische „fight or flight" Reaktion, die durch Freisetzung von Katecholaminen, Kreislaufstimulation und Mobilisation von Nährstoffen wie Glukose, Fett- und Aminosäuren gekennzeichnet ist. Dabei scheint die direkte Stimulation der Endorgane wichtiger zu sein als die Zunahme von zirkulierenden Katecholaminen durch Freisetzung aus dem Nebennierenmark. Die Ansprechbarkeit des sympathischen Nervensystems ist für das Überleben des Organismus im Streß von vitaler Bedeutung. Auf der anderen Seite aber kann, wie schon erwähnt, eine übertriebene und anhaltende Stimulation des Sympathikus schädlich sein. In der Behandlung handelt es sich also darum, eine optimale Aktivität des sympathischen Nervensystems zu gewährleisten.

Der Hypothalamus beherrscht aber nicht nur das vegetative Nervensystem, sondern über die Hypophyse auch andere endokrine Reaktionen des Organismus. Im Hypothalamus werden verschiedene sog. Faktoren aus den Neuronen sekretiert, die die Freisetzung der Hypophysenvorderlappenhormone stimulieren. Diese freisetzenden Faktoren oder Liberine, die Polypeptide sind, stehen wiederum unter monoaminergischer neuraler Kontrolle und deren Ausscheidung kann durch verschiedene zentrale und afferente Reize stimuliert werden. Für jedes der sechs Hypophysenvorderlappenhormone gibt es ein entsprechendes Liberin. So stimuliert Kortikoliberin (CRF) die Ausscheidung von Kortikotropin, Somatoliberin (GRF) die Ausscheidung von Somatotropin u.s.w. Dazu wird durch die Stimulation des Nucleus supraopticus und paraventricularis im Hypothalamus die Sekretion von Vasopressin und Oxytocin aus dem Hypophysenhinterlappen erhöht. Während die Axone der Zellen, die die Sekretion von Vasopressin und Oxytocin regulieren, direkt vom Hypothalamus bis in den Hypophysenhinterlappen hereinreichen, hören die Axone der Neuronen, die die Sekretion von Hypophysenvorderlappenhormonen regulieren, auf der Höhe der Eminentia medialis auf. In der äußeren Schicht der Eminentia medialis werden die freisetzenden Faktoren aus den Neuronen in der perivaskulären Raum des hypothalamischen Kapillarnetzes sezerniert und mit dem Blutstrom in den Vorderlappen transportiert. Hier teilt sich die Arterie in ein zweites Kapillarnetz, das die Liberine in Kontakt mit den verschiedenen Zellarten der Hypophyse bringt und die Sekretion der Hypophysenhormone auslöst. Außer den sechs erwähnten Liberinen sezerniert der Hypothalamus noch mindestens drei entsprechende Inhibitoren, die die Sekretion jener Hypophysenhormone bremsen, die nicht durch sekundär ausgeschiedene Hormone gebremst werden, wie z.B. Kortikotropin und Thyreotropin durch Nebennierenrindenhormone, bzw. durch Schilddrüsenhormone. Während der Streßreaktion wird jedoch die Wirkung der inhibitorischen Faktoren bzw. inhibitorischen Hormone sehr geschwächt, was zur vermehrten Ausscheidung von Hypophysenhormonen beiträgt.

Die Bedeutung dieser Hormone in der Abwehrreaktion ist noch nicht endgültig geklärt. Doch scheint die durch Kortikotropin hervorgerufene Freisetzung von Kortikosteroiden für die Mobilisation der Nährstoffe aus den Geweben und für die Kreislaufstimulation wesentlich zu sein. Dabei spielen die Kortikosteroide eine sog. permissive Rolle für die Wirkung der Katecholamine, indem sie die Anzahl oder die Reaktivität der β-Rezeptoren erhöhen sollen. Auch die Sekretion von Somatotropin wird erhöht. Obwohl Somatotropin durch seine Mobilisation der Fettlager und durch seinen glukose- und proteinsparenden Effekt den Organismus gegen Streß schützt, scheint seine Rolle in der Alarmreaktion unwesentlich zu sein. Gegen Ende der katabolischen Flowphase scheint Somatotropin aber für die Umstellung in die anabolische Phase wichtig zu sein. Auch die Rolle von Thyreotropin ist unklar. Es ist möglich, daß auch die Schilddrüsenhormone bei der Auslösung der anabolischen Phase mitwirken.

Zusätzlich zur Aktivierung des hypothalamischen Homeostats wird auch der Thermostat höher eingestellt, wodurch die Kerntemperatur des Organismus erhöht wird. Das muß hauptsächlich der vermehrten Sympathikotonie zugeschrieben werden, obwohl pyrogene Spaltprodukte mitwirken können.

Die geschilderten neuroendokrinen Funktionsveränderungen charakterisieren also die Alarmreaktion in verschiedenen Streßsituationen. Dazu gesellen sich viele andere Veränderungen, die nicht von geringerer Wichtigkeit für das Überleben zu sein brauchen, deren Bedeutung für das Gesamtgeschehen des Überlebens wohl aber weniger bekannt ist. Auch ihrer Mannigfaltigkeit wegen können sie hier nur stichwortartig erwähnt werden. So ruft z.B. die vermehrte Ausscheidung von Vasopressin Wasser- und Natriumretention hervor und sorgt somit für die Aufrechterhaltung des Wasserhaushalts. Allerdings ist dabei die Natriumretention weniger ausgeprägt, was verminderte Osmolalität zur Folge hat. Auch das Nebennierenrindenhormon Aldosteron fördert die Retention von Natrium und dazu die Ausscheidung von Kalium. Obwohl Kortikotropin in sehr hohen Konzentrationen auch die Ausscheidung von Aldosteron vermehren kann, sind in Verbindung mit Streß andere regulierende Mechanismen vermutlich von größerer Bedeutung wie z.B. Veränderungen im Wasser- und Elektrolytenhaushalt. Auch erhöhter Reningehalt im Plasma stimuliert die Ausscheidung von Aldosteron. Trotz Förderung der Natriumretention und Kaliumausscheidung durch Aldosteron wird während des Streß die Natriumretention auch durch andere Mechanismen reguliert. Die hohe Kaliumausscheidung im Streß scheint von anderen Veränderungen abhängig zu sein.

Auch die Ausscheidung von Glukagon, das von den Langerhanschen α-Zellen der Bauchspeicheldrüse sezerniert wird, wird durch Streß stimuliert. Die vermehrte sympathische Aktivität ist wohl der hauptsächliche Grund zur Hyperglukagonämie in Verbindung mit Streß. Ähnlich wie die Katecholamine ruft auch Glukagon Glykogenolyse und Inotropie hervor. Das Zusammenspiel zwischen Katecholaminen und Glukagon wird noch dadurch verstärkt, daß Glukagon seinerseits die Ausscheidung von Katecholaminen aus den Nebennieren stimuliert. Die Glykogenolyse wird außerdem noch durch die während der Alarmreaktion eintretende Insulinresistenz vermehrt.

Die Alarmreaktion wird auch von anderen metabolischen Veränderungen begleitet, die die Sicherung des erhöhten Energiebedarfs zum Ziel haben, wie z.B. der „six carbon – three carbon cycling", der Zwischenprodukte von Glukose mit drei Kohleatomen aus den Muskeln zur Leber bringt, wo sie Glukose bilden, die wiederum in den Muskeln zu 3 Kohleketten abgebaut werden. Der große Energiebedarf dieses Zyklus trägt zur Katabolie des Streß bei.

Alles in allem führt die Streßreaktion also zu negativem Stickstoffgleichgewicht, zum Verlust von Kalium und Körpergewicht. Tabelle 1 versucht einen Überblick über die Funktionsveränderungen im Streß darzustellen.

Das Ausmaß der erwähnten Veränderungen korreliert im großen und ganzen mit der Schwere und Länge der Streßsituation. Ist die Belastung oder das Trauma plötzlich und massiv, löst es anfänglich eine Lähmungsphase, die sog. „Ebb-phase", aus, die in ganz schweren Fällen direkt zum Tode führen kann, wobei die Streßreaktion nur teilweise, nicht voll oder gar nicht entwickelt wird.

Beim Operationsstreß dürfte dies nie der Fall sein, da die präoperative Angst und Spannung, gefolgt von der Nociception des Hautschnittes, gewöhnlich direkt zur Alarmreaktion ohne Lähmungsphase führen. Beim Operationsstreß werden diese Veränderungen noch dazu durch Anaesthesiemittel modifiziert. Eine allgemeine Anaesthesie kann jedoch die Streßreaktion nicht verhindern, eine hohe Epidural- bzw. Spinalanaesthesie dagegen kann die meisten Symptome der Streßreaktion beseitigen.

Tabelle 1. Alarmreaktion

Sympathikus	+++	Herzzeitvolumen	↑
		Gewebeperfusion	↑
Katecholamine	+++	Glukose	↑
		Glykolyse	↑
Glukagon	+++	Glukoneogenese	↑
		FFS	↑
Insulin	–	L-AS	↑
		O_2-Verbrauch	↑
Kortikosteroide	+++	Temperatur	↑
Somatotropin	?	Wasserretention	↑
		K^+-Ausscheidung	↑
Thyroxin	?	N-Gleichgewicht	↓
		Körpergewicht	↓
Vasopressin	+		
Aldosteron	+		

Literatur

1. Cannon WB (1939) The wisdom of the body. Norton, New York

Einfluß der Anästhesiemethode auf das Verhalten von Adrenalin und Noradrenalin während Anästhesie und Operation

R. Knitza, R. Ciasen, D. Theiß und U. Cordes

Jedes vom Organismus als Aggression empfundene Geschehen führt zu einer Aktivitätssteigerung der Hypothalamus-Hypophysen-Nebennierenachse. Durch die Untersuchungen von Cannon [1] und Levi [5] sowie neue Arbeiten von v. Euler [2] und anderen wurden die quantitativen Beziehungen zwischen verschiedenen Streßformen und der Antwort des sympatho-adrenergen Systems näher untersucht.

Bei unzureichender pharmakologischer Dämpfung des Systems kommt es während chirurgischer Eingriffe durch den operativen Schmerzreiz zu einer Ausschüttung von Adrenalin und Noradrenalin aus Nebennierenmark und anderen chromaffinen Zellen, den Endigungen postganglionärer sympathischer Fasern sowie aus vegetativen Zentren des Hypothalamus.

Adrenalin und Noradrenalin bedingen die häufig unerwünschten streßinduzierten hämodynamischen und metabolischen Veränderungen. Ziel zahlreicher Arbeitsgruppen war es daher, wegen der großen klinisch-praktischen Bedeutung den Einfluß verschiedener Anästhetika unter operativem Streß auf das sympathikoadrenale System zu untersuchen. Die dabei gefundenen Ergebnisse sind jedoch recht uneinheitlich und teilweise sogar widersprüchlich. Ursachen dafür können in unterschiedlichen Patientenkollektiven, unterschiedlichen Schweregraden des Operationstraumas, der Art der Probenentnahme und dem jeweiligen Bestimmungsverfahren begründet sein. Grundsätzlich besteht die Möglichkeit, Katecholaminanalysen im Harn oder im Plasma durchzuführen. Während die Harnbestimmung technisch weniger aufwendig ist, läßt sie doch immer nur Aussagen über größere Zeitintervalle zu, erfaßt also keine kurzfristig während des Beobachtungszeitraums auftretenden Konzentrationsschwankungen. Die Plasmabestimmungen der Katecholamine sind hingegen wegen der kurzen Halbwertszeit stets nur Momentaufnahmen, die den gerade zum Entnahmezeitpunkt herrschenden sympathikoadrenalen Aktivitätszustand widerspiegeln. Engmaschigen Meßkontrollen ist aber wegen des pro Bestimmung benötigten großen Blutvolumens eine Grenze gesetzt. Wir haben die Plasmakatecholamine spektralfluorimetrisch mit einer modifizierten Trihydroxyindolmethode bestimmt. Um die hormonellen und metabolischen Umstellungen zu erfassen, die sich unter starker psychischer Anspannung einstellen, wählten wir für unsere Untersuchung 14 stoffwechselgesunde Patienten, die sich einer diagnostischen Herzkatheteruntersuchung unterzogen. Dieser Eingriff erschien uns als geeignetes Modell, da eine Prämedikation oder Narkose nicht erfolgte und somit keine pharmakologische Dämpfung hypothalamischer Zentren vorlag. Wir untersuchten neben einigen anderen Hormonen und Stoffwechselgrößen, auf die in diesem Rahmen nicht näher eingegangen werden soll, das Verhalten von Adrenalin und Noradrenalin vor, während und 24 Stunden nach der Herzkatheterisierung.

Dabei fanden wir folgende Ergebnisse:

Die Adrenalinkonzentration im Serum stieg von im Mittel 30 ng/l vor der Katheteruntersuchung auf etwa das Dreifache während des Eingriffs an. 24 Stunden nach der Untersuchung lag sie geringgradig unter dem Ausgangswert. Die Noradrenalin-Konzentration zeigte im Prinzip ein ähnliches Verhalten. Sie stieg von 221 ng/l um 24% während der Katheterisierung an und lag am folgenden Tag geringgradig unter dem Ausgangswert (Abb. 1).

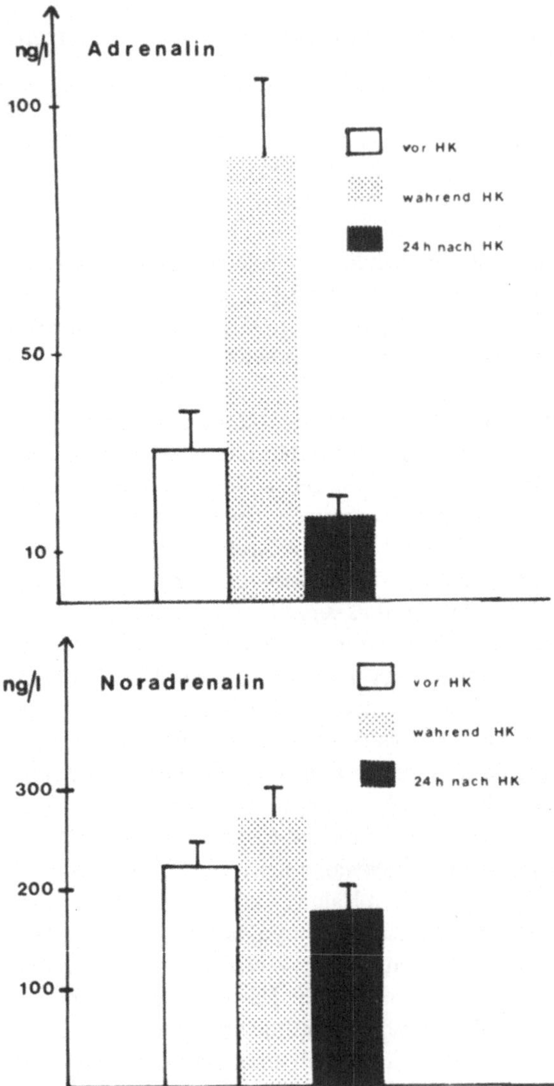

Abb. 1. Verhalten von Adrenalin und Noradrenalin vor, während und 24 Stunden nach Herzkatheterisierung

Die Veränderungen der Katecholaminkonzentration unter NLA und zusätzlicher chirurgischer Stimulation hat Tammisto [8] eingehend untersucht. Danach führt die Gabe von Fentanyl, Droperidol, Lachgas und Sauerstoff in klinisch üblicher Dosierung zu geringgradigen, statistisch jedoch nicht signifikanten Anstiegen von Adrenalin; die Noradrenalinkonzentration bleibt unverändert.

Eine Erklärungsmöglichkeit dafür wäre eine Zunahme der Adrenalinfreisetzung nach Fentanylgabe, wie etwa nach Morphininjektion, während die Noradrenalinfreisetzung nach Fentanylapplikation, wie aus tierexperimentellen Untersuchungen bekannt ist, offenbar unbeeinträchtigt bleibt [7]. Zusätzliche chirurgische Stimulation führt unter NLA stets zu einem erheblichen Anstieg der Katecholaminkonzentration, wobei das Ausmaß der Freisetzung vor allem von der nozizeptiven Reizintensität abhängig ist. Daß während der Operation dennoch meist recht stabile Kreislaufverhältnisse vorliegen, resultiert also nicht aus einer herabgesetzten Katecholaminfreisetzung, sondern aus einer verminderten Wirksamkeit, bedingt durch die α-Rezeptoren-blockierende Wirkung des DHB.

An 22 Patienten mit idiopathischer Trigeminusneuralgie, die durch partielle Elektrokoagulation des Ganglion Gasseri in Neurolepthypalgesie und Kommandoatmung operiert wurden, und einem starken, schmerzbedingten Streß ausgesetzt waren, konnten wir die unter unvollständiger Analgesie auftretenden Veränderungen besonders deutlich studieren.

Unmittelbar nach Operationsbeginn kam es bei allen Patienten (Gruppe A) zu einem schmerzbedingten, massiven Blutdruck- und Pulsanstieg (Abb. 2). Der Versuch, diese Kreislauf-

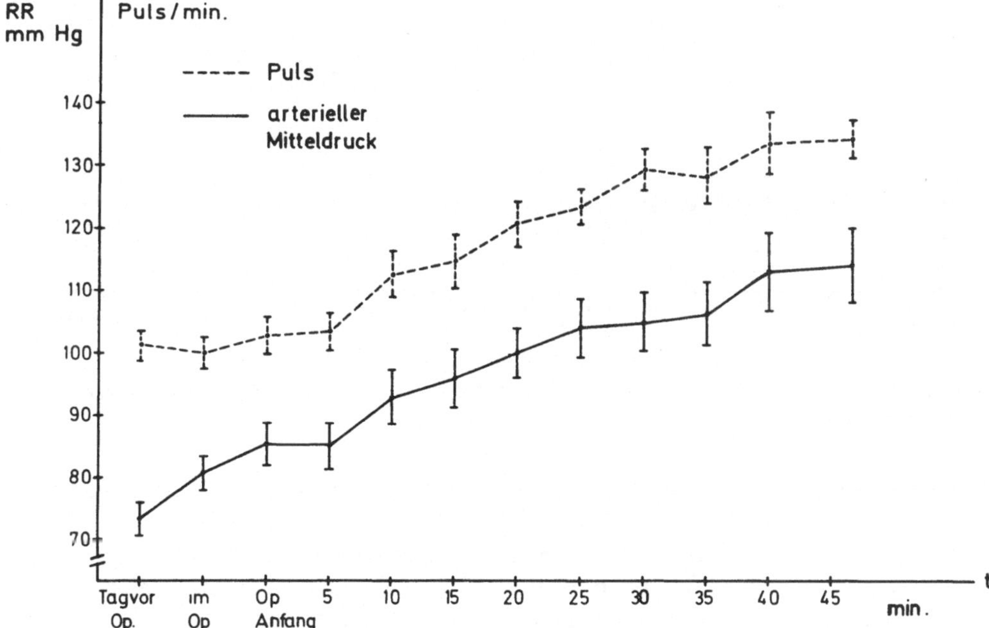

Abb. 2. Puls und arterieller Mitteldruck während partieller Elektrokoagulation des Ganglion Gasseri in Neurolepthypalgesie

parameter durch Steigerung der Analgetikazufuhr zu normalisieren, würde zu einer zunehmenden Atemdepression führen. Die dadurch bedingte Hypoxie und Hyperkapnie bewirken aber eine weitere Katecholaminausschüttung. Somit kann eine gesteigerte Analgetikazufuhr die Kreislaufsituation nicht normalisieren.

Wir gaben daher mit Operationsbeginn einer Patientengruppe B einen nichtselektiven Betarezeptorenblocker, um auf diese Weise die freigesetzten Katecholamine durch kompetitiven Antagonismus vom Rezeptor zu verdrängen. Die streßbedingten hämodynamischen Veränderungen ließen sich dadurch beseitigen (Abb. 3).

Die Adrenalinkonzentrationen waren am Operationsende um mehr als das Dreizehnfache angestiegen. Die Noradrenalinkonzentrationen hatten sich am Operationsende verdoppelt. Zwischen den beiden Patientenkollektiven A (ohne Betablocker) und B (mit Betablocker) fanden

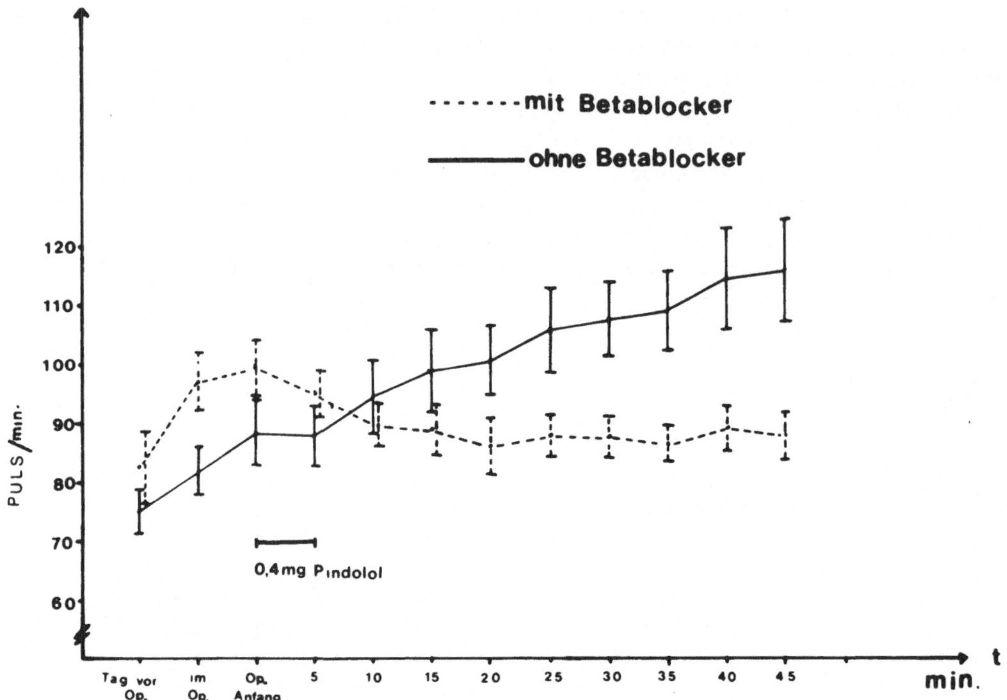

Abb. 3. Änderung der Herzfrequenz durch Gabe eines Betarezeptorenblockers bei der Elektrokoagulation des Ganglion Gasseri

sich keine statistisch signifikanten Unterschiede bezüglich der Adrenalin- und Noradrenalinkonzentrationen am Operationsende (Abb. 4).

Besondere Bedeutung kommt dem Verhalten von Adrenalin und Noradrenalin unter Halothannarkose zu, da dieses Anästhetikum zu einer „Sensibilisierung" des ventrikulären Reizleitungssystems gegenüber Katecholaminen führt. Ohne Operationsreiz senkt Halothan bereits in Konzentrationen von 0,5 Vol % die Sympathikusaktivität und führt zu einer geringgradigen Abnahme der Plasmaadrenalinkonzentration bei nahezu unveränderten Noradrenalinwerten.

Differierende Aussagen bestehen demgegenüber bei zusätzlichem Operationsreiz. Während einige Untersucher eine Abnahme der Harnkatecholaminausscheidung beobachteten, steigt nach neuen radioenzymatischen Plasmauntersuchungen von Halter et al. [4] besonders Noradrenalin während der Operation, gefolgt von einem zusätzlichen Adrenalinanstieg während der Ausleitung (Abb. 5). Die erhöhten Katecholaminkonzentrationen im Aufwachraum erklären sich aus dem nach der Operation rasch einsetzenden Wundschmerz.

Bei Spinal- bzw. Periduralanästhesie liegen vergleichsweise wenig Untersuchungen über das Verhalten von Adrenalin und Noradrenalin vor.

Hack [3] beobachtete unter Periduralanästhesie eine intraoperative Abnahme der Harnkatecholaminkonzentration mit postoperativer Steigerung der Adrenalinausscheidung (Abb. 6), während andere Untersucher bei Plasmabestimmungen meist nach der Blockade geringgradige Katecholaminanstiege fanden.

Wir haben daher an neun unfallchirurgischen Patienten, deren operative Eingriffe alle in Spinalanästhesie bei vollständiger Analgesie durchgeführt wurden, diese Frage nochmals ge-

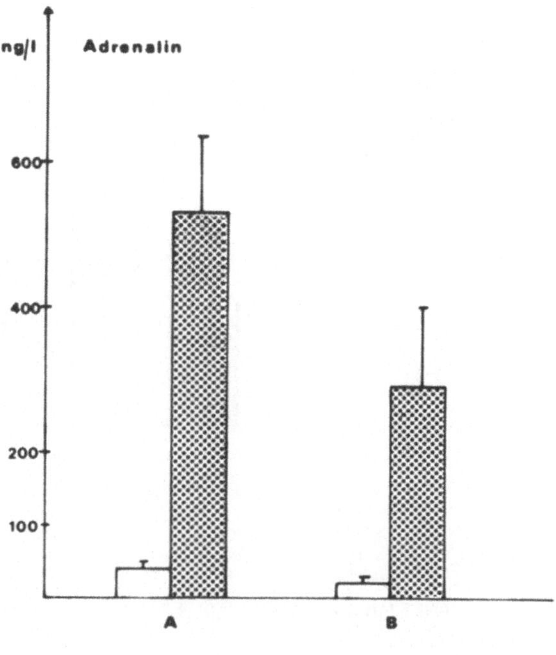

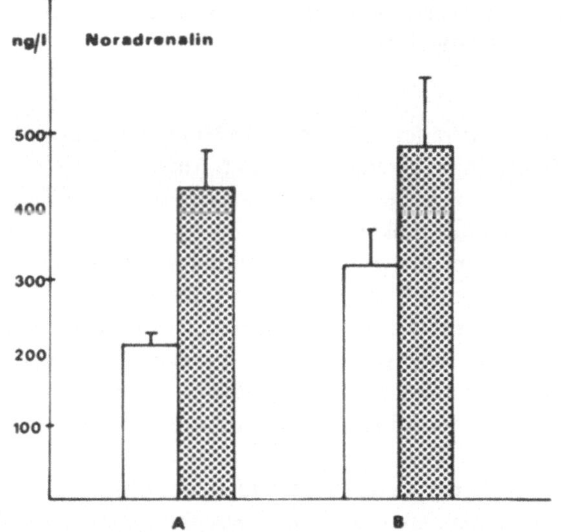

Abb. 4. Adrenalin- und Noradrenalinkonzentrationen vor Operationsbeginn ☐ und am Operationsende ▩ in Gruppe A und Gruppe B (mit Betablocker)

prüft. Als Infusionen wurden lediglich isotone Elektrolytlösungen verwandt, um durch Bestimmung der freien Fettsäuren auch katecholamininduzierte metabolische Veränderungen des Fettstoffwechsels mitzuerfassen.

Der lipolytische Wirkungsmechanismus ist in Abb. 7 schematisch dargestellt. Katecholamine steigern die Lipolyse. Sie aktivieren über die Adenylcyclase das zyclische 3-5′ AMP, welches die inaktive Lipase in die aktive Form überführt.

Die Blutentnahmen zu unserer Untersuchung erfolgten am Morgen der Operation gegen 7.00 Uhr auf Station, im Einleitungsraum vor Beginn der Anästhesie, nach vollständigem Wir-

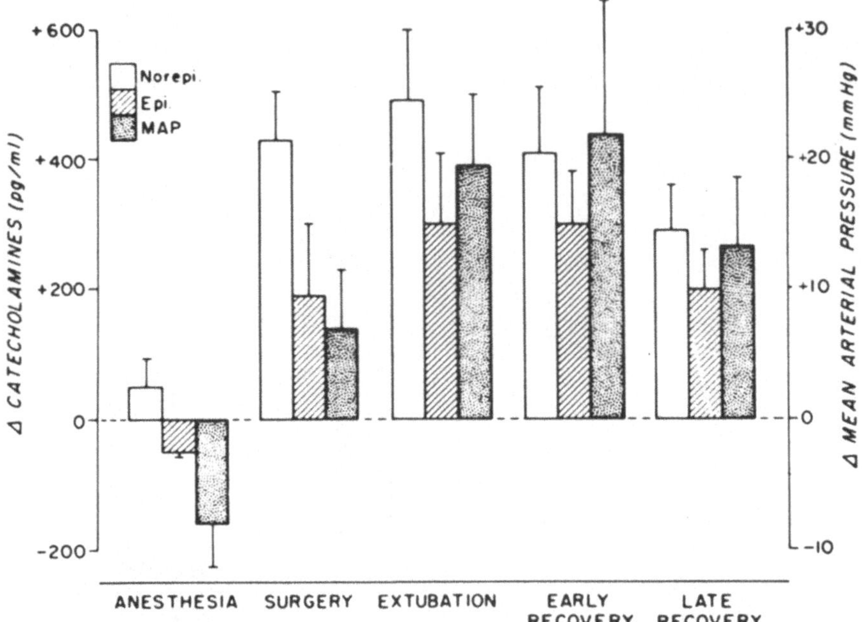

Abb. 5. Verhalten von Adrenalin, Noradrenalin und arteriellem Mitteldruck unter Halothannarkose und Operation (nach [4])

kungseintritt der Anästhesie, 30 Minuten nach Operationsbeginn, am Operationsende und 30 Minuten nach Operationsende im Aufwachraum. Abb. 8 zeigt das Verhalten von Blutdruck und Puls sowie die Konzentration der freien Fettsäuren und der Katecholamine zu den entsprechenden Zeitpunkten.

Im Einleitungsraum steigen Blutdruck und Puls aufgrund der praeoperativen Erwartungshaltung deutlich an. Infolge der Spinalanästhesie fällt dann der Blutdruck signifikant ab und die Herzfrequenz verlangsamt sich. Die nachfolgende Operation führt zu keiner wesentlichen Änderung dieser Größen. Die Plasmakonzentrationen von Adrenalin und Noradrenalin liegen im Normbereich. Die geringgradige Zunahme der Noradrenalinkonzentration und die minimale Abnahme der Adrenalinkonzentration zu den entsprechenden Zeitpunkten sind statistisch nicht signifikant.

Auch die Nichtesterfettsäuren des Plasmas, die wir als metabolische Parameter der sympathischen Aktivität gaschromatographisch bestimmten, zeigten bei relativ hohen Ausgangswerten keine signifikanten Änderungen.

Durch spinale Sympathikusblockade der präganglionären sympathischen Fasern und vollständige Unterbrechung afferenter Impulse aus dem Operationsgebiet zum ZNS läßt sich ein intraoperativer Anstieg der Katecholaminfreisetzung vermeiden. Auch in der postoperativen Phase, wo es durch das rasche Abfluten der volatilen Anästhetika schon bald infolge des auftretenden Wundschmerzes zu deutlichen Adrenalin- und Noradrenalinerhöhungen kommt, lassen sich bei geeigneter Auswahl des Lokalanästhetikums und der jeweiligen Anästhesiemethode der schmerzinduzierte Katecholaminanstieg und damit ungünstige hämodynamische und metabolische Veränderungen vermeiden.

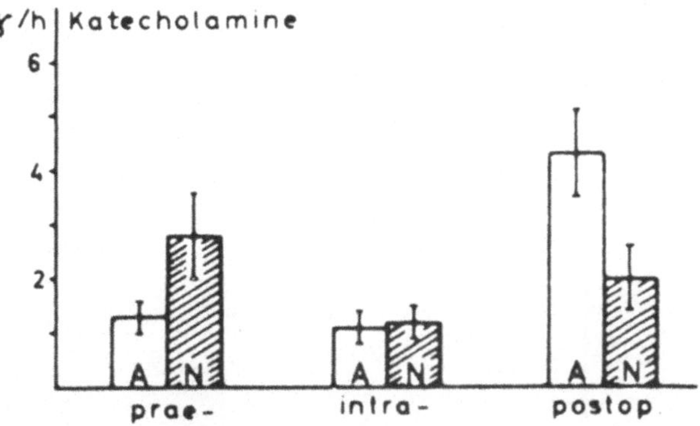

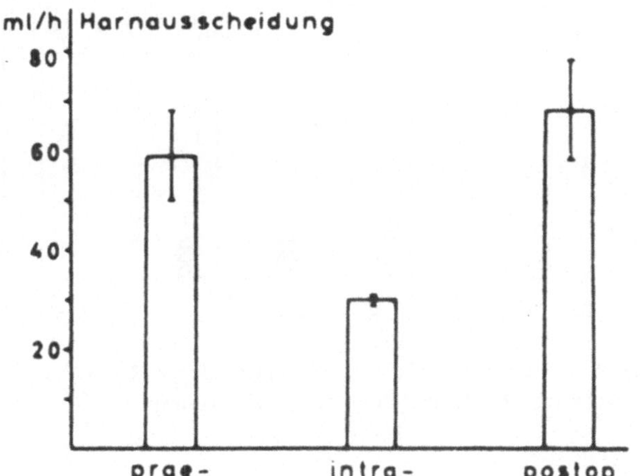

Abb. 6. Verhalten der Harnkatecholamine Adrenalin und Noradrenalin unter Periduralanästhesie (nach [3])

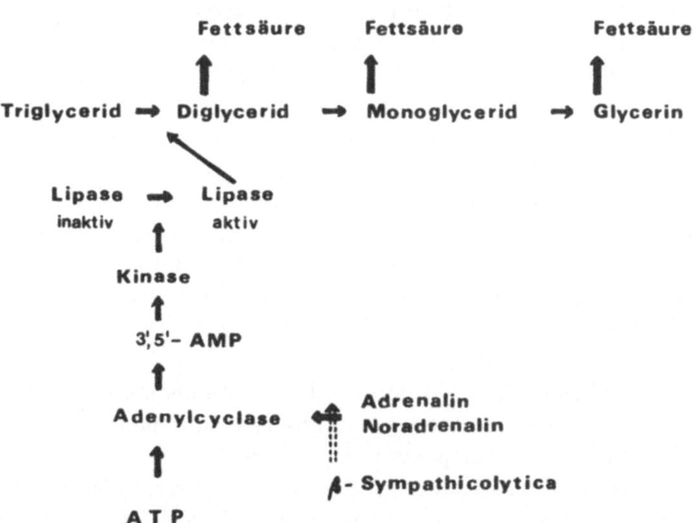

Abb. 7. Mechanismus der lipolytischen Wirkung der Katecholamine und Angriffspunkt der Beta-Sympathikolytica

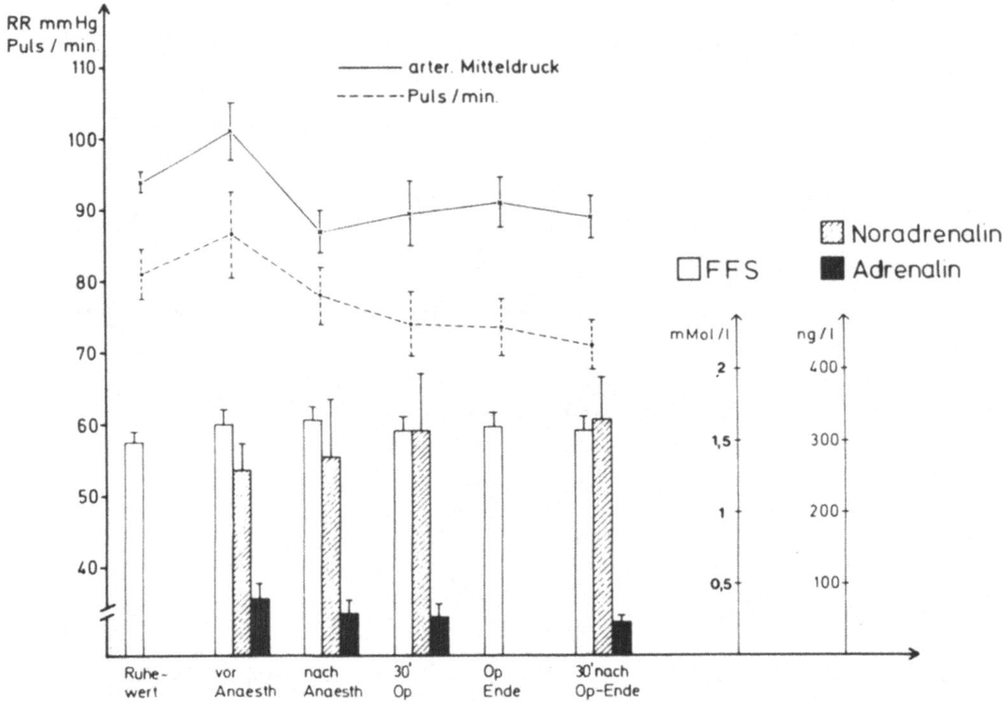

Abb. 8. Verhalten von Puls, arteriellem Mitteldruck, Adrenalin, Noradrenalin und freien Fettsäuren im Serum unfallchirurgischer Patienten unter Spinalanästhesie und Operation

Summary

Any event, which the organism perceives as aggression, induces an activation of the hypothalamus-hypophysis-adrenal axis. Under the irritation of surgical pain and under insufficient pharmacologic suppression, adrenalin and noradrenalin are liberated from the adrenal medulla and the ends of the adrenergic postganglionic nerve endings. Numerous teams examined the changes of the sympatho-adrenal system under variable anesthetic management and operative stress because of the great clinical importance of the catecholamine-induced hemodynamic and metabolic disorders. Variable samples of patients, varying severity of operative trauma, differing methods of sampling and of determination may be the reasons for the partly differing results. While the measurement of catecholamines in urine is technically less difficult, rapid changes cannot be recognized. Plasma level, however, are only snapshots because of the short half-life time. Frequent controls are limited by the great blood volumes which are necessary for fluorimetric methods.

According to Euler [2] emotional stress mainly induces a liberation of adrenalin, while an increase in noradrenalin excretion is observed with increased muscular work and in connection with circulatory and temperature regulation.

In metabolically healthy patients, who underwent diagnostic catheterization of the heart without any sedation or anaesthesia, plasma adrenalin concentrations rose due to psychic strain for 300%, noradrenalin for 24% of the precatheterization values.

According to numerous investigators, neuroleptanaesthesia suppresses the sympathico-adrenal system only insufficiently. After partial electrocoagulation of the Gasserian ganglion under neurolepthypalgesia and respiration on command, the concentration of adrenalin increased thirteenfold and those of noradrenalin twofold. These rises of adrenalin and noradrenalin levels were not prevented by additional administration of a beta blocking agent, while the hemodynamic and metabolic changes were impaired or influenced favorably.

Without the irritation of surgery halothane impairs the liberation of catecholamines in a concentration dependent way. Surgical manipulations, however, induce a statistically significant increase of noradrenalin, followed by increases of adrenalin immediately after the end of the operation with the perception of pain.

Trauma patients, who were operated under spinal anesthesia, had no essential changes in catecholamines or other metabolic stress parameters. The reason for this is the blockade of preganglionic sympathetic fibers and the interruption of somatic afferent impulses.

Literatur

1. Cannon W (1915) Bodily changes in pain, hunger, fear and rage. Appleton, New York
2. Euler US (1972) Pathophysiological aspects of catecholamine production. Clin Chem 18:1445
3. Hack G (1967) Über die Katecholaminfreisetzung bei großen abdominellen Eingriffen in Halothannarkose im Vergleich zur Periduralanästhesie. Inaugural-Dissertation, Universität Bonn
4. Halter BJ et al. (1977) Mechanism of plasma catecholamine increases during surgical stress in man. J Clin Endocrinol Metab 45:936
5. Levi L (1972) Stress and distress in response to psychosocial stimuli. Acta Med Scand [Suppl] 528
6. Schulte am Esch J, Kreppe E (1972) Veränderungen des Katecholaminstoffwechsels bei zentraler Sympathikusdämpfung durch Halothan. In: Hoder J, Jedlicka R, Pokomý J (eds) Anaesthesiology and Rexuscitation, vol I. Medical Press, Prague, pp 391-395
7. Starke K (1977) Regulation of Noradrenaline release by presynaptic receptor systems. Physiol Biochem Pharmacol 77:1-125
8. Tammisto T (1973) Effects of neuroleptanesthesia on catecholamines. Int Anesthesiol Clin 11:185

Diskussion

Frage: Um welche unfallchirurgischen Eingriffe handelte es sich?
Knitza: Es waren Patienten, die wegen Metallentfernungen am Unter- oder Oberschenkel und Frakturen im Bereich der unteren Extremität operiert wurden; stets also Eingriffe, bei denen kein Blut gegeben werden mußte, so daß keine größeren Verdünnungseffekte durch Infusionslösungen zu erwarten waren.
Frage: Eine echte Streßauslösung ist eigentlich nur bei wirklichen Oberbaucheingriffen zu erwarten. Bei Extremitäteneingriffen ist das nicht in der Form merkbar.
Knitza: Das ist die Frage. Es kam uns darauf an, durch die Sympathikusblockade eine völlige Analgesie zu erreichen. Wir haben parallel dazu an einem ähnlichen Patientengut die Veränderungen unter Neuroleptanaesthesie untersucht, wobei noch einige zusätzliche metabolische Parameter bestimmt wurden. Hierbei waren die Veränderungen noch deutlicher.
Frage: Zum Vorredner wollte ich nur sagen, daß es noch einige Untersuchungen gibt, nach denen selbst Extremitäteneingriffe auch diese Streßauswirkungen machen können. Das ist an Glukosetoleranztesten festgestellt worden. Kriterium dafür ist die Schwere des Eingriffes.
Frage: Haben die Patienten irgendwelche Prämedikation bekommen oder andere Medikamente, Valium z.B.?
Knitza: Ja. Die Patienten sind mit Promethazin und Pethidin (Atosil/Dolantin) prämediziert gewesen, im Mittel jeweils 50 mg. Intraoperativ haben wir bei der Hälfte der Patienten, da sie während des Eingriffs schlafen wollten, Valium in Fraktionen von jeweils etwa 2,5 mg nach Wirkung gegeben. 5 Patienten haben das nicht für nötig gefunden.

Influence of Neurogenic Blockade on the Endocrine-Metabolic Response to Surgery

H. Kehlet, and M.R. Brandt

Surgical stress or trauma leads to profound changes in the endocrine-metabolic balance towards a catabolic state. The release mechanisms have not been completely evaluated, although both humeral substances released from the area of trauma and afferent neurogenic stimuli mediated to the hypothalamus seem to be involved [8].

This study was performed to evaluate the role of neurogenic stimuli from the surgical area as a release mechanism of the endocrine-metabolic response to elective surgery in man.

Method

Twenty otherwise healthy premenopausal women scheduled for elective abdominal hysterectomy were studied. They received either general anaesthesia (halothane or ethrane) or epidural analgesia extending from T_4 to S_5 as described previously [4]. Analgesia, obtained with 0,5% bupivacaine (Marcaine) without adrenaline, was effective before skin incision and continued for 24 h. During the first 24 postoperative h the patients received only IV saline and tap-water orally. For nitrogen balance studies oral intake of calories and nitrogen as well as urinary excretion of nitrogen were recorded. Groups were comparable regarding age, weight, operation time, bleeding and fluid administration. Fourteen blood samples were taken before analgesia or anaesthesia and during the following 24 h. Blood was analyzed for cortisol, growth hormone, insulin, renin, aldosterone, thyroxine, triiodothyronine, glucose, alanine, glycerol, free fatty acids (FFA), lactate, beta-hydroxy-buturate and AMP.

Results

In an initial study the influence of the extent of the neurogenic blockade on the endocrine response to surgery was evaluated [4]. Using cortisol as the endocrine parameter, it was demonstrated that sensory blockade from S_5 to T_4 inhibited the cortisol response to surgery (Fig. 1), while surgery performed with lower levels of neurogenic blockade resulted in a per- and postoperative increase in plasma cortisol, despite the patients being free from pain. Patients operated under general anaesthesia plus epidural analgesia extending from S_5 to $T_{4\text{-}5}$ showed no peroperative increase in plasma cortisol, but after extubation plasma cortisol increased slightly – possibly due to the stress of extubation and awakening.

In the following studies all patients, therefore, underwent surgery under epidural analgesia, extending from T_4 to S_5, without general anaesthesia.

Hormones

Cortisol [2]

The normal peroperative increase in plasma cortisol was blocked by epidural analgesia (Fig. 2), the difference between groups being significant up to 9 h after skin incision.

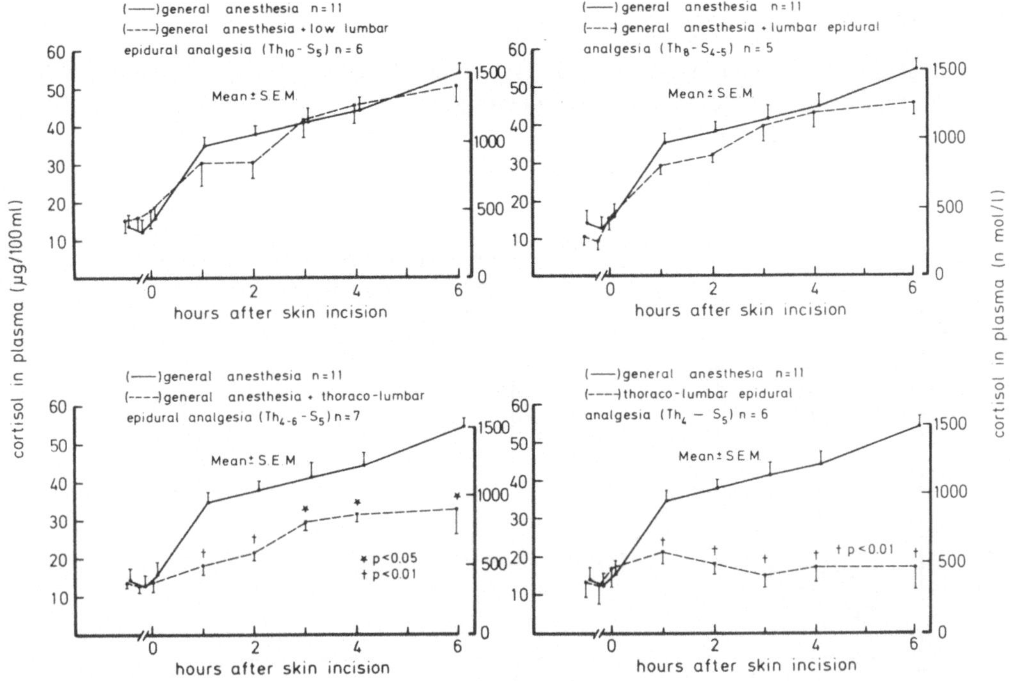

Fig. 1. Influence of the extent of sensory blockade by epidural analgesia on the adrenocortical response to hysterectomy [4]

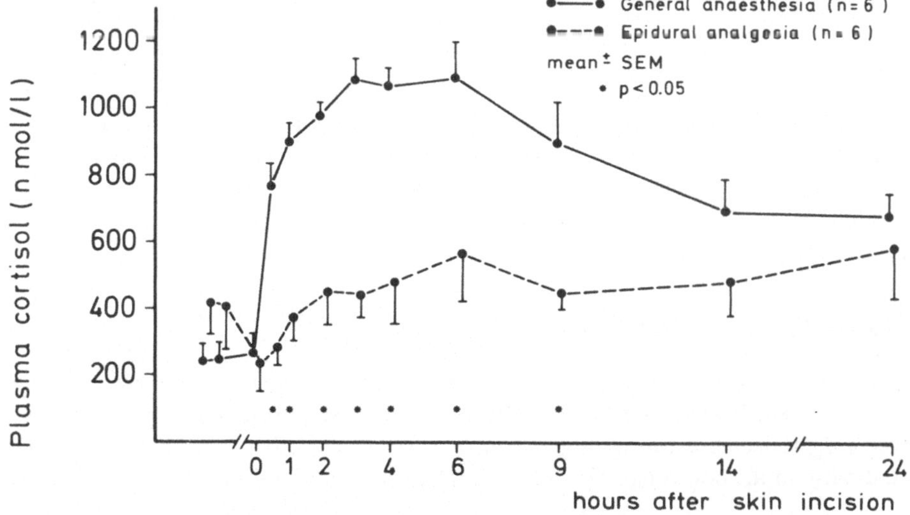

Fig. 2. Influence of epidural analgesia on the cortisol response to hysterectomy

Growth Hormone

The normal growth hormone response to surgery was also blocked by epidural analgesia (Fig. 3), but postoperatively no differences between groups could be demonstrated. Levels in the epidural groups fluctuated widely.

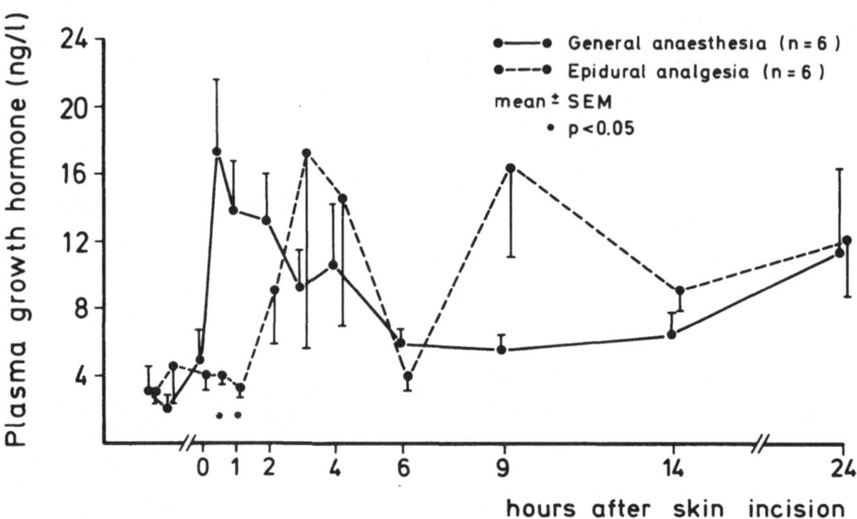

Fig. 3. Influence of epidural analgesia on the growth hormone response to hysterectomy

Renin and Aldosterone [3]

Plasma renin activity increased in the control group from 1.1 ± 0.3 ng/ml/h (mean ± SEM) to 1.8 ± 0.5 ng/ml/h during surgery. Plasma aldosterone in the control group increased from 15.8 ± 4.1 ng/100 ml (mean ± SEM) to 40.7 ± 8.9 ng/100 ml, and remained elevated for 9 h after skin incision. Epidural analgesia blocked both the renin and aldosterone response to surgery, since levels were constant throughout the study.

Thyroxine (T_4) and Triiodothyronine (T_3) [1]

T_4 increased during the operation, but returned to preoperative values 6 h after skin incision (Fig. 4). The peroperative increase is probably due to release from hepatic T_4 stores. T_4 levels showed a slight decrease during surgery under epidural analgesia. T_3 fell rapidly towards hypothyroid range in the control group and epidural analgesia did not influence these changes.

Insulin

Insulin in plasma was constant in both groups throughout the study (Fig. 5) despite hyperglycaemia in the control group (see below).

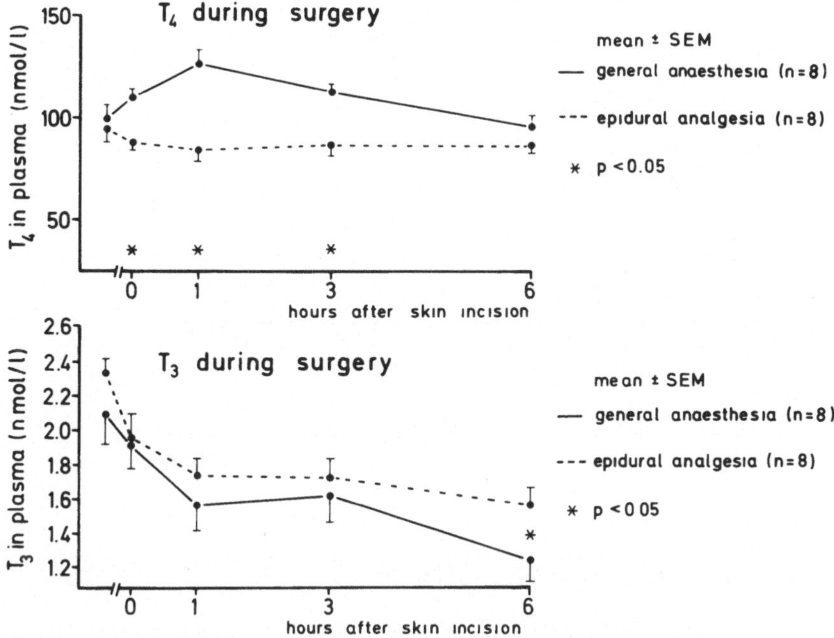

Fig. 4. Influence of epidural analgesia on Thyroxine (T_4) and Triiodothyronine (T_3) response to hysterectomy [1]

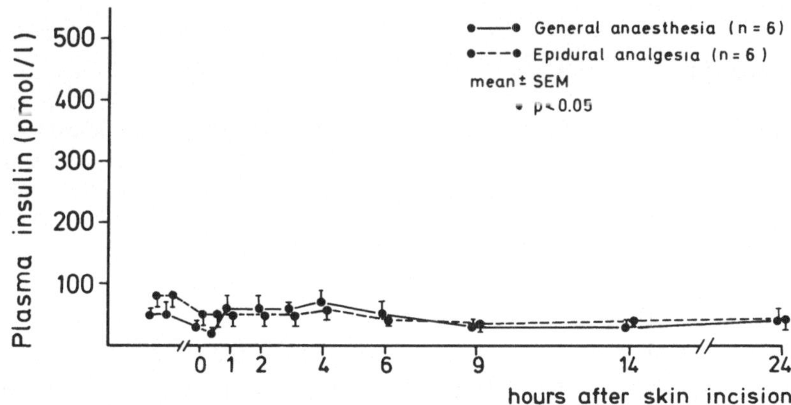

Fig. 5. Influence of epidural analgesia on the insulin response to hysterectomy

Metabolites

Glucose

The normal per- and postoperative increase in blood glucose was abolished during epidural analgesia (Fig. 6).

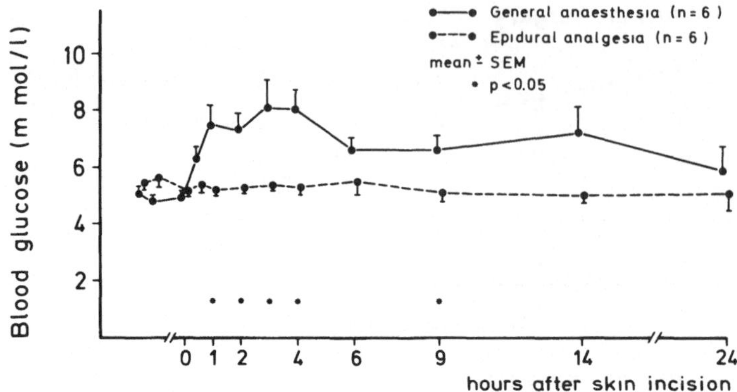

Fig. 6. Influence of epidural analgesia on the glucose response to hysterectomy

Free Fatty Acids (FFA) and Glycerol [5]

FFA and glycerol increased insignificantly during surgery under general anaesthesia, but during epidural analgesia FFA fell significantly from a preoperative value of 840 ± 118 mmol/litre (mean ± SEM) to 450 ± 62 mmol/litre ($p < 0.05$) 1 h after skin incision. Similarly, glycerol decreased from 0.101 ± 0.025 mmol/litre (mean ± SEM) to 0.051 ± 0.007 mmol/litre, respectively. Both FFA and glycerol increased to preoperative levels similar to the control group 4-6 h after skin incision.

Lactate [5]

Blood lactate increased peroperatively in the control group from 0.530 ± 0.051 mmol/litre (mean ± SEM) preoperatively to 1.057 ± 0.182 mmol/litre 30 min after skin incision. Preoperative level was gained 2 h after skin incision. Lactate levels were constant during surgery under epidural analgesia.

Beta-Hydroxybuturate [5]

Blood beta-hydroxybuturate increased immediately and steadily after skin incision in the control group, while epidural analgesia postponed this increase until 4 h after skin incision, at which time levels were similar in both groups.

Alanine [5]

Blood alanine decreased steadily from skin incision in both groups, and this decrease continued throughout the study without differences between groups.

Cyclic AMP [6]

The normal per- and postoperative increase in cAMP was prevented by epidural analgesia.

Nitrogen Balance [2]

Postoperative cumulative 5 day nitrogen balance was negative in both groups (Fig. 7), but patients operated under epidural analgesia were in nitrogen balance from the 2nd postoperative day. On the 5th postoperative day the control group had lost 22 ± 4 g (mean ± SEM) nitrogen compared to 10 ± 2 g in the epidural group ($p < 0.05$). Intake of calories and nitrogen was comparable within the two groups.

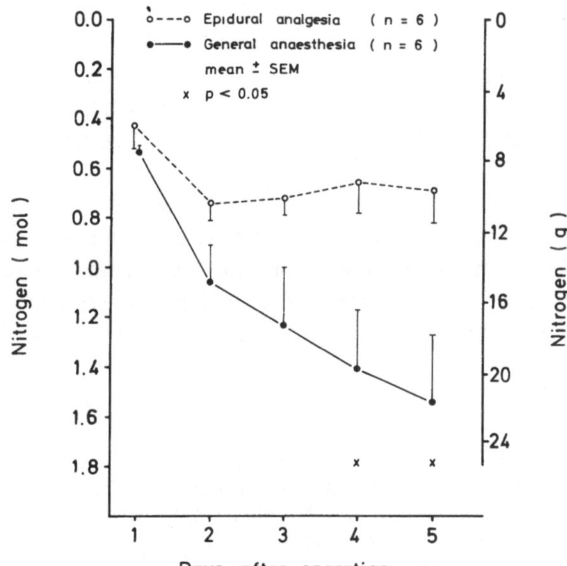

Fig. 7. Influence of epidural analgesia on 5 day cumulative nitrogen balance following hysterectomy [2]

Discussion

Our results clearly demonstrate that the main part of the endocrine-metabolic response to elective surgery in man is released by afferent neurogenic stimuli from the surgical area. Thus, epidural analgesia inhibited the normal surgically induced changes in cortisol, growth hormone, T_4, renin, aldosterone, cAMP, lactate, glucose, FFA, glycerol, beta-hydroxybuturate and nitrogen balance. In contrast, the normal decline in T_3 and alanine after surgery was unaffected by epidural analgesia. The underlying mechanism of this exception is unknown at present and deserves further evaluation.

The inhibition of the catecholamine response to surgery by epidural analgesia, as indirectly expressed by the inhibited cAMP response to surgery [6], plays a major role in the metabolic changes observed during epidural analgesia (inhibited lipolysis and glycogenolysis and lactate production).

No side-effects of the inhibited stress-response were observed.

Although release mechanisms other than the afferent limb may be acting in more severe forms of stress (i.e. burns and sepsis) [8], the inhibitory effect of neurogenic blockade on the endocrine-metabolic stress-response to elective surgery may have important theoretical and clinical implications. Thus, the results may question the necessity of the endocrine-metabolic response to trauma in man in conditions when blood, fluids and substrates are otherwise available. This hypothesis needs further evaluation. The influence of epidural analgesia on respiratory and cardiovascular function has been dealt with elsewhere in this symposium. In addition to the demonstrated improvement of nitrogen balance [2], and a shorter convalescence time reported by others [7], it remains to be established whether an inhibited stress-response may prevent other postoperative side-effects, such as, impaired immunocompetence and phagocytosis, and bleeding and thromboembolic complications. Such information may have important value in the future treatment of patients with high surgical morbidity.

Summary

The effect of epidural analgesia, extending from T_4 to S_5, on the per- and postoperative changes in blood concentrations of cortisol, growth hormone, insulin, renin, aldosterone, thyroxine, triiodothyronine, glucose, lactate, alanine, free fatty acids, glycerol, beta-hydroxybuturate and cyclic AMP, was investigated in connection with elective hysterectomy. The neurogenic blockade either blocked or postponed the surgically induced response in the various endocrine and metabolic parameters, except the rapid decline in triiodothyronine and alanine. Five day postoperative nitrogen balance was improved by neurogenic blockade. It is concluded that the endocrine-metabolic response to elective surgery in man is mainly released by neurogenic stimuli from the surgical area to the central nervous system.

References

1. Brandt MR, Kehlet H, Skovsted L, Hansen JM (1976) Rapid decrease in plasma-triiodothyronine during surgery and epidural analgesia independent of afferent neurogenic stimuli and of cortisol. Lancet 2:1333
2. Brandt MR, Fernandes A, Mordhorst R, Kehlet H (1978) Epidural analgesia improves postoperative nitrogen balance. Br Med J I:1106
3. Brandt MR, Ølgaard K, Kehlet H (1979) Epidural analgesia inhibits the renin and aldosterone response to surgery. Acta Anaesthesiol Scand 23:267
4. Engquist A, Brandt MR, Fernandes A, Kehlet H (1977) The blocking effect of epidural analgesia on the adrenocortical and hyperglycemic response to surgery. Acta Anaesthesiol Scand 21:330
5. Kehlet H, Brandt MR, Prange-Hansen A, Alberti KGMM (1979) Effect of epidural analgesia on metabolic profiles during and after surgery. Br J Surg 66:543
6. Nistrup-Madsen S, Brandt MR, Engquist A, Badawi I, Kehlet H (1977) Inhibition of plasma cyclic AMP, glucose and cortisol response to surgery by epidural analgesia. Br J Surg 64:669
7. Pflug AE, Murphy TM, Butler SH, Tucker GT (1974) The effects of postoperative peridural analgesia on pulmonary therapy and pulmonary complications. Anesthesiology 41:8
8. Wilmore DW, Long JM, Mason AD, Pruitt BA (1976) Stress in surgical patients as a neurophysiologic reflex response. Surg Gynecol Obstet 142:257

Zum Einfluß von Periduralanästhesie und Operation auf das Renin-Angiotensin-Aldosteron-System

G. Hack, M. Marx, F. Witassek und H. Vetter

Durch Operationsstreß und Narkose bedingte humorale Reaktionen können den intra- wie postoperativen Verlauf ganz erheblich beeinflussen, wobei die Nebenniere für viele dieser Veränderungen eine zentrale Bedeutung hat. Neben dem sympathikoadrenalen System und der Hypophysenvorderlappen-Nebennierenrinden-Achse ist hier als dritter Regelkreis das renoadrenokortikale System mit gesteigerter Renin-, Angiotensin- und Aldosteron-Aktivität am Streß-Ablauf beteiligt [8, 13, 14, 16].

Die Regulation der Reninfreisetzung ist bis heute nicht restlos geklärt. Sie wird durch Änderungen der Nierenhämodynamik, des Blutvolumens sowie des Wasser- und Elektrolythaushaltes beeinflußt und scheint darüber hinaus einer zirkadianen Rhythmik zu unterliegen [2, 11]. Auch für das Renin-Angiotensin-Aldosteron-System (RAAS) gilt, daß eine unter dem Operationsstreß gesteigerte Hormonsekretion durch rückenmarksnahe Regionalanästhesietechniken unter bestimmten Voraussetzungen und in gewissen Grenzen modifiziert werden kann. Die teleologische Frage nach der Bedeutung einer unter dem Operationsstreß gesteigerten Aktivität humoraler Regelkreise induziert für den Anästhesisten immer wieder die Entscheidung, ob man diesen Reaktionen therapeutisch entgegentreten soll oder ob sie unter Umständen pharmakologisch verstärkt werden müssen. Verständlicherweise kann es auf diese Frage keine globale Antwort geben.

Das RAAS spielt eine physiologisch wichtige Rolle bei der Aufrechterhaltung einer normalen Kreislaufhomöostase einschließlich der Wasser- und Elektrolytbilanz. Dies gilt besonders für die intra- und postoperative Phase, wo der Renin-Angiotensin-Aldosteron-Rückkopplungsmechanismus durch exogene Einflüsse gestört sein kann.

Andererseits muß damit gerechnet werden, daß eine überschießende, primär der Homöostase dienliche Sekretion von Renin und Aldosteron im weiteren Verlauf in einen postoperativen Hyperaldosteronismus einmündet, der vor allem bei älteren und kardial gefährdeten Patienten unerwünscht ist. Neben dem allgemeinen Operationsstreß einschließlich der intra- und vor allem unmittelbar postoperativ regelmäßig zu beobachtenden Stimulation des sympathikoadrenalen Systems kommen als disponierende Faktoren eine präexistente Hyponatriämie, eine Hypovolämie, lange prä- und postoperative Nahrungskarenz, Flüssigkeitssequestration sowie Flüssigkeitsverlust aus Wunden und Drainagen in Frage.

In früheren Studien fanden wir bei unter normotensiver Halothannarkose Operierten während und nach Oberbaucheingriffen eine dem Operationsstreß entsprechende Erhöhung der Plasma-Renin-, Aldosteron- und Cortisol-Werte [7]. In Weiterführung dieser Untersuchungen interessierte uns, inwieweit eine Periduralanästhesie (PDA) aufgrund der Unterbrechung der nervalen Rückkopplung zum Hypophysenvorderlappen (HVL) diese humorale Streß-Antwort zu modifizieren vermag. Dabei standen für uns zwei Fragen im Vordergrund:

1. Wie können die Sekretionsmuster im postoperativen Verlauf durch eine in diesem Zeitraum weitergeführte kontinuierliche PDA beeinflußt werden?
2. Wie verhalten sich Plasma-Renin, -Aldosteron und -Cortisol bei einer mittels Kombination von hoher PDA und Intubationsnarkose durchgeführten kontrollierten Hypotension?

Methoden

1. Patientengut, Operations- und Anästhesieverfahren

Untersucht wurden insgesamt 12 Patienten (9 Männer, 3 Frauen) mit einem Durchschnittsalter von 36,5 Jahren (20-75 Jahre), die präoperativ keinerlei endokrinologische Störungen oder Elektrolytentgleisungen aufwiesen. Zur Prämedikation wurden ausnahmslos 10-20 mg Diazepam p.o. am Vorabend sowie 0,5 mg Atropin und 2 ml Thalamonal 1 Stunde vor Anästhesiebeginn gegeben. Bei 3 Patienten, bei denen eine Alloarthroplastik des Hüftgelenks vorgenommen werden sollte, führten wir eine normotensive kontinuierliche PDA durch. Nach Punktion des Periduralraumes in Höhe L_2/L_3 wurde der Periduralkatheter 3-4 cm proximal vorgeschoben. Die Initialdosis bestand aus 200 mg Mepivacain 2%, danach wurden im Mittel 5-6 ml einer Mepivacainlösung 2%/Stunde kontinuierlich über eine Motorspritze instilliert. Zur postoperativen Analgesie wurde an Stelle des Mepivacains eine Bupivacainlösung 0,25% kontinuierlich über 14-18 Stunden zugeführt. Zur intraoperativen psychovegetativen Dämpfung erhielten die Patienten im Durchschnitt 10-20 mg Diazepam/Stunde. Bei 6 kreislaufgesunden Patienten, die sich einer bilateralen transabdominalen Lymphadenektomie wegen Hodenkarzinom bei Zustand nach Semikastration unterziehen mußten, kam eine kontrollierte Hypotension mittels hoher, den regulativen Sympathikotonus ausschaltender single-shot PDA nach Intubation und Beatmung mit einem Stickoxydul-Sauerstoffgemisch und niedrigen Halothankonzentrationen in der von Havers et al. [10] beschriebenen Technik zur Anwendung. 3 weitere Patienten, die wegen eines Ulcus ventriculi gastrektomiert werden mußten, erhielten eine normotensive Intubationsnarkose unter Verwendung von Propanidid, Halothan, N_2O/O_2 und Alloferin. Sekretionsstudien bei diesem Anästhesieverfahren sollen als Vergleich zu den unter normotensiver wie hypotensiver PDA gewonnenen Ergebnissen herangezogen werden.

2. Zeitpunkte der Blutentnahmen und Bestimmungsmethoden

Allen Patienten wurden präoperativ am Vortag zur Operation zwei Blutproben (Probe 1 nach Bettruhe um 8.00 Uhr morgens, Probe 2 nach körperlicher Belastung 2 Stunden später) zur Ermittlung der Plasma-Renin-Aktivität (PRA), des Plasma-Aldosterons (PA) und Plasma-Cortisols (PC) entnommen. Am Operationstag erfolgten Bestimmungen während Anästhesie und Operation in 1/2 stündigem Abstand, postoperativ bis 17.00 Uhr in 1 stündigem Abstand (Tabelle 1). Alle Blutproben wurden über einen Venenverweilkatheter entnommen. Weitere Blutentnahmen

Tabelle 1. Zeitpunkte der Blutentnahmen für die Bestimmung von Renin, Aldosteron, Cortisol

Präop. Tag:	8 Uhr (nach Bettruhe) und 10 Uhr (nach körperlicher Belastung)
OP.-Tag:	jede 1/2 Std. ab Anästhesiebeginn bis 1 Std. nach Anästhesieende; dann jede volle Std. bis 17 Uhr
1., 2., 6. und 9. Postop. Tag	jeweils 8 und 17 Uhr
Zusätzlich:	24 Std. Sammelurin am präop. sowie 2., 6. und 9. postop. Tag

führten wir jeweils nach einer nächtlichen Ruheperiode am 1., 2., 6. und 9. postoperativen Tag durch. Natrium- und Kalium-Bestimmungen erfolgten präoperativ, am Operationstag sowie am 1. und 9. postoperativen Tag. Die Analysen für Plasma-Renin, -Aldosteron und -Cortisol wurden im Endokrinologischen Labor der Medizinischen Universitätspoliklinik Bonn (Direktor: Prof. Dr. F. Krück) durchgeführt. Die Plasma-Renin-Aktivität (PRA) wurde radioimmunologisch nach Haber et al. [5] ermittelt. Als Normwert gelten 0,3-3 ng/ml/3 Std. Plasma-Aldosteron (PA) bestimmten wir ebenfalls mittels Radioimmunoassay nach Vetter et al. [15], Normbereich 20-120 pg/ml. Die Plasma-Cortisol-Bestimmung (PC) erfolgte nach der Methode von Murphy u. Pattee [12], Normbereich 2-25 µg/ml (Tabelle 2).

Tabelle 2. Angewendete Bestimmungsmethoden und Normbereich für Plasma-Renin, Plasma-Aldosteron und Plasma-Cortisol

	Autor	Normbereich
Renin (PRA)	Haber et al. [5]	0,03-3 ng/ml/3 hr
Aldosteron (PA)	Vetter et al. [15]	20-120 pg/ml
Cortisol (PC)	Murphy u. Pattee [12]	2- 25 µg/100 ml

Ergebnisse

In einer Übersicht (Abb. 1) ist das Verhalten der PRA, des PA sowie des PC bei allen Patienten unter den 3 verschiedenen Anästhesieverfahren dargestellt. Während der Gesamtphase der nor-

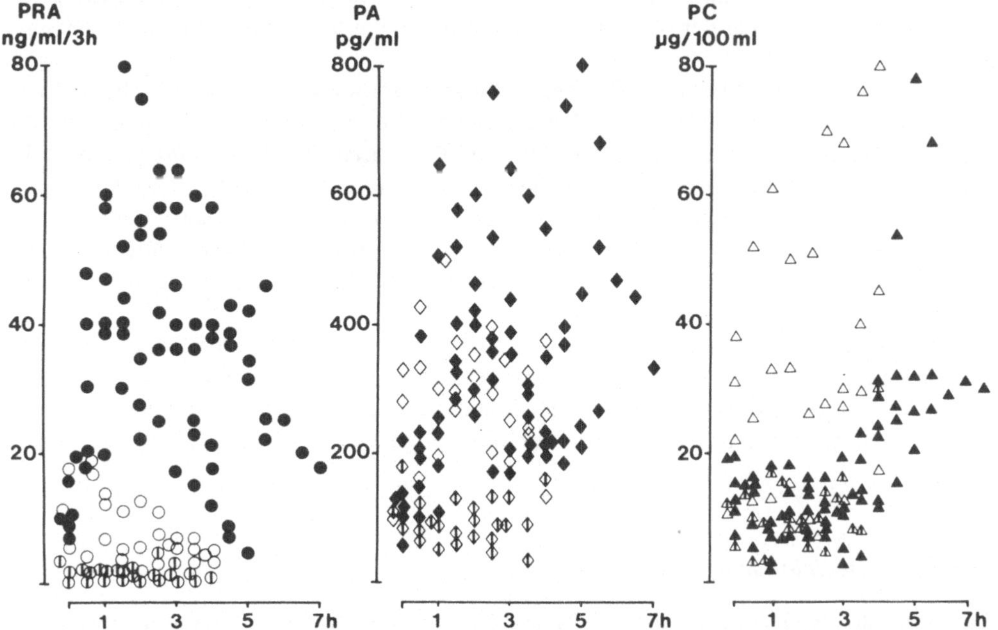

Abb. 1. Übersicht über das Verhalten der Plasma-Renin-Aktivität (PRA), des Plasma-Aldosterons (PA) und des Plasma-Cortisols (PC) in der intra- und unmittelbaren postoperativen Phase. Symbole mit Längsbalken: normotensive kontinuierliche PDA; schwarze Symbole: hypotensive PDA; helle Symbole: normotensive Halothannarkose

motensiven kontinuierlichen PDA lagen die Sekretionsraten für Renin (PRA), Aldosteron (PA) und Cortisol (PC) im Normbereich. Im Gegensatz hierzu wurden unter hypotensiver single shot PDA nach einem steilen Initialanstieg extrem hohe Plasma-Renin-Aktivitäten bis zu 80 ng/ml/ 3 Std. gemessen, wobei die Werte in der unmittelbaren postoperativen Phase eine eher abfallende Tendenz aufwiesen. Auch die PA-Spiegel waren bei diesem Anästhesieverfahren stark erhöht, während die PC-Werte für die Dauer der PDA im Normbereich lagen und erst mit Abklingen der Blockade nach durchschnittlich 3 1/2 Stunden auf übernormale Werte anstiegen. Unter normotensiver Halothannarkose wurden mäßige Erhöhungen der PRA bis maximal 19 ng/ml/ 3 Std., mittlere Anstiege des PA und besonders starke Zunahme des PC mit großer Streuung der Einzelwerte gefunden.

In Abb. 2 sind die Befunde der unter normotensiver kontinuierlicher PDA operierten Patienten im einzelnen wiedergegeben. Es wird ersichtlich, daß auch über die eigentliche Operationsphase hinaus PRA und PA im Normbereich bleiben, während der Cortisolanstieg bei Patient L in der frühen postoperativen Phase am ehesten auf eine unzureichende sympathische Blockade bei ausreichender Analgesie zu diesem Zeitpunkt zurückgeführt werden muß. Der 1. Cortisolwert bei Patient K war, wohl bedingt durch den präoperativ trotz Prämedikation bestehenden emotionalen Streß, noch erhöht, fiel jedoch nach Applikation der PDA prompt ab.

Abb. 3 verdeutlicht das inverse Verhalten der PRA zum Blutdruckverlauf bei allen unter hypotensiver PDA operierten Patienten. Die Maxima wurden 1-2 Stunden nach Beginn der Blutdrucksenkung, die bis zu einem arteriellen Mitteldruck von 60-70 mm Hg vorgenommen wurde, bzw. nach Durchführung der single shot PDA gemessen und lagen teilweise um das zehnfache über den zu Beginn der Anästhesie ermittelten Werte. Die Aldosteron-Sekretion verhielt sich durchweg gleichsinnig mit der PRA, während, wie auch aus Abb. 1 hervorgeht, die Cortisolwerte für die Dauer der PDA im Normbereich lagen und erst mit deren Abklingen anstiegen.

Postoperativ (Abb. 4) fanden sich unter und nach normotensiver kontinuierlicher PDA am 1. postoperativen Tag normale Renin-Werte, die nach Entfernen des PDA-Katheters nur unwesentlich über den Normbereich anstiegen. PA und PC zeigten über die gesamte postoperative Phase Normalwerte. Demgegenüber wiesen die unter hypotensiver PDA operierten Patienten eine Steigerung der Renin-Sekretion über den 9. postoperativen Tag hinaus auf, während die PA- und PC-Werte bis zum 6. postoperativen Tag normalisiert waren. Nach normotensiver Halothannarkose blieben in erster Linie die PRA, zum Teil auch die Sekretion von PC bis zum 6. postoperativen Tag gesteigert.

Die parallel zu den Hormonbestimmungen durchgeführten Analysen des Serum-Natrium und -Kalium erbrachten intra- wie postoperativ außer einer nicht relevanten Erniedrigung der Kalium-Werte unter den Bedingungen der normotensiven Halothannarkose und der hypotensiven PDA keine Abweichungen der Serum-Elektrolytspiegel von der Norm (Tabelle 3).

Diskussion

1. Normotensive Halothannarkose

Durch normotensive Halothananästhesie lassen sich intraoperative Streß-Reaktionen vonseiten des HVL-NNR wie des RAAS nicht verhindern. In Übereinstimmung mit anderen Autoren [16] konnten auch wir einen bereits durch die Narkose allein ausgelösten Hyperreninismus nachweisen. Diese Tatsache legt die Vermutung nahe, daß ähnlich dem Myokard auch der juxtaglomeruläre Apparat gegenüber unter flacher Halothananästhesie vermehrt freigesetzten endogenen

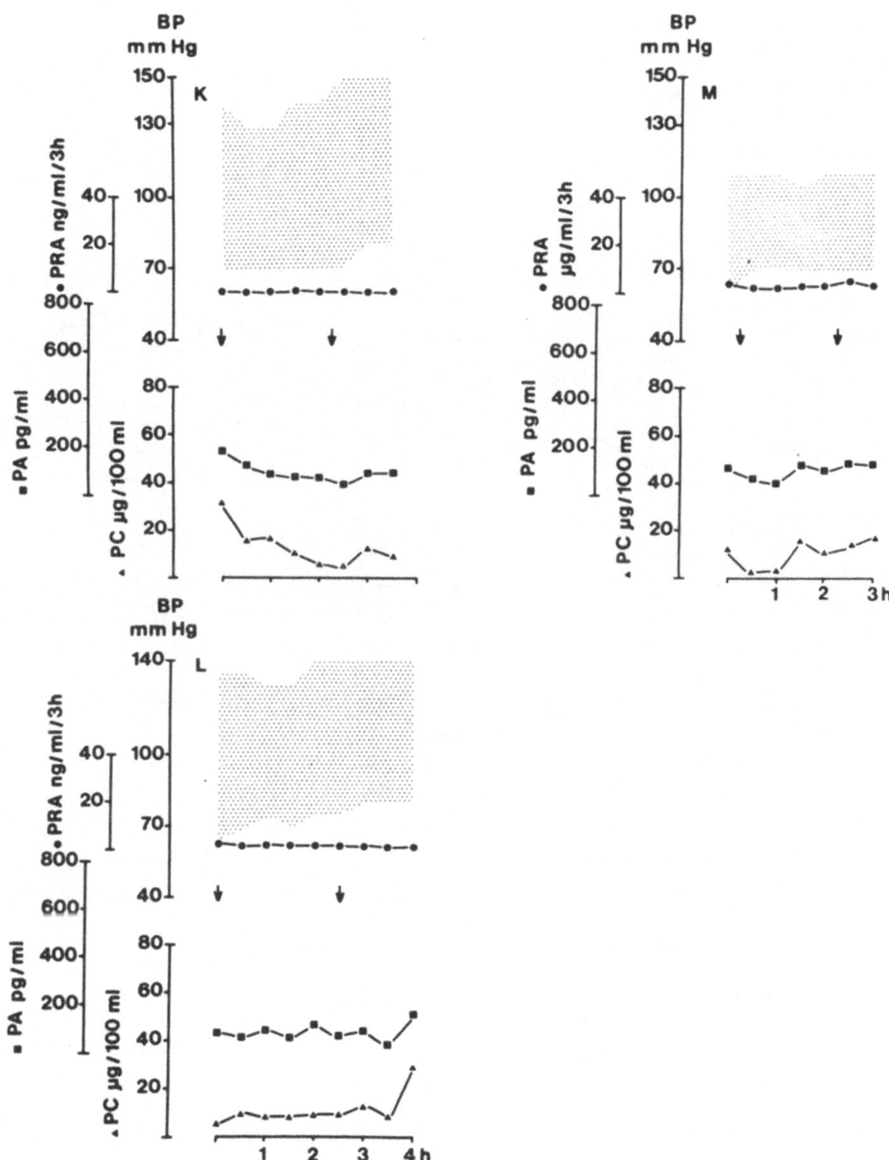

Abb. 2. Sekretionsstudien der 3 unter normotensiver kontinuierlicher PDA operierten Patienten (K, L, M). Von oben nach unten sind jeweils aufgezeichnet: Plasma-Renin-Aktivität (PRA), Plasma-Aldosteron (PA) und Plasma-Cortisol (PC). Der Blutdruckverlauf ist durch Raster markiert, die Pfeile kennzeichnen Operationsbeginn und -ende

Katecholaminen [9] sensibilisiert wird. Vor allem die stark erhöhten Plasma-Cortisol-Werte geben einen Hinweis auf eine gesteigerte NNR-Aktivität, wie sie bei jedem Streß-Ablauf beobachtet werden kann. Hierbei ist die vermehrte Cortisolfreisetzung ACTH-getriggert und auch der Hyperaldosteronismus kann durch eine Streß-bedingte ACTH-Überproduktion erklärt werden. Eine Ursache für den Hyperreninismus dürfte in der bei flacher Halothannarkose fehlenden

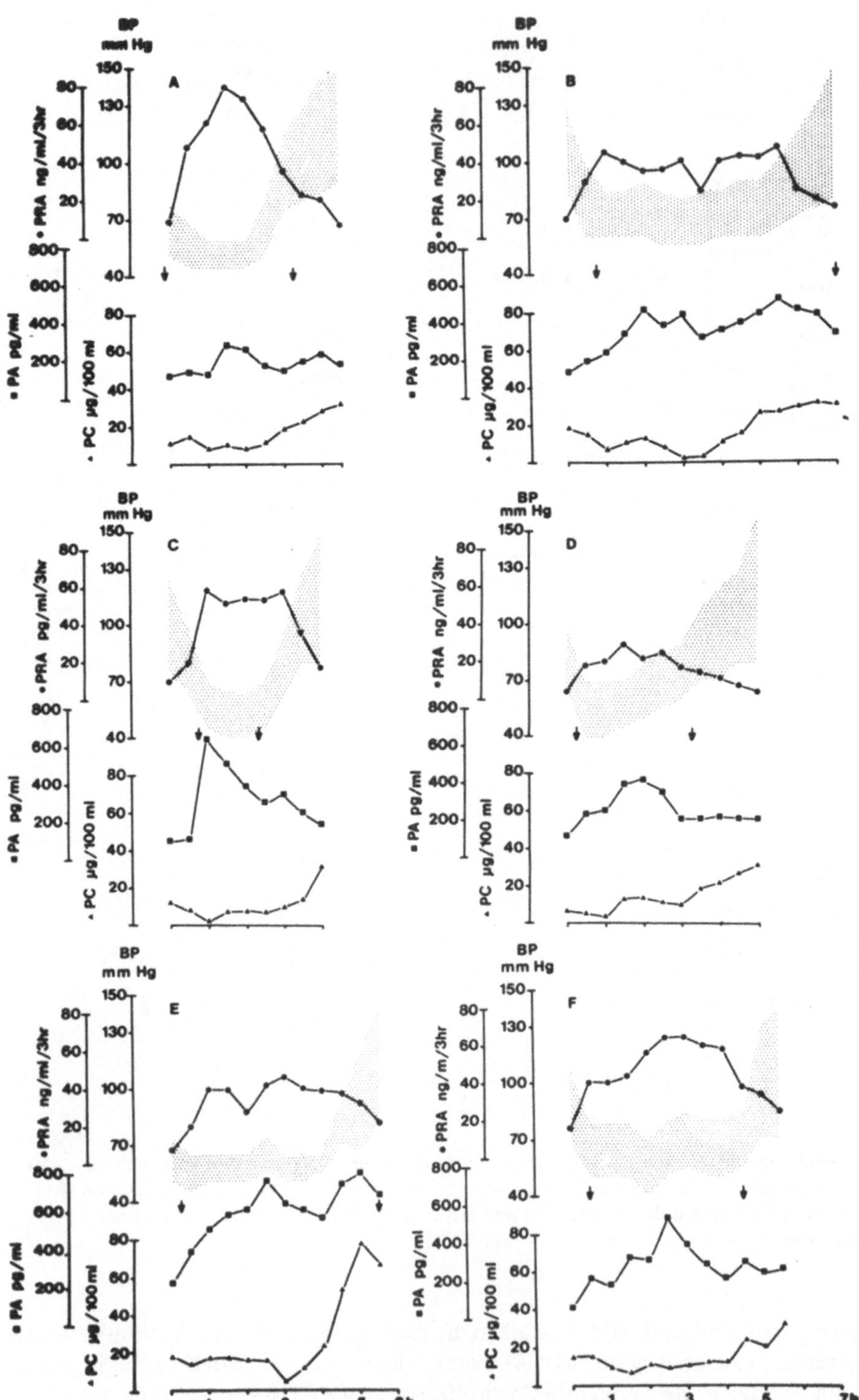

Abb. 3. Sekretionsstudien der 6 unter hypotensiver PDA operierten Patienten (A, B, C, D, E, F). Die Aufzeichnung der Parameter erfolgte in gleicher Anordnung wie auf Abb. 2 (siehe Legende zu Abb. 2)

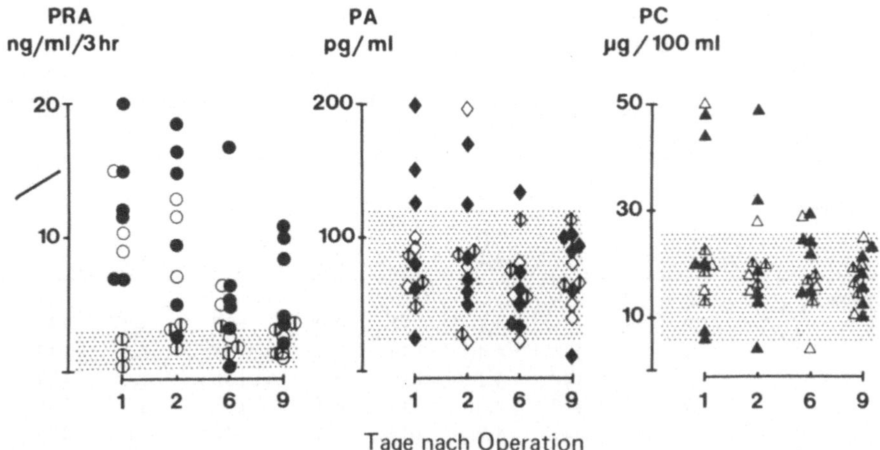

Abb. 4. Zusammenfassende Darstellung der Plasma-Renin-Aktivität (PRA), des Plasma-Aldosterons (PA) sowie des Plasma-Cortisols (PC) am 1., 2., 6. und 9. postoperativen Tag. Der Normbereich ist durch Raster markiert; Symbole mit Längsbalken: normotensive kontinuierliche PDA; schwarze Symbole: hypotensive PDA; helle Symbole: normotensive Halothannarkose

Sympathikusdämpfung mit teilweise erhöhter Katecholaminfreisetzung liegen. Auch im weiteren postoperativen Verlauf scheint die Stimulation der Reninsekretion durch den in diesem Zeitraum gesteigerten Sympathikustonus zu erfolgen. Während der eigentlichen Narkoseperiode muß dagegen zusätzlich eine durch die Anästhetika ausgelöste Minderperfusion der Nieren als die Reninsekretion steigernder Faktor in Betracht gezogen werden. Bihler [1] sowie Deutsch et al. [3] wiesen nach, daß die meisten Anästhetika zu einer Perfusionseinschränkung der Nieren mit Absinken der PAH- und Inulin-Clearance sowie einem Anstieg des renalen Gefäßwiderstandes führen.

2. Normotensive kontinuierliche PDA

Die unter normotensiver kontinuierlicher PDA und intraoperativer Sedierung mittels Diazepam gewonnenen Sekretionsmuster für Renin, Aldosteron und Cortisol verhalten sich dagegen grundlegend anders. Die Nervenblockade unterbricht die Rückkopplung zum HVL, eine erhöhte ACTH-Ausschüttung unterbleibt und somit liegen die Werte für Cortisol und Aldosteron, dessen episodische Sekretion ja ebenfalls ACTH-getriggert wird, für die Dauer der PDA im Normbereich. Auch die Reninfreisetzung steigt nicht an, weil eine Stimulierung des juxtaglomerulären Apparates bei Normotension und unter PDA verminderter Katecholaminfreisetzung [6] vermieden wird.

Bei kontinuierlicher PDA kann diese Dämpfung des HVL-NNR- wie auch des Renin-Angiotensin-Aldosteron-Systems für die Dauer der Weiterführung des Verfahrens im postoperativen Verlauf verlängert werden. Im Hinblick auf die Prophylaxe eines postoperativen Hyperaldosteronismus darf dieses Regionalanästhesieverfahren gerade bei Risikopatienten somit als besonders geeignet bezeichnet werden. In diesem Zusammenhang gewinnen selbstverständlich auch weitere wesentliche Maßnahmen zur Vermeidung negativer Streß-Auswirkungen wie Elektrolyt- und Volumensubstitution, präoperativ durchgeführte Kalium- und Magnesium-reiche Ernährung sowie die Anwendung von Aldosteron-Antagonisten an Bedeutung.

Tabelle 3. Prä-, intra- und postoperative (1. und 9. postoperativer Tag) Serumspiegel für Natrium und Kalium bei allen untersuchten Patienten

		präoperativ		intraoperativ		1. postop. Tag		9. postop. Tag	
Anästhesiemethode	Patient	Na^+	K^+	Na^+	K^+	Na^+	K^+	Na^+	K^+
normotensive kontinuierliche PDA	K	140	4,1	135	3,8	136	3,7	136	3,9
	L	135	4,0	139	3,8	139	3,5	144	4,0
	M	142	4,1	145	3,7	140	3,4	139	4,0
hypotensive Single shot PDA	A	139	4,1	131	3,9	137	3,8	138	4,1
	B	145	4,4	139	3,9	137	4,4	142	4,1
	C	140	4,1	139	3,5	138	4,4	137	4,0
	D	137	4,2	135	4,4	133	3,9	135	3,8
	E	142	4,9	133	3,4	140	4,6	139	4,4
	F	136	4,3	133	3,9	138	4,8	140	4,1
Normotensive Halothan-Narkose	G	137	4,1	131	3,5	133	4,3	138	4,0
	H	136	3,9	131	4,0	131	4,1	132	4,5
	I	138	4,9	140	3,6	140	4,8	138	4,4

3. Hypotensive single shot PDA

Unsere Untersuchungen der Reninsekretion bei Patienten, die unter hypotensiver PDA operiert wurden, sollten zur weiteren Klärung der Regulation des RAAS unter PDA beitragen. Während erwartungsgemäß aufgrund der Unterbrechung der nervalen Rückkopplung zum HVL auch hier die Cortisolsekretion für die Dauer der PDA im Normbereich bleibt, steigen die Aldosteron-, vor allem aber die Renin-Sekretionsraten mit Beginn der Blutdrucksenkung stark an. Die vermehrte Aldosteron-Aktivität ist demnach hier nicht ACTH-bedingt, sondern allein auf einen durch die kontrollierte Hypotension induzierten Hyperreninismus zurückzuführen. Als weitere Ursache für den erhöhten Plasma-Aldosteron-Spiegel muß aber auch eine erniedrigte metabolische Clearance-Rate der Leber für dieses Hormon aufgrund einer Minderperfusion dieses Organs während der Blutdrucksenkung diskutiert werden. Gerbershagen et al. [4] wiesen in diesem Zusammenhang eine Lidocain-spezifische Einschränkung der Leberperfusion unter PDA nach und erklären dies mit den kardiovaskulär stimulierenden Eigenschaften und einer Erhöhung des Lebergefäßwiderstandes durch dieses Lokalanästhetikum. Unsere eigenen unter normotensiver kontinuierlicher PDA ermittelten Aldosteron-Spiegel geben dagegen keinen indirekten Hinweis auf eine Einschränkung der Leberdurchblutung.

Unsere Befunde machen deutlich, daß im Gegensatz zu allen anderen humoralen Regelkreisen das RAAS unter PDA eine Stimulation erfährt, wenn gleichzeitig durch diese PDA eine länger dauernde Hypotension induziert wird. Bei der Frage nach der Ursache für diese Aktivitätssteigerung sei auf die Regulation der Reninfreisetzung schlechthin hingewiesen, die nach heutiger Auffassung im Wesentlichen unter Vermittlung des sympathikoadrenalen Systems, der Macula densa sowie der renalen Barorezeptoren im Bereich der afferenten Arteriolen erfolgt [2, 11]. Bei der unter PDA nachgewiesenen Dämpfung bzw. Blockierung des sympathikoadrenalen Systems [6] kommt eine Induktion der Reninsekretion sowohl durch endogene Katecholamine als auch durch sympathische Nervenfasern außer Betracht. Im Hinblick auf die nur geringfügigen, klinisch nicht relevanten Abweichungen der Serum-Natrium- und -Kalium-Spiegel scheint auch eine Stimulation unter Vermittlung der Macula densa eher von untergeordneter Bedeutung zu sein. Als Hauptursache für die unter hypotensiver PDA gesteigerte PRA muß somit eine infolge der Hypotension verminderte Wandspannung der afferenten Arteriolen im Bereich des juxtaglomerulären Apparates angenommen werden. Der erniedrigte renale Perfusionsdruck führt zu einer Erregung der myoepithelialen Zellen mit konsekutiver vermehrter Renin-Freisetzung. Die starken Auswirkungen einer länger dauernden kontrollierten Hypotension sind auch im weiteren postoperativen Verlauf dokumentiert: Während nach normotensiver Allgemeinanästhesie die Sekretionsraten für Renin, Aldosteron und Cortisol bis spätestens zum 6. postoperativen Tag normalisiert sind, bleibt die Renin-Aktivität über den 9. postoperativen Tag hinaus nach Hypotension deutlich gesteigert. Insgesamt ist die Steuerung der Reninsekretion im postoperativen Verlauf, nach Abklingen der PDA, komplexer durch Zusammenwirken der Regelmechanismen Barorezeptoren, sympathikoadrenales System und Macula densa. Die postoperativ über 9 Tage gesteigerte Renin-Sekretion nach hypotensiver PDA unterstreicht die Forderung, diese Narkosetechnik, wie überhaupt alle Verfahren zur kontrollierten Hypotension, sofern sie sich über einen längeren Zeitraum von 1-2 Stunden und mehr erstrekken, nur aus strenger Indikation bei kreislauf- und nierengesunden jungen Patienten anzuwenden, wo lange Operationsdauer und ein zu erwartender hoher intraoperativer Blutverlust diese Verfahren rechtfertigen.

Abschließend sei für das Verhalten des RAAS unter PDA nochmals hervorgehoben, daß eine Steigerung dieses humoralen Regelkreises nur dann verhindert werden kann, wenn während der PDA eine normotensive Kreislauflage aufrecht erhalten wird (Tabelle 4).

Tabelle 4. Zusammenfassende Darstellung der Beeinflussung der Plasma-Renin-Aktivität (PRA), des Plasma-Aldosterons (PA) und Plasma-Cortisols (PC) durch die untersuchten Anästhesieverfahren während operativer Eingriffe

	Halothan (Normotension)	PDA (Hypotension)	Katheter-PDA (Normotension
PRA	+	++	–
PA	+	++	–
PC	++	-bis (+)	–

+ = Erhöhung; ++ = Starke Erhöhung; – = Keine Erhöhung

Summary

Blockade of afferent neurogenic stimuli from the surgical area induced by epidural anaesthesia inhibits most parameters of the endocrine-stress-response. The present study was undertaken to investigate the effect of epidural anaesthesia and surgery on renin-angiotensin-aldosterone-system (RAAS) and on the adrenocortical function as judged from plasma cortisol levels.

Twelve patients were studied before, during and after surgery. Three of them undergoing total hip replacement received normotensive continuous epidural block (normotensive PDA). Six patients with malignant testicular tumour underwent lymphadenectomy under high single shot epidural anaesthesia plus light general anaesthesia (nitrous oxide/oxygen and low doses halothane) in association with induced hypotension by PDA (hypotensive PDA). Three patients received light general anaesthesia alone (halothane, nitrous oxide/oxygen) for gastrectomy. Plasma-renin-activity (PRA), plasma aldosterone (PA) and plasma cortisol (PC) were determined at short time intervals.

In the group receiving normotensive continuous PDA no significant elevation in PRA, PA or PC was noted during surgery and the postoperative period demonstrating the inhibitory effect of normotensive epidural block on the stress-response of RAAS. In contrast under induced hypotension (hypotensive PDA) the fall of systolic blood pressure was combined with increased PRA and PA while PC was within normal range until the epidural blockade began to wear off. In the three patients receiving light general anaesthesia alone, PRA, PA and PC was significantly higher during surgery and the postoperative period than it had been preoperatively. The almost parallel secretion of PC and PA indicates that in these patients hyperaldosteronism results from surgical stress with concomitant ACTH excess. Comparing these findings with the results of the hypotensive PDA group it is apparent that PRA and PA are higher in patients undergoing hypotensive PDA. This result indicates that a distinct and persistent decrease in blood pressure stimulates the RAAS more than major surgery (gastrectomy). The metabolic clearance rate of aldosterone could however, be lower during hypotension than in surgery with almost normal blood pressure. Our data suggests that the stress-response of RAAS is inhibited only by normotensive epidural anaesthesia and not by deliberate hypotension induced by high single shot PDA.

Literatur

1. Bihler K (1969) Anästhesiebedingte Veränderungen der Nierenfunktion und renale Elektrolytexkretion. Anästhesist 18:396
2. Davis JO, Freeman RH (1976) Mechanisms regulating renin release. Physiol Rev 56:1
3. Deutsch S, Bastron RD, Pierce EC, Vandam LD (1969) The effects of anaesthesia with thiopentone, nitrous oxide, narcotics and neuromuscular blocking agents on renal function in man. Br J Anaesth 41:807
4. Gerbershagen HU, Kennedy WF Jr, Bonica JJ, Everett GB, Cobb LA, Allen GD, Sawyer TK, Cutler RE (1972) Hämodynamische Einflüsse der Peridural- und Spinalanästhesie auf andere Organe. In: Nolte H (Hrsg) Die rückenmarksnahen Anästhesien. Thieme, Stuttgart
5. Haber E, Koerner T, Page LB, Kliman B, Purnode A (1969) Application of a radioimmunoassay for angiotensin I to the physiologic measurements of plasma renin activity in normal human subjects. J Clin Endocrinol Metab 29:1349
6. Hack G, Freiberger KU, Schulte am Esch J, Havers L (1975) Zum Problem der Stress-Reaktion in der unmittelbaren postoperativen Phase. Fortschr Med 93:212
7. Hack G, Marx M, Bayer JM, Vetter H (1975) Zum Einfluß von normo- und hypotensiver Anästhesie auf das Renin-Angiotensin-Aldosteron-System. Vortrag ZAK Bremen
8. Hackl JM, Skrabal F (1975) Das Verhalten von Plasmareninaktivität, Plasmaaldosteron und Elektrolytbilanz in der postoperativen Phase. Anästhesist 24:477
9. Havers L, Kreppel E, Hack G (1972) Das Verhalten der Katecholamine bei langdauernden Eingriffen in Peridural-, Halothan-, Methoxyfluran- und Neuroleptanästhesie. Medical Press, Prague
10. Havers L, Hack G, Vollmar A, Etzel F (1975) Die kombinierte Periduralanästhesie und ihre Indikation. In: Bergmann H, Blauhut B (Hrsg) Intensivtherapie. Anästhesiologie und Wiederbelebung, Bd 94, S. 58. Springer, Berlin Heidelberg New York
11. Meurer KA (1975) Das Renin-Angiotensin-Aldosteron-System. Kurzmonografien Sandoz, Nürnberg
12. Murphy BEP, Pattee CJ (1964) Determination of plasma corticoids by competitive protein-binding analysis using gel filtration. J Clin Endocrinol Metab 24:919
13. Oyama T, Kimura K, Sato K, Demura H (1972) Effects of anaesthesia and surgery on plasma aldosterone levels in man. Anesth Analg Curr Res 52:31
14. Robertson D, Michelakis AM (1972) Effect of anaesthesia and surgery on plasma renin activity in man. J Clin Endocrinol Metab 34:831

15. Vetter W, Vetter H, Siegenthaler W (1973) Radioimmunoassay for aldosterone without chromatography. Acta Endocrinol (Kbh) 74:548
16. Wernze H, Hilfenhaus M, Rietbrock I, Schüttke R, Kühn K (1975) Plasmareninaktivität und Plasma-Aldosteron unter Narkose und Operationsstreß und Beta-Receptoren-Blockade. Anästhesist 24:471

Podiumsdiskussion: Streß und Endokrinium während Narkose und Operation

Vorsitz: H. Lennartz, Marburg und T. Tammisto, Helsinki
Teilnehmer: G. Hack, H. Kehlet und R. Knitza

Lennartz: Wie wir bei den Referaten zum Thema der Podiumsdiskussion gehört haben, greifen wir mit unseren Anästhesiemethoden sehr unterschiedlich in den humoralen Mechanismus unseres Organismus ein, was wiederum (z.T. rückwirkend) Folgen auf die postoperative Phase haben kann. Man wundert sich gelegentlich, wenn man Ihre Bilder gesehen hat, Herr Hack, daß das Herz diesen Renin-Ausscheidungen überhaupt noch folgen kann, daß es überhaupt noch pumpen kann und nicht ständig bei unseren Narkosen insuffizient wird. Ich darf jetzt als Advocatus diaboli fragen: was haben diese Befunde für die Anästhesie für eine Bedeutung, sollen wir darauf überhaupt achten?

Zuerst vielleicht aber, Herr Tammisto, einige klärende Worte noch zur Adrenalinsekretion bzw. -ausscheidung. Ich erinnere mich, daß wir in Düsseldorf eine Untersuchungsreihe durchgeführt haben, eine Doktorarbeit über Vanillin und Vanillin-Mandelsäureausscheidung. Es wurde dabei zwischen Halothan und Neuroleptanalgesie verglichen, dabei schnitt die Neuroleptanalgesie sehr schlecht ab. Es kam nämlich bei der NlA zu einer sehr hohen Ausscheidung von Vanillin und Vanillin-Mandelsäure im Urin.

Tammisto: Eine Antwort darauf habe ich leider nicht. Ich habe mich selber über diese Renin Sekretion gewundert. Zweifelsohne ist diese sympathische Reaktion nicht vergebens da. Wir brauchen sie, um diesen Streß zu überleben, und nun scheint es, daß die Dämpfung dieser Reaktion Vorteile hat, wie wir aus den Vorträgen gesehen haben. Wir sollten wenn möglich Anästhesiemethoden verwenden, die diese Reaktion dämpfen und zu denen gehört vielleicht die Neuroleptanalgesie nicht. Sie dämpft zwar die zirkulatorischen Reaktionen, aber die Katecholamine steigen mehr an als bei manchen anderen Allgemeinnarkoseverfahren. Es könnte sein, daß wir trotz unserer heutigen Lebensweise immer noch mit dieser Alarmreaktion ausgestattet sind. Wir können damit vielleicht viel größerem Streß entgegentreten, als die hier vorgeführten Operationen bedeuten. Wenn in der postoperativen Phase schwere Komplikationen eintreten, ist es sehr wichtig, daß unser Organismus auf diesen Katecholamin-Response getrimmt und verteidigungsfähig ist. Ich würde deswegen gern die Meinung der Diskussionsteilnehmer hören. Soll man dämpfen oder nicht, denn diese Reaktionen können eventuell doch sinnvoll sein.

Kehlet: The main question is: is this stress response an inherited reflex for which we have no use in the hospital, where we can get blood transfusions and fluids if we need them, or is it a response which increase our chances of survival? I think we have to do further studies. Epidural anaesthesia is one technique and I think the data shows that it may be valuable. There are other data showing that this stress response may not be necessary. If you give morphine in doses of 4 mg/kg body wt. you also abolish the stress response and in normal risk patients it does not matter whether the stress response is present during elective procedures or not. In patients with an increased morbidity however, I think you may precipitate cardiopulmonary complications because of the stress response. So future scientific work will study if there is a beneficial effect in inhibiting this stress response.

Lennartz: Ich danke Herrn Kehlet für diese aufklärenden Worte, denn man konnte allgemein heute nachmittag doch den Eindruck gewinnen, es gehe also nur noch mit einer hohen kontinuierlichen Periduralanaesthesie, alles andere könnten wir vergessen. Ich meine wir haben auch noch andere Narkosemethoden und Sie erwähnten also jetzt schon das Morphin; das ist sehr erfreulich und ich bin der Meinung, daß man auch eine tiefe Halothannarkose machen kann. Die Narkose sollte ja nicht so sein, daß dem Patienten die Augen tränen, wenn er operiert wird. Vielleicht könnten Sie noch etwas dazu sagen, Herr Hack. Sie haben ja jetzt die Methode von Havers mit der hypotensiven Periduralanaesthesie in Kombination mit Halothan, Lachgas und Diazepam untersucht. Was würden Sie dazu sagen? Stehen wir jetzt wirklich hier und müssen sagen: alles andere weg, nur noch Periduralanaesthesie oder dürfen wir auch noch anderes?

Hack: Selbstverständlich darf über manchen Vorzügen einer rückenmarksnahen Regionalanästhesie für das Endokrinium die für den anästhesiologischen Alltag mit einem gemischten Operationsprogramm quantitativ größere Rolle der Allgemeinnarkose nicht vergessen werden, wobei auch hier bestimmte Substanzen wie z.B. Morphin oder Enfluran die Streß-Antwort zu modifizieren vermögen. In meinen Ausführungen bin ich kurz auf die physiologische Bedeutung der intra- wie postoperativ erhöhte Aktivität humoraler Regelkreise eingegangen. In diesem Zusammenhang dürfen wir Anästhesisten uns selbst wohl ohne Übertreibung als streßtrainiert bezeichnen. Dies gilt sowohl für die Katecholamine als auch für das Renin-Angiotensin-Aldosteron-System, zumal wenn wir uns die an arbeitsreichen Tagen im Operationssaal oft sicher unzureichende Flüssigkeitszufuhr vor Augen halten. Eine vermehrte Freisetzung von Katecholaminen ebenso wie von Renin, Aldosteron oder etwa Cortisol als Reaktion auf einen operativen Eingriff oder adäquate andere Streß-Einwirkungen dürfte für einen nicht vorgeschädigten Organismus ohne bleibende Folgen sein. So ließen sich auch bei den 6 jüngeren Kranken, deren Renin-, Aldosteron- und Cortisol-Spiegel unter hypotensiver PDA von uns untersucht wurden, klinisch keinerlei bleibende Schädigungen trotz der stark erhöhten Plasma-Renin-Aktivität nachweisen. Andererseits sollten im Hinblick auf den bis zum 9. postoperativen Tag bei diesem Anästhesieverfahren nachgewiesenen Hyperreninismus bei älteren Patienten mit eingeschränkter Leistungsbreite des kardiovaskulären Systems länger dauernde hypotensive Phasen in Verbindung mit einer PDA vermieden werden.

Lennartz: Herr Knitza, wir haben heute morgen gehört, daß es unter der postoperativen Periduralanalgesie zu einem Abfall der Sauerstoffaufnahme des Organismus kommt, wenn man das Muskelzittern mit Dolantin aufhebt. Eine Frage, die ich an Sie stellen möchte, ist das alles auch im Zusammenhang mit Adrenalin- Noradrenalinfreisetzung zu sehen? Die gesteigerte oder die abnehmende Sauerstoffaufnahme, wenn ich nun also das Muskelzittern vermeide?

Knitza: Es ist bekannt, daß Adrenalin und Noradrenalin den O_2-Verbrauch steigern. Deswegen ist es wichtig, auch die hormonellen Veränderungen, die sich während der Anaesthesie und der postoperativen Phase einstellen, zu beachten. Ich habe versucht, an einem Beispiel den Zusammenhang zwischen der hormonellen und metabolischen Seite, also den Mechanismus der Lipaseaktivierung, darzustellen. Die Tatsache, daß im Organismus während einer Streß-Situation eine gesteigerte Lipolyse einsetzt, führt zu einem wesentlich erhöhten Verbrauch an Sauerstoff. Deshalb sollte man sich überlegen, welche Möglichkeiten man hat, auch während der Anaesthesie diese hormonell bedingten Veränderungen zu steuern. Es ist heute doch häufig so, daß man irgendeine Lösung, die sich gerade bietet, dem Patienten infundiert. Man sollte überlegen, wie durch geeignete Wahl der Hohlenhydrate die metabolische Situation gebessert werden kann. Bekanntlich kommt es im Postaggressionssyndrom, welches seinen Ursprung bereits während der Anaesthesie hat, zu einem Glukoseanstieg und die Insulinkonzentration verändert sich, wie Herr Kehlet gezeigt hat, nicht. Manchmal ist es sogar so, daß der Insulinspiegel trotz erhöhter Glukosekonzentration absinkt und dann die Ketonkörper ansteigen. Dies kann dann sogar bis zu einer metabolischen Azidose führen. Durch Infusion von Xylit oder Sorbit beispielsweise könnte man dieses Problem angehen, weil diese auch in Streß-Situationen insulinabhängig in den Stoffwechsel eingeschleust werden können und damit der Zelle ausreichend alpha-Glycerophosphat zur Reveresterung der Fettsäuren bereitsteht. Auf diese Art wären möglicherweise die massiven streß-induzierten Veränderungen zu mindern. Man sollte daher überlegen, ob man in Streß-Situationen, bedingt durch den Schweregrad der Operation oder die jeweilige Anaesthesietechnik, schon intraoperativ mit der Gabe einer Kombination von Zuckeraustauschstoffen beginnt.

Lennartz: Es hat den Vorschlag gegeben, zur Verhinderung des Anstiegs an freien Fettsäuren als Ausdruck der Streßreaktion Glukose mit Insulin zu infundieren, präoperativ schon. Würden Sie das für sinnvoll halten?

Knitza: Dies ist sicher gewagt, und zwar aus zweierlei Gründen. Insulininfusionen verlangen gerade bei einem bewußtlos anaesthesierten Patienten eine sehr engmaschige Kontrolle. Die Gefahr einer Hypoglykämie sollte nicht unterschätzt werden. Zum anderen ist die Möglichkeit einer Resistenzbildung gegen Insulin gegeben, so daß die Dosis bei Gabe über längere Zeit gesteigert werden müßte.

Lennartz: Ich möchte zur Diskussion stellen, ob diese Streß-Situationen wirklich so bedenklich sind. Wir haben uns ja angewöhnt, bei Streß immer gleich an Furchtbares zu denken. Diese geringen Anstiege von Aldosteron oder Cortisol oder Änderungen des Fettsäurespiegels – ist das denn wirklich so bedrohlich oder dieser Renin-Anstieg, der relativ flüchtig ist? Das einzige, was wir zu fürchten haben, ist eigentlich die Wirkung der Katecholamine auf den Kreislauf und das Herz. Sind die übrigen Dinge denn so beängstigend, daß Sie deswegen eine Periduralanaesthesie machen müssen?

Knitza: Gerade bezüglich der Fettsäurespiegel gibt es sehr interessante Untersuchungen. Wesentliche Anstiege von freien Fettsäuren können zu einer gesteigerten Thrombozytenaggregation führen. Ich denke an die Arbeiten von Stremmel in Freiburg. Vielleicht gewinnen diese Veränderungen auch im Zusammenhang mit einer Thromboseprophylaxe an Bedeutung. Diese Zusammenhänge sind noch nicht ausreichend systematisch untersucht worden. Gezielte Langzeituntersuchungen könnten relevante Zusammenhänge zeigen.

Lennartz: Zu der letzten Anregung von Herrn Knitza, der vorschlug, evtl. intraoperativ schon Zuckeraustauschstoffe zu geben, man kommt da etwas in Schwierigkeiten, weil man die vorgeschriebenen Infusionszeiten unterschreitet und dann sicher Verwertungsstörungen auftreten. Bei 500 ml Infusion pro Stunde bei eröffnetem Abdomen hat man nämlich die Infusionszeiten sicher unterschritten. Ich weiß nicht, ob man das Problem irgendwie lösen kann. Ich hätte aber an das Podium die Frage, ob der Vorschlag, der gelegentlich gemacht wird, wegen des intra- und postoperativen Hyperaldosteronismus natriumreiche Infusionen zu geben, dazu führen sollte, daß man tatsächlich ein erhöhtes Natriumangebot bereits intraoperativ geben soll?

Hack: Hackl und Skrabal (1975, zitiert im Vortrag) haben in ihren Untersuchungen zum Verhalten der Plasma-Renin-Aktivität, des Plasma-Aldosterons und der Elektrolytbilanz in der postoperativen Phase zeigen können, daß sich Anstiege des Plasma-Renins und des Plasma-Aldosterons trotz Positivierung der Natriumbilanz um 250 mval nicht unterdrücken ließen. In der intra- wie postoperativen Phase dürfte eine Beeinflussung der Plasma-Renin-Aktivität durch Schwankungen des Blutdrucks und des Blutvolumens mit dem Einfluß des Serum-Natrium-Spiegels auf die Reninfreisetzung und somit auch auf den Aldosteron-Spiegel interferieren, so daß trotz normaler oder sogar erhöhter Natrium-Werte eine Hypovolämie zu einer verstärkten Renin-Freisetzung führt und umgekehrt.

Knitza: Das Problem hierbei sind sicher die mit etwa 0,125 g/kg/h sehr niedrigen Umsatzraten. Es ist also nicht gedacht, den Patienten jetzt nur Xylit oder Sorbit zu infundieren, aber man könnte beispielsweise eine gewisse Menge im Bypass zu einer Vollelektrolytlösung anbieten. Ich dachte nicht an massive Xylitininfusionen, da sonst sicher die Laktatkonzentration ansteigt und andere Komplikationen eintreten.

Hack: Ich darf nochmals betonen, daß wir trotz des bis zum 9. postoperativen Tag nachgewiesenen Hyperreninismus nach hypotensiver PDA keinerlei Komplikationen von seiten der Blutdrucksenkung, welche hier über eine Dauer von 2 1/2 bis 3 Stunden und bis zu systolischen Blutdruckwerten von 60 mm Hg vorgenommen wurde, bei Kreislaufgesunden beobachtet haben. Bei der von Ihnen angesprochenen Indikation dürften derart niedrige Werte über einen längeren Zeitraum wohl kaum in Frage kommen. Gerade die kontinuierliche PDA bietet aber die Möglichkeit, unter vorsichtiger Dosierung des Lokalanästhetikums eine mäßige Drucksenkung auf tolerable Werte beim Hypertoniker mit Nierenarterienstenose zu erreichen. Dabei sollte aber auch hier an die Möglichkeit eines sekundären postoperativen Hyperaldosteronismus gedacht und eine Prophylaxe mit Aldosteron-Antogonisten betrieben werden.

Lennartz: Meine Frage geht in folgende Richtung. Könnte man die Streß-Situation einigermaßen objektivieren? Wir sehen, daß alle biochemischen Parameter eine sehr breite Streuung haben, auch die 10fachen Werte werden als noch normal bezeichnet. Eine weitere Frage sind die Tagesprofile in den biochemischen Parametern. Wir haben in Basel Untersuchungen mit Prolactin durchgeführt und bei jeder Streß-Situation steigen die Prolactinwerte an; schon die Berührung der Mamille bei freiwilligen Studentinnen führt zu einer Streß-Situation. Zusammengefaßt: Gibt es echte biochemische Parameter für den Streß? Es wird behauptet, daß alle biochemische Parameter breite Streuungen haben und daß die 10fachen Werte noch im Normbereich liegen.

Hack: Die Plasma-Renin-Aktivität und das Plasma-Aldosteron können sicherlich weite Streuungen innerhalb des Normbereiches aufweisen. Die Sekretion dieser Hormone unterliegt zudem einer zirkadianen Rhythmik und darüber hinaus gibt es Patienten mit einem sogenannten „low-renin", welche auf einen gleichwertigen Streß-Faktor mit deutlich geringerer Renin-Freisetzung reagieren wie ein anderer Kranker auf den gleichen Stimulus. Neben der Tatsache, daß wir ein nur kleines Kollektiv von 12 Patienten untersucht haben, war dies für uns der Hauptgrund, Einzelstudien wiederzugeben, bei denen wir allerdings mittels Kurzzeitblutentnahmen einen besonders engmaschigen Überblick gewinnen konnten.

IV. Veränderung der Atmung bei postoperativer Schmerzbekämpfung durch Opiate und Periduralanaesthesie

Vorsitz: H. Nolte, Minden und K. Falke, Düsseldorf

Postoperative Periduralanästhesie (Technik und Indikationen)

H.P. Siepmann, H.J. Wüst und G. Liebau

Die kontinuierliche Periduralanalgesie zur postoperativen Schmerzbekämpfung bietet gegenüber den herkömmlichen Verfahren folgende Vorzüge:

1. Drastische Reduktion des Verbrauchs an Analgetika (insbesondere Opiate) und Sedativa [2].
2. Senkung der pulmonalen Komplikationsrate durch Vermeidung der postoperativen Hypoventilation (zentrale Atemdepression, Schon-Atmung) [1, 5].
3. Senkung der Nachbelastung des Herzens durch Sympathikolyse [4].
4. Steigerung des Blutflusses im Bereich von Gefäßanastomosen nach Operationen wegen peripherer Durchblutungsstörungen [3].
5. Günstige Beeinflussung der Darmmotilität (Atonie-Prophylaxe).

Technik

Der Patient wird auf die rechte oder linke Seite gelagert und aufgefordert, die Beine anzuziehen und den Kopf auf die Brust zu nehmen („Katzenbuckel").

Die Rückenhaut wird zuerst mit einem chirurgischen Händedesinfektionsmittel abgewaschen, getrocknet und im Thorax-, Lenden- und Kreuzbeinbereich mit einem nichtjodhaltigen Hautdesinfektionsmittel eingesprüht.

Während der Einwirkzeit von 3 Minuten zieht sich der Arzt sterile Kleidung an (Kopfbedeckung, Mundschutz, steriler Kittel, Handschuhe) und nimmt hinter dem Rücken des Patienten Platz. Mit dem Mittel- und Zeigefinger der linken Hand (bei Rechtshändern) wird die Haut des Patienten über der beabsichtigten Punktionsstelle zwischen zwei Dornfortsätzen gestrafft und ein Lokalanästhetikum in die Haut, die Subkutis und in die unmittelbare Nachbarschaft des Ligamentum interspinosum injiziert, um die Tuohy-Nadel schmerzfrei vorschieben zu können.

Ohne die linke Hand von der Punktionsstelle wegzunehmen, nimmt man sich mit der rechten Hand die Tuohy-Nadel, stößt sie im Zentrum der Hautquaddel durch die Haut und schiebt sie ca. 4 cm vor, und zwar im Lumbalbereich senkrecht zur Haut, im Thoraxbereich in einem nach kaudal offenen Winkel von ca. 40°.

Man entfernt nun den Mandrin der Tuohy-Nadel, setzt eine mit physiologischer Kochsalzlösung gefüllte Spritze auf und umfaßt mit den Fingern der linken Hand die Kanüle wie einen Bleistift. Dabei stützt sich der Kleinfingerballen auf dem Rücken des Patienten ab. Während nun die Finger der linken Hand die Tuohy-Nadel millimeterweise an den Periduralraum heranführen, übt der Daumen der rechten Hand einen ständigen Druck auf die Glasspritze aus.

Solange man sich noch im Ligamentum interspinosum oder Ligamentum flavum befindet, spürt man mit dem Daumen einen gummiartig-federnden Widerstand. Perforiert nun die Spitze der Tuohy-Nadel das Ligamentum flavum, so kommt es zum plötzlichen Druckverlust, der dieser Methode zur Identifizierung des Periduralraumes den Namen „Widerstandsverlust-Methode" eingebracht hat.

Da im Augenblick des Widerstandsverlustes nur etwa das vordere Drittel der Öffnung der Tuohy-Nadel im Periduralraum liegt, empfiehlt sich ein vorsichtiges Vorschieben der Kanüle um weitere 1-1,5 mm.

In dieser Position wird nun mit der rechten Hand der Katheter in die Nadel eingeführt und bis zur Spitze vorgeschoben. Daß man die Spitze erreicht hat, erkennt man an einem leichten Widerstand.

Wenn man ihn überwindet, läßt sich der Katheter nahezu rechtwinklig zur Achse der Tuohy-Nadel nach oben in den Epiduralraum vorschieben. Wenn auf diese Weise die vorderen 3-4 cm des Katheters in den Periduralraum eingebracht wurden, zieht man die Tuohy-Nadel unter stopfenden Bewegungen über den Katheter zurück, wobei darauf zu achten ist, daß der Katheter bei dieser Manipulation nicht wieder zurückgezogen bzw. noch weiter vorgeschoben wird. Nach Entfernen der Tuohy-Nadel wird das äußere Katheterende mit einer passenden, vorne flachgeschliffenen Kanüle verbunden und ein Bakterienfilter aufgesetzt. Über diesen Bakterienfilter injiziert man dann 5 ml 0,5%-iges Bupivacain als Testdosis, von denen ca. 3 ml, entsprechend 15 mg, im Periduralraum ankommen.

Läge der Katheter versehentlich subdural, also im Liquorraum, so würde diese Menge sicher ausreichen, um innerhalb von 5 Minuten eine Spinalanästhesie anzuzeigen.

Während dieser Wartezeit wird die Punktionsstelle mit sterilen Platten abgedeckt, der Katheter nach cranial über die Schulter geführt und mit Pflaster fixiert. Um eine Dekonnektion zwischen Katheter, Nadel und Bakterienfilter zu verhindern, werden diese Teile auf einem Mundspatel befestigt.

Dosierung

Nachdem man sich mit der Testdosis davon überzeugt hat, daß der Katheter nicht versehentlich subdural liegt (Gefahr der totalen Spinalanästhesie), erhält der Patient initial 8 ml 0,125%-iges Bupivacain. Danach werden im Mittel 6 ml/Std 0,125%-iges Bupivacain kontinuierlich von einer Motorspritze injiziert. Im allgemeinen erreicht man damit eine ausreichende Analgesie für etwa 14 Stunden. Danach wird eine weitere Bolus-Injektion von 8 ml 0,125%-iges Bupivacain und eine Erhöhung der kontinuierlich verabreichten Lokalanästhetika-Menge auf 11 ml/Std notwendig sein.

Sollte nach ca. 14 Stunden wegen der inzwischen eingetretenen Tachyphylaxie eine 2. Repetitionsdosis erforderlich werden, so empfiehlt sich eine Bolus-Injektion von 8 ml 0,25%-igem Bupivacain und eine kontinuierliche Verabreichung von 6 ml/Std einer 0,25%-igen Lösung; nach weiteren 10-12 Stunden wird im allgemeinen eine Erhöhung der Zufuhr auf 12 ml/Std notwendig werden.

Insgesamt überbrückt man mit diesem Dosierungsschema einen postoperativen Zeitraum von 2 Tagen.

Einstichhöhe

Die Höhe der Einstichstelle richtet sich danach, welches Dermatom (Headsche Zone) im Zentrum des zu anästhesierenden Bezirks liegen soll. Dabei ist allerdings zu berücksichtigen, daß die Katheterspitze ein Segment oberhalb der Einstichstelle liegt. Für Oberbaucheingriffe genügt deshalb als Punktionsstelle Th 8-10, für Mittelbaucheingriffe Th 10-12 und für Unterbauch und Extremitäteneingriffe Th 12-L 4.

Vorsichtsmaßnahmen

1. Die Regeln der Asepsis beim Legen des Katheters, bei Nachinjektionen und beim Wechseln von Spritzen sind streng einzuhalten.
2. Nach jeder Bolus-Injektion werden Kreislauf und Atmung für 20 Minuten überwacht.
3. Ein- bis zweimal täglich werden die motorischen Funktionen kontrolliert zum Ausschluß einer unnötigerweise zu hohen Dosierung oder einer zwischenzeitlich aufgetretenen Nervenkompression durch ein peridurales Hämatom.
4. Alle Maßnahmen werden zeitgerecht in einem Protokoll vermerkt.

Indikationen

- Respiratorische Risikopatienten,
- kardiovaskuläre Risikopatienten,
- Eingriffe mit hohem postoperativem Schmerzmittelverbrauch,
- Gefäßeingriffe.

Kontraindikationen

- Lokale Infekte; Sepsis,
- Rückenmarkserkrankungen,
- Gerinnungsstörungen (Quick-Wert unter 50%). Eine prophylaktische Heparinisierung darf erst nach Legen des Periduralkatheters eingeleitet werden.

Literatur

1. Bromage PR (1967) Physiology and pharmacology of epidural anesthesia. Anesthesiology 28:592
2. Meridies R, Siepmann H, Maar K (1977) Schmerzbekämpfung nach retroperitonealer Lymphadenektomie mit Hilfe der kontinuierlichen Epiduralanalgesie. Urologe [A] 16.219
3. Sandmann W, Kremer K, Wüst HJ, Florack G, Ruf S (1977) Funktionskontrolle von rekonstruierten Arterien durch postoperative elektromagnetische Strömungsmessung. Thoraxchir Vask Chir 25:427
4. Wüst HJ, Sandmann W, Florack G, Lennartz H (1976) Kreislaufveränderungen während und nach aortofemoralen Bypass-Operationen unter kontinuierlicher Epiduralanästhesie. Langenbecks Arch Chir 342:594
5. Wüst HJ, Sandmann W, Richter O (to be published) Effect of neuroleptanaesthesia on haemodynamics and postoperative respiratory function in patients undergoing minor and major vascular surgery. Proc R Soc Med

Diskussion

Frage: Legen Sie einen Patienten mit einem Periduralkatheter auf eine Allgemeinstation oder behalten Sie ihn auf der Wachstation?

Zweite Frage: Ist Ihnen ein solcher Katheter schon einmal abgerissen und wenn ja, wie haben Sie sich dann verhalten?

Siepmann: Unsere Patienten kommen in der Regel auf die Normalstation. Allerdings muß man dazu sagen, daß die Schwestern und die Chirurgen dort mit der Methode vertraut sind.

Zur zweiten Frage: Es ist zu zwei derartigen Abrissen gekommen, und zwar schert der Katheter dann ab, wenn man versucht, den nicht ausreichend weit vorgeschobenen Katheter wieder zurückzuziehen und ihn dann noch einmal – in einer vielleicht etwas günstigeren Position der Tuohy-Nadel – vorzuschieben. Bei dieser Manipulation schert dann der Katheter an der relativ scharfen Kante der Nadelöffnung ab. Ist diese Komplikation eingetreten, konsultieren wir unsere Neurochirurgen, die bisher immer von einem Eingriff abrieten mit der Bemerkung, daß sie bei ihren Operationen viel mehr Nahtmaterial zurücklassen als es einer kurzen Katheterspitze entspricht.

Frage: Ich möchte doch davor warnen, sich auf die Testdosis zu verlassen. Mir sind zwei Fälle bekannt, wo nach der Testdosis die Hauptdosis gegeben wurde und eine totale Spinalanaesthesie auftrat. Wir geben grundsätzlich keine Testdosis und ich meine, man sollte das auch künftig bei Gutachten durchaus berücksichtigen. Hier wird viel zu viel Wert auf diese Testdosis gelegt. Bromage gibt grundsätzlich keine Testdosis, das sollte man einmal bedenken.

Siepmann: Ich bin Ihnen dankbar für diesen Hinweis. Wie so oft in der Medizin gibt es natürlich keine absolute Sicherheit. Trotzdem werden wir nicht auf diese Testdosis verzichten wollen. Allerdings muß man genug geben; das sind 15-20 mg Bupivacain! Nur wenn man eine Menge verabreicht, die sicher für eine Spinalanaesthesie ausreichen würde, kann man von einer Testdosis sprechen. Sie haben jedoch recht, wenn Sie betonen, daß sich der Arzt trotz des negativen Tests nicht in einem falschen Sicherheitsgefühl wiegen darf.

Frage: Meine Frage zielt auf die Thromboseprophylaxe. Wie lange lassen Sie die Katheter liegen? Dürfen die Patienten bald schon wieder aufstehen?

Siepmann: Die Katheter bleiben in der Regel zwischen 2-4 Tage liegen. Aber schon am nächsten Tag können die Patienten mit einem Katheter aufstehen.

Frage: Meine Frage betrifft den Filter. Es wurde vor einigen Monaten in der Zeitschrift „Anesthesiology" publiziert, daß die Filter gar nichts nützen. Hat sich die Meinung hierzu geändert, oder soll man ein schlechtes Gewissen haben, wenn man keinen Filter verwendet?

Siepmann: Wir haben selbst nicht untersucht, ob diese Filter notwendig sind. Bei uns sind sie eingeführt und werden benutzt. Schließlich schaden sie dem Patienten nicht, und wenn sich in Zukunft ihr Nutzen doch herausstellen sollte, dann umso besser! Außerdem gibt es noch den Gesichtspunkt der forensischen Absicherung für den Fall, daß es einmal zu einer Infektion kommt und man beweisen muß, daß man alle möglichen Vorsichtsmaßnahmen ergriffen hat.

Frage: Wie verhält es sich mit dem Blasenkatheter? Muß man einen Blasenkatheter so lange liegen lassen, wie die Periduralanaesthesie läuft?

Siepmann: Nein, man muß nicht. Es gibt gelegentlich Blasenentleerungsstörungen, u.a. weil der Patient den Füllungszustand der Blase nicht mehr wahrnimmt. Daneben können noch echte Innervationsstörungen vorkommen, die dann ebenfalls eine einmalige oder auch wiederholte Katheterisierung notwendig machen.

Pathophysiology of Postoperative Pulmonary Complications

H. Pontoppidan

Introduction

The general architecture and physiology of the normal lung including the large and small airways, vasculature, innervation, lymphatic drainage, and basic blood gas exchange functions are assumed to be familiar to most participants. In the following sections particular attention will be directed to those structural and physiological changes which seem principally altered in postoperative respiratory complications and in the "Adult respiratory distress syndrome" (ARDS). For a review of those aspects of normal pulmonary structure and functions which will not be covered, the recent book by Murray [7] is recommended.

Despite major advances over the past decade in the understanding of the pathophysiology and treatment of acute lung disease, pulmonary complications remain the most common cause of postoperative morbidity and mortality [1, 8, 9]. Many factors may be responsible for this continued high frequency; the most probable are the steady increase in both age and sickness in our surgical patient population with the associated greater hazard of pulmonary complications occurring intra- and postoperatively. It is also now recognized that non-pulmonary medical and surgical complications, most notably septicemia, is associated with a high incidence of secondary acute lung injury and may in fact initially present with pulmonary manifestations, e.g., hypoxemia, tachypnea and hypocapnia [9].

The mortality from advanced respiratory failure has been found to be higher than generally realized. This is well illustrated in an 18-month study of acute respiratory failure sponsored by the National Heart, Lung and Blood Institute (NHLBI) [17]. In this collaborative study at 9 medical centers in the United States of America, 680 patients of 12 years and older requiring, [1] intubation, [2] mechanical ventilation for 24 h or more, and [3] an inspired oxygen concentration of 50% or more, were the subject of detailed data collection for a 3-week period beginning from 2 days prior to tracheal intubation. The mortality rate in patients having respiratory failure only (and no non-pulmonary complications) was 41%, and rose to between 75% and 100% in patients where complications from other non-pulmonary organ systems were present either on admission to the study or subsequently developed.

This study emphasizes that until we learn more about the mechanisms of pulmonary injury and respiratory failure it is essential that physicians, nurses and respiratory therapy personnel be aware of the factors which promote pulmonary complications and/or secondary lung injury in order to pay scrupulous attention to their prevention, early detection, and prompt treatment. Unnecessary delay in diagnosis and treatment may add to the damage owing to the need for high inspired oxygen concentrations, large tidal volumes, and high airway pressures necessary to achieve adequate gas exchange.

Generally, the pathophysiological and morphological manifestations of acute respiratory failure are lung-specific and not disease- or injury-specific [6]. The pathophysiological hallmarks, detectable by bedside pulmonary function and hemodynamic studies, are [1] diminished lung volume, [2] reduction in dynamic and static compliance causing an increased work in breathing, and [3] derangement of the normal distribution of ventilation perfusion ratios, with resultant increase in right-to-left interpulmonary shunting ($\dot{Q}_S/\dot{Q}_T$), alveolar-arterial oxygen tension difference ($AaDO_2$), and dead space to tidal volume ratio (V_D/V_T) [8]. In patients with severe respiratory failure these changes in lung volume, mechanics and blood gas exchange are accompanied by [4] an increase in the pulmonary vascular resistance [9, 14, 15]. However in patients with the most common variety of postoperative lung complications, such as atelectasis and pulmonary edema (in the absence of microcirculatory leakage) and in early stages of ARDS, pulmonary vascular resistance is usually normal [9].

Classification of Postoperative Lung Complications

The description of pulmonary pathophysiology is facilitated by examining changes as they develop within alveoli and small airways, in the alveolar wall itself, the pulmonary circulation and in the interstitial space. This morphological classification is employed primarily for didactic reasons; it does not imply that distinct anatomic features can be documented in all cases. Organization of effective preventive and therapeutic programs are facilitated by the recognition that most surgical patients with acute lung disease fall into broad categories: [1] Those with "classical" non-ARDS, postoperative lung complications (by far the largest population), and [2] the smaller category of "capillary leak" or "diffuse alveolar-capillary injury syndromes" commonly referred to as "adult respiratory distress syndrome" (ARDS).

While clinical and physiological manifestations are well defined in man, their anatomic basis has largely been arrived at by study of animal models of human lung injury and disease. There is no agreement on how faithfully these models mimic mechanisms, morphologic features, and pathophysiology of human ARF [6]. Within the last few years open lung biopsy has been performed with increasing frequency in patients with severe ARF and has yielded much information on this type of lung injury [4, 15]. However with few exceptions we must rely on autopsy observations in patients dying of or with advanced ARF.

The "Common" Typical Postoperative Lung Complications

These complications are characterized by preservation of basic pulmonary architecture. As a rule changes are preventable and reversible provided effective treatment is instituted early.
Atelectasis and Airway Closure. The fundamental changes manifest at the level of the large and small airways and the gas exchanging units they supply [8]. Apart from the recognition of small airway closure as an important predisposing event, little has been added to the concept of atelectasis since it was first developed 20 or 30 years ago [1, 8]. Segmental or lobar collapse secondary to partial or complete obstruction of a major airway is readily diagnosed on the chest roentgenogram. In contrast, diffuse airspace collapse is usually a presumptive diagnosis in a patient who presents evidence of impaired oxygenation, clear lung fields, and a variable degree of reduction in lung volumes (provided positive end-expiratory pressure is not in use). Although often referred to as "diffuse" it is a regional phenomenon confined to dependent lung regions where lung volumes are smaller and therefore the tendency to small airway closure greater. This propensity for dependent small airway closure and alveolar collapse is especially prominent during mechanical ventilation where most of the inspired volume is distributed to the non-dependent regions of the lung; whereas during spontaneous ventilation the tidal volume is preferentially distributed to the dependent lung regions [10]. The accumulation of interstitial lung water also promotes small airway closure and atelectasis [12]. Since both hypoventilation and interstitial pulmonary edema accumulation have a predilection for

dependent lung regions, it is clear that pre- and postoperative physical therapy including frequent changes in posture are the most important preventive and therapeutic measures. Adjunctive therapy such as intermittent positive pressure breathing, incentive spirometry, and short-term or long-term use of continuous positive airway pressure (CPAP) administered with a face mask or via an endotracheal tube, are in common use. At the present time it would seem that the most promising and physiological techniques are incentive spirometry and continuous positive airway pressure. Adequate postoperative pain relief is, of coûrse, essential. Use of regional techniques for intra- and postoperative analgesia have a major role in management of postoperative pain following abdominal and thoracic surgery.

Influence of Inspired Oxygen Concentration (F_IO_2). It has been postulated that even mild-moderate degrees of ARF are associated with the presence of gas exchanging units having very low but finite ventilation/perfusion ratios, in the range of 0.05-0.1 [9, 12, 13]. In such units minimal amounts of fresh gas enter with each breath and presumably only at or near the peak of transpulmonary pressure and inspiratory volume. The rise in $AaDO_2$ and $\dot{Q}_S/\dot{Q}_T$ observed in patients following breathing of 100% oxygen may in part result from absorption atelectasis [12, 13]. Airspace collapse will occur if the amount of oxygen entering the alveoli per min is too small to replenish that taken up by the mixed venous blood. Some protection against absorption atelectasis is offered by the presence of an inert gas, which is not taken up in the pulmonary capilliaries. Prevention and therapy of atelectasis must not only incorporate measures aimed at maintaining normal lung volumes, but also use of F_IO_2 ranges which delay onset of atelectasis in low $\dot{V}/\dot{Q}$ units, supplied by partially or completely obstructed airways.

Pulmonary Edema. In the absence of microvascular injury causing an increased permeability to plasma protein and red cells, pulmonary edema can be assumed to have a hemodynamic basis and be present when the amount of fluid filtered across the microvascular bed exceeds the drainage capacity of the pulmonary lymphatics. This type of pulmonary edema is most often caused by fluid overload, with or without a detectable increase in left atrial and pulmonary vascular pressures. As mentioned above, gravity promotes accumulation of lung water in the lower lung regions. This mechanism presumably accounts for the "down-lung syndrome" used to describe the intra- and postoperative occurrence of pulmonary edema in the dependent lung, be it secondary to hypoventilation and/or fluid overload. Prevention consists of careful fluid replacement, maintenance of adequate functional residual capacity and ventilation of the dependent lung (including use of PEEP), and frequent change of posture (if possible) to prevent prolonged dependency of the same lung regions.

Derangement of Pulmonary Defense Mechanisms. Many factors in the pre-, intra- and postoperative phase may interfere with adequate pulmonary defenses. Anesthetic drugs, hypoxia, hyperoxia, prolonged administration of dry gases, and presence of an endotracheal tube impair ciliary function and mucus transport. Inadequate coughing follows pharmacologic depression of the cough reflex, pain, splinting, abdominal muscle weakness or instability of the chest wall. Appropriate use of regional analgesia techniques in conjunction with chest physical therapy will lead to improved coughing. Pulmonary macrophage function may transiently be impaired by the action of anesthetic drugs, narcotics, and hyperoxia.

Colloid Osmotic Pressure and Pulmonary Edema. It is commonly assumed that a decline in plasma colloid osmotic pressure (PCOP) and/or in the difference between PCOP and pulmonary artery wedge pressure (PAWP) are important determinants of pulmonary edema formation. However, several recent studies have failed to document a causal relationship of pulmonary edema and a reduction in PCOP and the PCOP to PAWP gradient. Furthermore, use of deliberate hemodilution with associated large decreases in PCOP has not been shown to result in clinically detectable pulmonary edema. These observations probably pertain to both the intact and the injured pulmonary vascular bed and would lead to the conclusion that extensive use of albumin or plasma fractions for the purpose of raising PCOP is of no value, or may on occasion be harmful, as preventive or therapeutic measures in pulmonary edema. Regardless of the integrity of the small vessels walls (50-200 micron diameter), the most important, and probably the only determinants of the balance of pulmonary extra-vascular fluid is the transmural hydrostatic pressure within these vessels. (It has recently been demonstrated that capillaries only account for part of fluid movement. As much as one-half may leave the vascular bed via walls of small extra-alveolar arteries and veins.) [3]

In summary, the "classical," common postoperative pulmonary complications involve pathophysiological and morphological changes which usually are preventable and reversible with adequate prophylactic and therapeutic measures. If undetected and untreated they may progress to severe acute respiratory failure and cause a marked increase in mortality.

Acute Alveolar-Capillary Lung Injury, the ARDS Syndrome

The ARDS syndrome differs from the pulmonary complications described above by being rarely preventable, and by causing far more profound changes in pulmonary morphology and physiology. Severe derangement of basic pulmonary architecture is a characteristic feature in more advanced stages of disease. Depending on etiology, the mortality ranges from 40%-75% for patients with extensive disease meeting the NHLBI criteria for entry in the NHLBI Randomized, Controlled Study of ECMO [17].

As discussed earlier most of the data on pathophysiologic and morphologic changes in the ARDS syndrome are based on animal models mimicking the syndrome in man. More extensive investigations, focusing on the etiological role of coagulopathies, studies of pulmonary metabolic and other nonventilatory functions, greater use of open lung biopsy, and careful morphometric examination of biopsy and autopsy material will be necessary to elucidate the mechanisms of lung injury in human ARDS [6]. At present most evidence favors the concept that the injury is "lung specific" and not disease specific, since there are few distinct physiological and morphological changes which characterize patients with ARDS of diverse etiologies.

Numerous conditions may produce the ARDS syndrome as shown in Table 1. Many are apt to occur in the surgical setting.

Changes in Early ARDS (Hours to days)

Vasculature. Several recent studies of pulmonary hemodynamics in early ARDS have failed to demonstrate an elevated pulmonary vascular resistance within 24 h of injury [9]. However, with progression of time most patients develop a fixed pulmonary artery hypertension (PAH) (usually defined as a mean pulmonary artery pressure exceeding 20 mmHg). Pulmonary vascular resistance (PVR) is two to three times normal and there is an inverse relationship of PVR and cardiac index [9, 14]. Therefore, sequential measurements of PVR must be referred to a specific cardiac index or a PVR cardiac index curve constructed before changes in PVR can be interpreted as representing true changes in the status of pulmonary circulation.

Biopsies from patients within one week following injury show considerable venous and capillary congestion, endothelial cell death and frequent thrombi in small arterioles [2, 4]. Following trauma or amniotic fluid embolization intravascular marrow elements or components derived from the amniotic fluid may be observed. (R. Trelstad, . . . , personal communication).

Table 1. Conditions Associated with ARDS and Microvascular Plasma Leak

Severe trauma
Fat Embolization
Endotoxemia
Aspiration Pneumonia
Smoke or gas inhalation
Surface burns
Long-chain hydrocarbon ingestion
Drug overdose, heroin
Neurogenic pulmonary edema
Viral, mycoplasma, bacterial pneumonia
Legionnaire's disease
Acute vasculitis
Goodpasture's syndrome
Anaphylactic reaction to drugs and blood
Radiation
Immunosuppression
Oxygen toxicity

Interstitial and vascular wall edema, reflex vasoconstriction, or release of mediators, e.g., arachidonic acid and its derivatives may account for the elevated PVR in early ARDS. Use of vasodilators (isoproterenol, nitroprusside, alpha blockade) has failed to alter the course of PAH in ARDS suggesting that vascular smooth muscle contraction may not be an important factor [9]. Pulmonary microthrombosis and small vessel emboli are commonly observed in human lung biopsy and autopsy material, but whether in man it is a primary pathogenetic event, as commonly assumed [2, 11], or a secondary phenomenon following acute lung injury remains to be established. There is no well documented effective treatment of the pulmonary microthrombosis/emboli syndrome.

Alveolar Lining and Alveolar Space. Hyaline membranes form readily within the first few days of injury and are a consistent finding within 3-4 days following onset of ARF. Hyaline membranes consist of necrotic alveolar lining cells, probably principially the Type I alveolar epithelial cell, the principal lining cell of the alveolar space. This cell is highly vulnerable to injury and is incapable of reproduction. Dead Type I cells are replaced by hyperplasia of the Type II epithelial cell, which is thought to be the progenitor of the Type I cell. Hyaline membranes also include coagulated intra-alveolar proteins derived from the exudate which may flood the intra-alveolar airspace following loss of vascular and alveolar wall integrity.

Interstitium. Swelling and edema of the interstitial space in both the distal airway and in lobular septy is a universal early feature. Perivascular and peribronchial hemorrhage is also present, implying a major loss of vascular functional integrity. By the end of the first week following injury the fibroblasts in the interstitium reveal cytological features consistent with an activated secretory cell with a large increase, e.g., in amount of endoplasmic reticulum. Inflammatory cells are not a characteristic feature in most cases of early ARDS. Macrophages are commonly present.

In summary, the major changes occurring during the first few days of lung injury in ARDS are intra-alveolar and interstitial edema and hemorrhage, necrosis of the alveolar lining epithelium, and appearance of microthrombi in the small vessels. The changes at this time do not suggest substantial alterations in the underlying architecture of the lung. The basic normal pattern of alveolar spaces and interstitial matrix has been retained. (R. Trelstad, . . . , personal communication). Reversibility of morphologic changes in this early stage would seem likely were effective therapeutic measures available.

Late Changes in ARDS (Days to Weeks)

Vasculature. There are now readily identifiable thrombi in small and medium sized arteries. Intact megakaryocytes may be prominent in small vessels. Postmortem perfusion studies show substantial obliteration of the normal alveolar capillary network [16]. Endothelial cell necrosis is commonly observed but neovascularization is not readily detected.

At this stage PAH is usually more pronounced, with mean pressures frequently exceeding 30-40 mmHg. The PVR is often elevated more than threefold and evidence of right ventricular dysfunction, with a decrease in right ventricular ejection fraction and an increase in right ventricular end-diastolic volume, has recently been observed in several patients with severe advanced ARDS [9]. Unfortunately, no therapy has proven effective in reversing these profound pulmonary vascular changes.

Alveolar Lining and Alveolar Space. The alveolar lining now features multilayered cuboidal epithelium, representing vigorous hyperplasia of Type II epithelial cells and presumably reflecting regenerative efforts by the alveolar lining. Accumulation of plump Type II cells in conjunction with intra-alveolar hyaline membranes cause a marked interference with the normal ventilation/perfusion relationships and blood gas exchange. This is further aggravated as the disease process advances and intra-alveolar fibrosis with production of an obliterative matrix becomes a consistent finding.

Interstitium. Light and electron microscopy show a substantial increase in connective tissue matrix particularly in respect to fibrillar collagen. These changes can also be confirmed by biochemical analysis of total lung collagen content, which in some cases may increase to two or threefold of normal. Concomitant increase in total lung mass is generally apparent. In addition to the extensive interstitial fibrosis there appears to be a change in the character of the interstitial matrix in that elastic tissue, as detected by routine light microscopic methods, is diminished. The overall alveolar architecture is severely disrupted and it seems likely that turnover or degradation of matrix components go hand in hand with substantial deposition of new matrix. (R. Trelstad, . . . , personal communication). These changes of the matrix turnover have a profound effect on the architecture of the gas exchanging units and it is questionable whether such changes are reversible.

Although pulmonary morphologic changes are frequently described as being diffuse, they have, in fact, a distinct focal distribution with areas of relatively well preserved lung interspersed between areas of profound destruction of normal architecture. Such nonuniform disease distribution presumably has profound effects on the distribution of ventilation and blood flow. The conventional description of distribution of ventilation and perfusion relationships in three relatively distinct geographic zones may no longer be pertinent. Instead, numerous "minizones" may be present throughout the lungs. At this stage of illness optimal therapy of the profound derangement of blood gas exchange and pulmonary mechanics is disputed. The role of conventional controlled mechanical ventilation with moderate end-expiratory pressures, versus use of intermittent mandatory ventilation with extremely high levels of end-expiratory pressure, or extracorporeal membrane oxygenation still needs definition [9]. However, unless the overwhelming changes in normal morphology and basic architecture can be modified by therapy, it is unlikely that manipulation of mechanical ventilation patterns or temporary pulmonary bypass will reverse the inexorable progression of disease.

Summary

Pulmonary complications remain the most important cause of increased morbidity following major abdominal or thoracic surgery and trauma. Small airway closure, atelectasis, impaired pulmonary defenses, and hemodynamic pulmonary edema are common features of "classical" postoperative complications. Response to preventive and therapeutic measures with return to normal lung function are the rule. In contrast, the ARDS syndrome which may develop as a primary or secondary complication of surgery and trauma is not readily preventable, lung pathology is poorly reversible and the mortality rate is high – probably exceeding 50%. Profound changes of basic lung architecture and function are the rule and affect the alveolar space, the alveolar-capillary membrane, the vasculature and the interstitial matrix. The precise mechanism of progressive lung destruction in the ARDS syndrome is unknown and therapy remains largely symptomatic.

References

1. Bendixen HH, Egbert LD, Hedley-Whyte J, Laver MB, Pontoppidan H (1965) Respiratory care. Mosby, St. Louis
2. Blaisdell FW, Lewis FR Jr (1977) Respiratory distress syndrome of shock and trauma. Major Probl Clin Surg 21:
3. Butler J, Culver BH, Huseby J, Albert R (1977) The hemodynamics of pulmonary edema. Am Rev Respir Dis 115:173
4. Hill JD, Ratliff JL, Parrott JCW, et al (1976) Pulmonary pathology in acute respiratory insufficiency: Lung biopsy as a diagnostic tool. J Thorac Cardiovasc Surg 71:64
5. Jardin F, Delille F, Gurjian F, Blanchet F, Margairaz A (1977) Hemodynamic profile in acute respiratory distress syndromes in the adult. Nouv Presse Med 37:3401
6. Murray JF (1977) Conference report: Mechanisms of Acute Respiratory Failure. National Heart, Lung and Blood Inst. Am Rev Respir Dis 115:1071
7. Murray JR (1976) "The normal lung". Saunders, Philadelphia
8. Pontoppidan H, Geffin B, Lowenstein E (1973) Acute respiratory failure in the adult. Brown, Boston
9. Pontoppidan H, Wilson RS, Rie M, Schneider RC (1977) Respiratory intensive care. Anesthesiology 47:96
10. Rehder K, Sessler AD, Marsh HC (1975) State of the art; general anesthesia and the lung. Am Rev Respir Dis 112:541
11. Saldeen T (1976) The microembolism syndrome. Microvasc Res 11:227
12. West J (1977) Pulmonary Pathophysiology: The Essentials. Williams & Wilkins, Baltimore
13. Wilson RS, Pntoppidan H (1974) Acute respiratory failure: Diagnostic and therapeutic criteria. Crit Care Med
14. Zapol WM, Snider MT (1977) Pulmonary hypertension in severe acute respiratory failure. N Engl J Med 296:476
15. Zapol WM, Snider MT, Schneider RC, Rie MA (1976) Pulmonary hypertension in severe acute respiratory failure. In: Zapol WM, Qvist J (eds) Artificial lungs for acute respiratory failure. Hemispehre Publishing, Washington D.C., p 435
16. Zapol WM, Kobayashi K, Snider MT, et al (1977) Vascular obstruction causes pulmonary hypertension in severe acute respiratory failure. Chest 71:306
17. Final Report of the National Heart, Lung, and Blood Institute (to be published) Collaborative Study entitled "Extracorporeal Support for Respiratory Insufficiency"

Intra- und postoperative kardiopulmonale Komplikationen bei transurethralen Prostataresektionen in Intubationsnarkose und rückenmarksnaher Leitungsanästhesie

W. Tolksdorf, G. Raiss, J.-P. Striebel und H. Lutz

Einleitung

Kardiopulmonale Komplikationen sind die häufigsten intra- und postoperativen Todesursachen beim geriatrischen Patienten [9, 18, 21]. Dies gilt auch für urologische Patienten, die sich einer transurethralen Prostataresektion unterziehen müssen.

Bandhauer u. Madersbacher [3] konnten anhand eines Krankengutes von 1 444 Patienten zeigen, daß über 40% der aufgetretenen Todesfälle nach TUR der Prostata auf kardiopulmonale Komplikationen zurückzuführen waren.

Da die Meinungen noch immer geteilt sind, wenn um die Frage „Allgemeinanästhesie oder rückenmarksnahe Leitungsanästhesie beim alten und damit meist Risikopatienten" diskutiert wird, versuchten wir, anhand eines ausgesprochen geriatrischen Krankengutes – Patienten, die sich einer transurethralen Prostataresektion unterziehen mußten – einer Lösung dieses Problems näher zu kommen. Aus Gründen der Standardisierung führten wir unsere Studie bei nur einem Operationsverfahren durch. Wir sind dennoch der Meinung, anhand unserer Untersuchung Aussagen über die Auswahl des Anästhesieverfahrens beim geriatrischen Patienten allgemein machen zu können.

Dem Hauptargument für die Anwendung rückenmarksnaher Leitungsanästhesien bei TUR der Prostata, der Früherkennung operationsspezifischer Komplikationen [3, 11, 12] soll in dieser Arbeit weniger Beachtung geschenkt werden, dagegen muß auf die Einschwemmung von Spülfküssigkeit in den Patientenkreislauf durch eröffnete periprostatische Venensinus, einer nahezu obligaten Komplikation dieses Operationsverfahrens, aufgrund seiner eminenten Bedeutung für die kardiopulmonale Funktionen eingegangen werden.

Material und Methode

Die Studie wurde in einem Zeitraum von 9 Monaten bei 78 Patienten durchgeführt, wobei die Zuordnung zu den Verfahren der Allgemeinanästhesie und den rückenmarksnahen Leitungsanästhesien nach einem zuvor festgelegten Randomisierungsplan zufällig erfolgte.

36 Patienten mit einem Altersmedian von 70 Jahren erhielten eine Allgemeinanästhesie, 42 Patienten mit einem Median von 72 Jahren eine Regionalanästhesie, davon 12 eine Spinal- und 30 eine Periduralanästhesie. Die beiden Gruppen unterschieden sich weder im Alter noch hinsichtlich ihrer Vorerkrankungen und präoperativ erhobenen laborchemischen Befunden (Tabelle 1). Anhand der in unserem Institut verwendeten Risiko-Checkliste mußten wir die Patienten in die Risikogruppen III-V einordnen, nach der ASA-Risikonomenklatur in die Risikogruppen II-IV. Alle 78 Patienten wurden aus Gründen der Standardisierung lediglich mit 0,5 mg Atropin i.m. prämediziert.

Die Allgemeinanästhesie wurde als sog. modifizierte Neuroleptanalgesie durchgeführt (Tabelle 2): Nach Gabe von 2 ml Alloferin verwendeten wir zur Narkoseeinleitung Diazepam, Flunitrazepam, Etomidate oder Thiopental, wobei wegen unzureichender Einschlafwirkung der beiden Benzodiazepine in einigen Fällen die zusätzlichen Gaben von Thiopental in geringer

Tabelle 1. Anamnestisch erhobene Vorerkrankungen, Laborchemische Parameter, mittleres Lebensalter und Altersmedian

Praeoperative Befunde	Anaesthesieverfahren		Statistik
	JTN	RA	
1. Anamnese (+ EKG + Rö Thorax)	n = 36	n = 42	
a) Herz-Kreislauf-Gefäßsyst.			
Herzinfarkt i.d.A. > 2 J	17%	7%	∅
Rekomp. Herzinsuff. + Rhythmusstrgn.	86%	86%	∅
Hypertonus	39%	33%	∅
Gefäßerkr.	28%	24%	∅
b) Bronchopulm. Vorerkr.			
vorw. obstruktiv	22%	21%	∅
vorw. restriktiv	67%	57%	∅
c) Lebererkr.	17%	10%	∅
d) Nierenerkr.	25%	17%	∅
e) Diabetes mell.	17%	24%	∅
f) Allergien	3%	2%	∅
g) Erkrgn. ZNS + Psyche	8%	5%	∅
2. Laborchemische Param.			
Hb:	14,0 ± 2,0	14,0 ± 1,8	∅
Hkt:	40 ± 6	41 ± 5	∅
Na	141 ± 8	143 ± 6	∅
K:	4,4 ± 0,2	4,2 ± 0,5	∅
Ges. Ew.	67 ± 6	66 ± 8	∅
3. Alter			
MW.	68,2 J	71,6 J	∅
Median	70 J	72 J	∅

Dosierung notwendig war. Nach Relaxation mit Succinylcholin und Intubation wurde die Anästhesie mit Fentanyl bzw. Fentanyl und Droperidol unterhalten. Die Beatmung erfolgte im halbgeschlossenen Kreissystem mit einem Lachgas-Sauerstoff-Gemisch im Verhältnis 2:1 bis 1:1. Die weitere Relaxation erfolgte mit Alloferin. Alle Patienten wurden vor Ausleitung der Narkose mit Levallorfan, Pyridostigmin und Atropin antagonisiert und konnten nach Extubation ausreichend wach und spontan atmend in den Aufwachraum verbracht werden.

Die Spinalanästhesie, ebenso wie die Periduralanästhesie, legten wir in Höhe L 3 bis L 5 an, wobei 2 ml Mepivacain 4%ig hyperbar bzw. Bupivacain 0,5%ig mit oder ohne CO_2 als Lokalanästhetika zur Anwendung kamen.

Tabelle 2. Angewendete Verfahren der Allgemeinanästhesie (ITN) (siehe Text)

Alloferin (2 mg) ↓	Succinylcholin (1 mg/kg KG) ↓	Alloferin (10-20)	Pyridostigmin 5-10 mg 1/2 im Atropin 0,5 mg 1(2 iv Levallorphan 1 mg iv ↓	n
		Intubation ↓	Extubation ↓	
Diazepam (15-20 mg)		Fentanyl (0,15-0,45 mg)		2
Diazepam (-15 mg) + Thiopental (1,5-3 mg/kg KG)		Fentanyl (0,15-0,35 mg)		3
Flunitrazepam (),8-1 mg)		Fentanyl (0-0,15 mg)		5
Flunitrazepam (0,6-0,8 mg) + Thiopental (1,5-3 mg/kg KG)		Fentanyl (0,1-0,5 mg)		11
Hypnomidate		Fentanyl (0,4-0,5 mg) + Droperidol (5-10 mg)		4
Thiopental (2,5-5 mg/kg KG)		Fentanyl (0,15-0,6 mg) + Droperidol (5-12,5 mg)		11

Alle weiteren Meßnahmen waren in beiden Gruppen standardisiert: Die Infusion von 500 ml Ringer-Lactat, 500 ml einer Halbelektrolytlösung, die Gabe von 2 g trans-AMCHA und 500.000 I.E. Trasylol zur Hyperfibrinolyseprophylaxe, sowie der Infusionszusatz von 40 mval Natriumchlorid zur Vermeidung des TUR-Syndroms.

Sowohl die Anästhesie als auch die Lungenfunktionsprüfung wurden von jeweils 1 Person durchgeführt.

Die Blutdruckmessung erfolgte nach Riva-Rocci, EKG und Herzfrequenz wurden kontinuierlich abgeleitet, der zentrale Venendruck über einen zentralen Venenkatheter in mindestens 10-minütigen Abständen mit einem Flüssigkeitsmanometer gemessen.

Die Spirometrie führten wir am Abend präoperativ, am Operationstag ungefähr 4-10 Stunden postoperativ und am Abend des 1. postoperativen Tages durch.

Als intraoperative Komplikationen von seiten des Kreislaufs sahen wir Hypotensionen mit einem Abfall des arteriellen Mitteldrucks um mehr als 30% vom Ausgangswert (Meßzeitpunkt 1) sowie Hypertensionen mit einem Anstieg des arteriellen Mitteldruckes um mehr als 30% vom Ausgangswert an. Als intraoperative Kreislaufkomplikation betrachteten wir ebenfalls Anstiege des zentralen Venendrucks um mehr als 12 cm H_2O [8]. Abb. 1 zeigt ein für eine transurethrale Prostataresektion typisches Narkoseprotokoll, in dem die kritischen Kreislaufphasen verdeutlicht werden können. Mit römischen Ziffern sind die von uns gewählten Meßzeitpunkte für Blutdruck, Puls und zentralen Venendruck gekennzeichnet:

Meßzeitpunkt I: Eintreffen im Operationssaal, Flachlagerung mit mäßig erhobenem Oberkörper.

Meßzeitpunkt II: Steinschnitt-Lage.

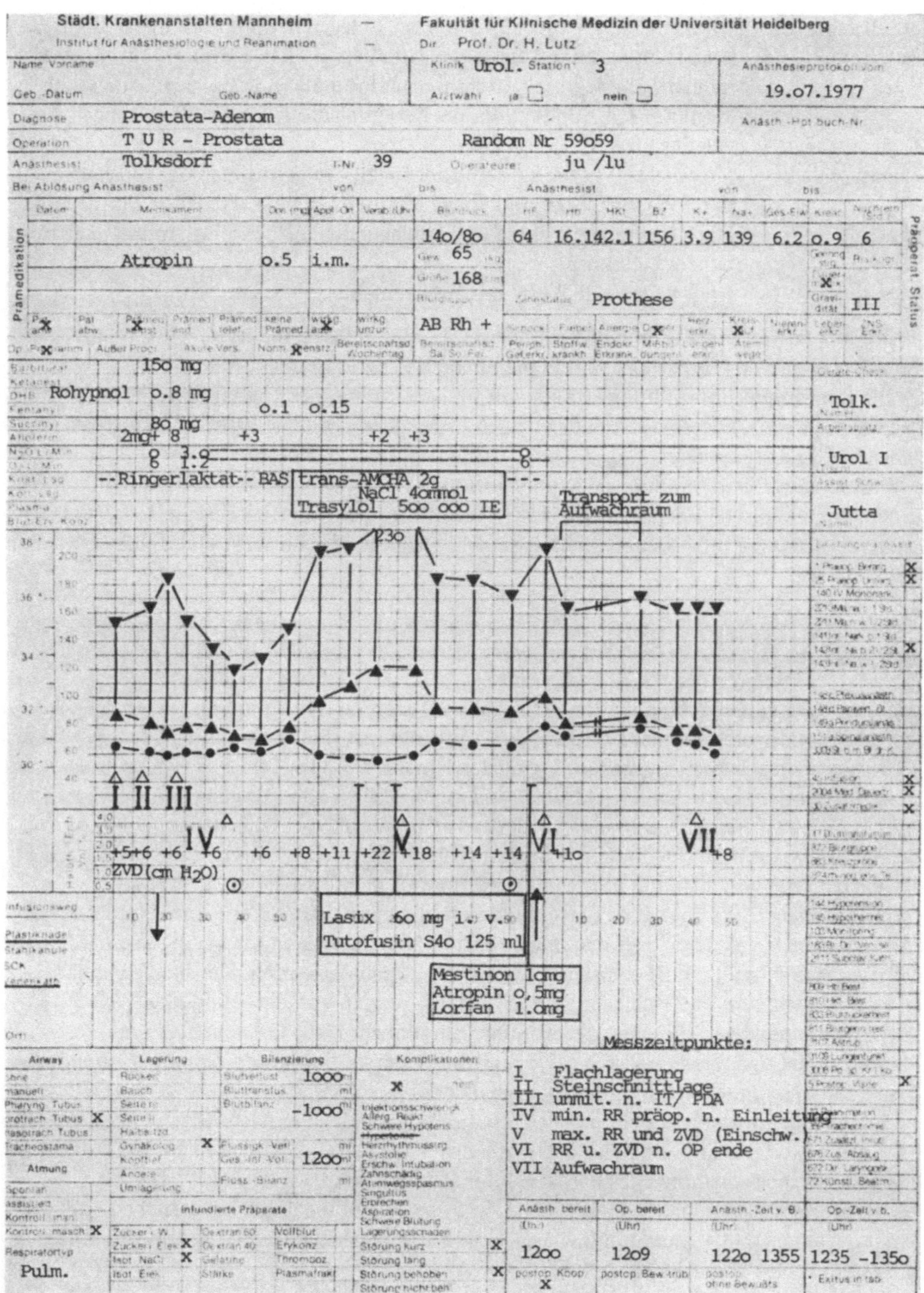

Städt. Krankenanstalten Mannheim – Fakultät für Klinische Medizin der Universität Heidelberg

Institut für Anästhesiologie und Reanimation – Dir. Prof. Dr. H. Lutz

Klinik Urol. Station 3

Anästhesieprotokoll vom 19.o7.1977

Diagnose: Prostata-Adenom

Operation: T U R - Prostata

Random Nr 59o59

Anästhesist: Tolksdorf

Operateure: ju /lu

Prämedikation: Atropin o.5 i.m.

140/80 64 16.1 42.1 156 3.9 139 6.2 o.9 6

Gew. 65

Größe 168

Prothese

AB Rh +

III

150 mg

Rohypnol o.8 mg

o.1 o.15

80 mg

2mg+ 8 +3 +2 +3

3.9

1.2

--Ringerlaktat-- BAS

trans-AMCHA 2g

NaCl 4ommol

Trasylol 5oo ooo IE

Transport zum Aufwachraum

230

Tolk.

Urol I

Jutta

I II III IV V VI VII

+5+6 +6 +6 +6 +8 +11 +22 +18 +14 +14 +1o +8

ZVD (cm H_2O)

Lasix 6o mg i. v.

Tutofusin S4o 125 ml

Mestinon 1mg

Atropin o,5mg

Lorfan 1.omg

Messzeitpunkte:

I Flachlagerung

II Steinschnittlage

III unmit. n. IT/ PDA

IV min. RR präop. n. Einleitung

V max. RR und ZVD (Einschw.)

VI RR u. ZVD n. OP ende

VII Aufwachraum

Airway – Lagerung – Bilanzierung – Komplikationen

Blutverlust 1ooo ml

Blutbilanz -1ooo ml

Ges.-Inf.-Vol. 12oo ml

Atmung

Infundierte Präparate

Respiratortyp: Pulm.

Anästh. bereit (Uhr) 12oo

Op. bereit (Uhr) 12o9

Anästh.-Zeit v. B. (Uhr) 122o 1355

Op.-Zeit v. b. (Uhr) 1235 -135o

Abb. 1. Narkoseprotekoll mit den für TUR-P. kritischen Kreislaufphasen. Meßzeitpunkte: siehe Text

Meßzeitpunkt III: Unmittelbar nach Intubation bzw. Anlegen der Regionalanästhesie.
Meßzeitpunkt IV: Tiefste Hypotension zu den anästhesietypischen Zeitpunkten: in Allgemeinanästhesie bis zu 10 min. nach Intubation, in Spinalanästhesie bis 10 min. nach Applikation, bei Periduralanästhesie bis 30 min. nach Anlegen der PDA.
Meßzeitpunkt V: Maximale Hypertension und zentraler Venendruck (in der Regel erreicht der ZVD sein Maximum einige Minuten vor dem arteriellen Blutdruck).
Meßzeitpunkt VI: Nach Narkoseausleitung und Umlagerung in Rückenlage mit mäßig erhobenem Oberkörper.
Meßzeitpunkt VII: Erste gemessene Werte im Aufwachraum.

Alle intraoperativen Kreislaufkomplikationen traten zu den Meßzeitpunkten IV (Hypotension) und Meßzeitpunkt V (Hypertension und maximale ZVD) auf.

Die Lungenfunktionsprüfung erfolgte mit dem elektronischen Digital-Spirometer SPIROTRON (Fa. Dräger). Dieses Gerät hat sich nach Untersuchungen von Klose et al. [13] als ausreichend zuverlässig erwiesen.

Postoperative kardiopulmonale Komplikationen während des Krankenhausaufenthaltes wurden durch klinische Untersuchung, EKG und Röntgenbildvergleich gesichert.

Als statistische Prüfverfahren dienten der Chi-Quadrat-Test für vier Feldertafeln sowie der Wilcoxon-Test.

Ergebnisse

Intraoperative Kreislaufkomplikationen (Tabelle 3): Hypotensionen mit einem Abfall des arteriellen Mitteldruckes um mehr als 30% vom Ausgangswert (Meßzeitpunkte II und IV) fanden sich in Allgemeinanästhesie 7 mal, in Regionalanästhesie nicht ($p \leqslant 0.05$). Hypertensionen mit einem Anstieg des arteriellen Mitteldruckes um mehr als 30% vom Ausgangswert (Meßzeitpunkt II und V) waren in Allgemeinanästhesie 6 mal und in Regionalanästhesie 2 mal zu verzeichnen. Keinen Unterschied fanden wir auch im Auftreten von Arrhythmien, welche wir in Allgemeinanästhesie 3 mal und in Regionalanästhesie 1 mal registrierten. Einen Anstieg des zentralen Venendrucks über 12 cm H_2O fand sich in Allgemeinanästhesie 7 mal, in Regionalanästhesie 3 mal ($p \leqslant 0.05$). Der maximale zentrale Venendruck wurde in Allgemeinanästhesie im Mittel nach 43 min., in Regionalanästhesie nach 33 min. gemessen. Kreislaufkomplikationen im Aufwachraum unterschieden sich in beiden Gruppen mit einer Häufigkeit von 3 bzw. 2 nicht. Intraoperative Störungen der Atmung konnten wir nicht feststellen.

Sowohl die Anästhesie als auch die Operationsdauer unterschieden sich mit 77 min. bzw. 84 min. und 63 min. bzw. 59 min. nicht voneinander.

Zu postoperativen kardiopulmonalen Komplikationen kam es nach Allgemeinanästhesie in 4 Fällen (11,2%) und in Regionalanästhesie in 1 Fall (2,4%). 2 Patienten aus der Allgemeinanästhesie-Gruppe verstarben aus kardiopulmonaler Ursache.

Die Hospitalisationsdauer unterschied sich in beiden Gruppen um einen halben Tag, wobei der mittlere Krankenhausaufenthalt nach Allgemeinanästhesie 12,4 Tage und nach Regionalanästhesie 11,9 Tage betrug.

Bei der Auswertung der spirometrisch bestimmten Ventilationsparameter fanden wir folgende Ergebnisse, wobei wegen der nicht immer zu erwartenden Kooperation der Patienten am Operationsabend nur die präoperativ und am ersten postoperativen Tag gemessenen Werte verglichen werden:

Tabelle 3. Häufigkeit der intraoperativen Kreislauf- und Atemkomplikationen, Anästhesie- und Operationsdauer, postoperative cardiopulmonale Komplikationen, Hospitalisationsdauer und Anzahl der Exitus

Intraoperative Kreislauf-komplikationen	JTN	RA	Statistik
1.) Hypotension: $\bar{p}_a\downarrow > 30\%$	7 n = 36	0 n = 42	$p \leqslant 0{,}05$
2.) Hypertension: $\bar{p}_a\uparrow > 30\%$	6 n = 36	2 n = 42	∅
3.) Arrhythmien:	3 n = 36	1 n = 36	∅
4.) ZVD↑ > 12 cm H_2O	7 43 ± 15 n = 17	3 33 ± 19 n = 17	$p \leqslant 0{,}05$
5.) Hypotension im AWR	3 n = 36	2 n = 42	∅
Intraoperative Strgn. der Atmung	∅	∅	∅
Anaesthesiezeit (mittl.)	77	84 min.	∅
Operationsdauer (mittl.)	63	59	∅
Postoperative cardiopulmonale Komplikationen	4 (11,2%)	1 (2,4%)	∅
Exitus aus cardiopulmonaler Ursache	2	0	∅
Hospitalisationsdauer	12,4 Tge	11,9 Tge	∅

Die forcierte Vitalkapazität fiel von 101 ± 24% auf 78 ± 24% in Allgemeinanästhesie, dagegen in Regionalanästhesie von 95 ± 32% auf 84 ± 26% ($p \leqslant 0.01$) (Abb. 2).

Die absolute Ein-Sekunden-Kapazität fiel in Allgemeinanästhesie von 101 ± 26% auf 82 ± 25%, in Regionalanästhesie von 98 ± 30% auf 87 ± 27% (Abb. 3).

Die relative Ein-Sekunden-Kapazität (Tiffeneau-Test) blieb als Quotient aus absoluter Ein-Sekunden-Kapazität und forcierter Vitalkapazität nahezu unverändert. In Allgemeinanästhesie fanden wir präoperativ 73 ± 18% und am 1. postoperativen Tag 74 ± 20%, die entsprechenden Ergebnisse in Regionalanästhesie waren 73 ± 17% und 70 ± 17% (Abb. 4). Der maximale exspiratorische Atemstrom (peak flow) fiel nach Allgemeinanästhesie von 121 ± 46% auf 93 ± 39%, in Regionalanästhesie von 101 ± 31% auf 92 ± 31% ($p \leqslant 0{,}01$) (Abb. 5).

Für die forcierte Vitalkapazität verwendeten wir die von Morris et al. [20] angegebenen Sollwerte unter Berücksichtigung der normalerweise vorhandenen Minderung der inspiratorischen Vitalkapazität um 10-20% [1]. Sollwert und Normgrenze für die absolute Ein-Sekunden-Kapazität übernahmen wir von denselben Autoren. Bei der Beurteilung des maximalen exspiratorischen Atemstroms kamen die Sollwerte von Leiner et al. [16] zur Anwendung, wobei als Marke zwischen normalen und pathologischen Werten die 73%-Grenze nach Anderhub et al. [1] Anwandung fand.

Bei 9 Patienten, die in Allgemeinanästhesie operiert wurden und präoperativ eine normale Vitalkapazität hatten, kam es am 1. postoperativen Tag zu pathologischen Werten, während dies nach Regionalanästhesie nur in 4 Fällen beobachtet werden konnte. Eine entsprechende

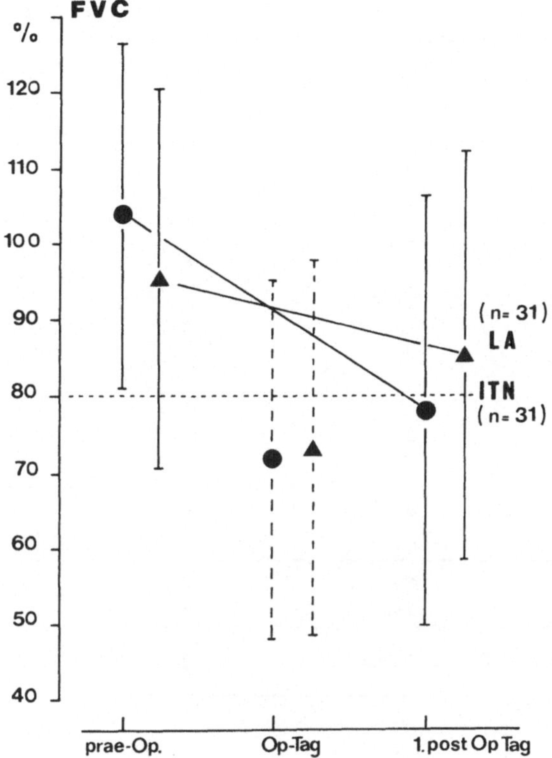

Abb. 2. Forcierte Vitalkapazität praeoperativ, am OP-Tag und am 1. postop. Tag in Prozent der Normalwerte.
▲ = LA = Lokal (Regional)anästhesie
= ITN = Intubationsnarkose
• (= Allgemeinanaesthesie)

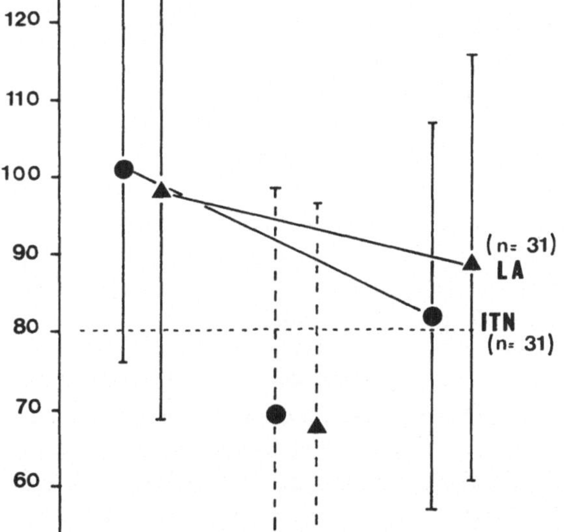

Abb. 3. Einsekundenkapazität (absolut) in Prozent der Normalwerte. Testzeitpunkte und Symbole wie in Abb. 2

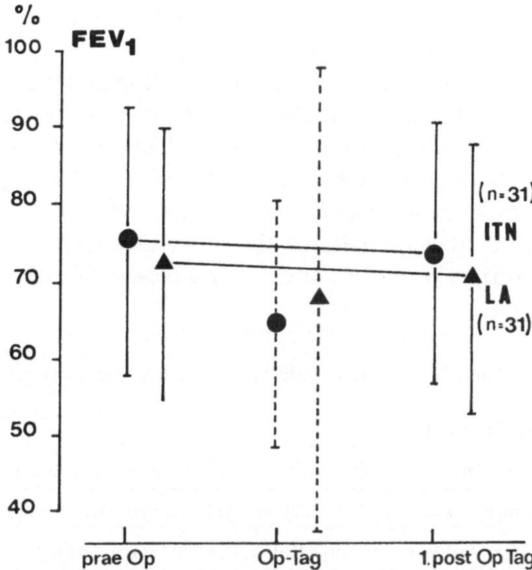

Abb. 4. Einsekundenkapazität (relativ) in Prozent der forcierten Vitalkapazität (Tiffenau-Wert) zu den Testzeitpunkten wie in Abb. 2

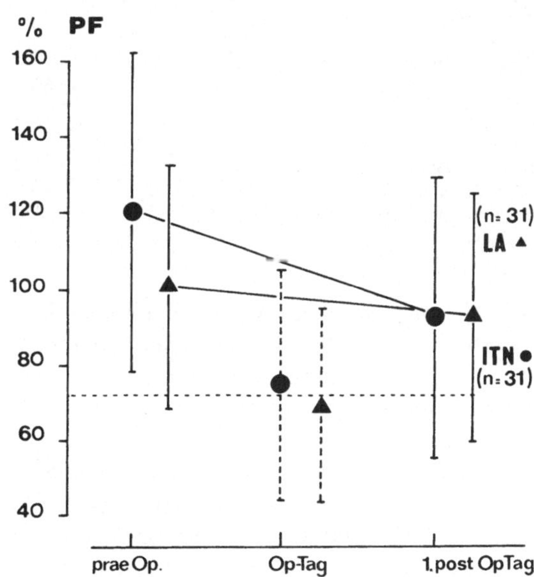

Abb. 5. Maximaler exspiratorischer Atemstrom (Peak flow = PF) in Prozent der Normalwerte zu den in Abb. 2 angegebenen Meßzeitpunkten

Abnahme des peak flow fanden wir nach Allgemeinanästhesie in 6 Fällen, nach Regionalanästhesie bei nur zwei Patienten.

Postoperative cardiopulmonale Komplikationen fanden wir nach Regionalanästhesie bei 1 Patient (Tabelle 3): Hier kam es am 2. postoperativen Tag zu einer Lungenembolie, die szintigraphisch objektiviert wurde. Im EKG zeigte sich ein deutlich verstärkter Rechtsschenkelblock. Bei vorbestehender rekompensierter Herzinsuffizienz und Altersemphysem waren der Anästhesie- und Operationsverlauf unauffällig. Am 1. postoperativen Tag fanden wir die forcierte Vitalkapazität, die absolute und die relative Ein-Sekunden-Kapazität bei präoperativ normalen Werten unter der Norm liegend (Tabelle 4).

Tabelle 4. Postoperative cardiopulmonale Komplikationen nach TUR-Prostata in Regionalanaesthesie

Pat. 1: (75 J)

2. postop. Tag: Lungenembolie (Lu-szintigraphie!) deutl. verstärkter RSB

Vorerkrankungen: Komp. Herzinsuff. (RSB) Altersemphysem

PDA u. OP-Verlauf: Unauffällig. (Sediert mit Diazepam 5 mg)

Ventilation:		praeop.	OP-Tag	1. postop. Tag
FVC	(l):	2,5	2,3	2,2
	(%):	83	77	73
FEV_1	(l/sec):	2,0	1,3	1,4
	(%):	100	65	70
FEV_1	(%):	80	57	64
PF	(l/sec):	3,7	2,2	3,6
	(%):	76	45	73

Nach Allgemeinanästhesie kam es in 4 Fällen (Pat. 2-5) zu schweren kardiopulmonalen Komplikationen im weiteren postoperativen Verlauf (Tabelle 5): Patient 2 verstarb am 28. postoperativen Tag am Herzkreislaufversagen. Eine genauere Diagnose war wegen Sektionsverweigerung nicht möglich. Bei vorbestehender Herzinsuffizienz und eingestelltem Hypertonus gestaltete sich der Narkoseverlauf unauffällig. Am 1. postoperativen Tag war die forcierte Vitalkapazität signifikant niedriger als präoperativ und lag unter der Norm.

Bei Patient Nr. 3 kam es am 2. postoperativen Tag zu einer Pneumonie, am 3. Tag zur Sepsis, am 5. zum akuten Nierenversagen und am 7. postoperativen Tag zum Exitus durch Linksherzversagen. An Vorerkrankungen waren neben dem Prostatakarzinom eine interstitielle Nephritis, Koronarsklerose und Lungenemphysem bekannt. Nach Einleitung der Narkose kam es zu einem Abfall des arteriellen Mitteldruckes um 58% vom Ausgangswert und intraoperativ zu einem Anstieg des zentralen Venendrucks um 7 cm H_2O. Am 1. postoperativen Tag waren die forcierte Vitalkapazität und der peak flow signifikant erniedrigt und lagen unter der Norm.

Bei unauffälligem Narkoseverlauf kam es bei Patient Nr. 4 am 1. postoperativen Tag zu retrosternalen Schmerzen, wobei im EKG eine deutliche Verschlechterung im Sinne einer Koronarinsuffizienz diagnostiziert werden konnte. Eine deutliche Abnahme der forcierten Vitalkapazität sowie der absoluten Ein-Sekunden-Kapazität und des peak flow konnten ebenfalls am 1. postoperativen Tag festgestellt werden.

Tabelle 5. Postoperative cardiopulmonale Komplikationen bei TUR-Prostata in Allgemeinanaesthesie

Pat. 2: (72 J)

Exitus am 28. Tag postop. Herz-Kreislaufversagen

Vorerkrankungen: Herzinsuffizienz (Belastungsdyspnoe)
Hypertonus (eingestellt)
Prostataadenom

Narkoseverlauf: unauffällig

Ventilation:		praeop.	OP-Tag	1. postop. Tag
FVC	(1):	3,6	1,8	2,2
	(%):	116	58	71
FEV_1	(1/sec):	2,0	1,8	1,7
	(%):	95	86	81
FEV_1	(%):	60	100	77
PF	(1/sec) (%):	4,7	4,2	5,0
	(%):			

Pat. 3: (86 J)

2. postop. Tag: Pneumonie/3. po.T.: Sepsis/5. po.T. ak. Nierenvers.
7. postop. Tag: **Exitus** durch Linksherzversagen

Vorerkrankungen: Prostatakarzinom, Interstitielle Nephritis, Koronarsklerose, Lungenemphysem

Narkoseverlauf: Nach N.einleitung $\bar{p}_a\downarrow$ um 58%
Intraop. ZDV↑ um 7 cm H_2O

Ventilation:		praeop.	OP-Tag	1. postop. Tag
FVC	(1):	1,9	1,4	1,3
	(%):	70	52	48
FEV_1	(1/sec):	1,5	1,4	1,4
	(%):	88	82	82
FEV_1	(%):	79	100	100
PF	(1/sec):	4,1	3,6	3,2
	(%):	87	77	68

Pat. 3: (68 J)

1. postop. Tag: retrosternale Schmerzen: Im EKG deutl. Verschlechterung im Sinne einer Koronarinsuffizienz

Entlassung nach Hause

Vorerkrankungen: Komp. Herzinsuff.

Narkoseverlauf: unauffällig

Ventilation:		praeop.	OP-Tag	1. postop. Tag
FVC	(1):	3,2	1,8	1,6
	(%):	107	60	53
FEV_1	(1/sec):	1,8	1,6	1,4
	(%):	86	76	67
FEV_1	(%):	56	89	89
PF	(1/sec) (%):	5,6	4,9	4,0
	(%):	112	98	80

Tabelle 5. Fortsetzung

Pat. 5: (70 J)

3. postop. Tag wegen persist. Ruhedyspnoe Verlegung in Med.Kl.				
Diagnose: Cor pulmonale bei chron. Lungenemphysem				
Entlassung nach Hause.				
Vorerkrankungen: Komp. Herzinsuff., Lungenemphysem.				
Narkoseverlauf:	Anstieg des ZVD um 8 cm auf 15 cm H_2O			
Ventilation:		praeop.	OP-Tag	1. postop. Tag
FVC	(l):	2,5	1,9	2,1
	(%):	83	63	73
FEV_1	(l/sec):	1,3	0,6	0,6
	(%):	65	30	30
FEV_1	(%):	51	32	34
PF	(l/sec):	3,1	1,8	1,4
	(%):	63	37	29

Patient Nr. 5 mußte am 3. postoperativen Tag wegen vorher nicht bestehender persistierender Ruhedyspnoe in die Medizinische Klinik verlegt werden. Die Diagnose lautete „Cor pulmonale bei chronischem Lungenemphysem". An Vorerkrankungen wies der Patient eine kompensierte Herzinsuffizienz und ein Lungenemphysem auf. Während der Operation kam es zu einem Anstieg des zentralen Venendrucks um 8 cm auf 15 cm H_2O. Am 1. postoperativen Tag war eine deutliche Abnahme aller Lungenfunktionswerte festzustellen.

Diskussion

Kardiopulmonale Komplikationen sind die häufigsten Todesursachen beim geriatrischen Patienten. Während intraoperativ kardiozirkulatorische Komplikationen im Vordergrund stehen, gewinnen die respiratorischen Störungen in der postoperativen Phase an Bedeutung [9]. Schwere Hypotensionen um mehr als 30% vom Ausgangswert fanden wir in Allgemeinanästhesie statistisch auffällig häufiger als in rückenmarksnaher Leitungsanästhesie. Abfälle des arteriellen Mitteldruckes dieses Ausmaßes können beim geriatrischen Patienten mit sklerosierten Gefäßen und evtl. vorhandenen Stenosen, insbesondere der Koronar- und Hirngefäße [24] durch Minderperfusion und daraus resultierender Gewebsischämie und Hypoxie deletäre Folgen haben. Nach Lutz et al. [18] kommt der Hypotension die größte Bedeutung als pathogenetischer Faktor der intra- und postoperativen Mortalität zu.

Hypertensionen um mehr als 30% vom Ausgangswert sahen wir in Allgemeinanästhesie ebenfalls häufiger als in Regionalanästhesie, doch konnte dieser Unterschied statistisch nicht gesichert werden. Anstiege des zentralen Venendrucks über 12 cm H_2O bei im Mittel annähernd gleichen Ausgangswerten von 3,5 bzw. 4,8 cm H_2O konnten wir ebenfalls in Allgemeinanästhesie statistisch auffällig häufiger feststellen als in Regionalanästhesie. Im wesentlichen beeinflussen 4 Faktoren den zentralen Venendruck:

1. das Blutvolumen,
2. die Lagerung,

3. die intrathorakalen Druckverhältnisse und
4. die Herzleistungsfähigkeit.

Beim Vergleich der beiden Anästhesieverfahren können wir die Lagerung und die intrathorakalen Druckverhältnisse als Ursache des Venendruckanstiegs ausklammern, da wir bei identischer Steinschnittlage und während der Allgemeinanästhesie in Beatmungspause gemessen haben. Im wesentlichen führen wir den Anstieg des zentralen Venendrucks auf Hypervolämie zurück: Bei transurethralen Resektionen der Prostata kommt es regelmäßig zur Einschwemmung von Spülflüssigkeit über eröffnete periprostatische Venensinus in den Patientenkreislauf. Die in der Literatur angegebenen Durchschnittswerte [19] eingeschwemmter Volumina betragen zwischen 1.225 und 1.990 ml. Dieselbe Autorin beschreibt Einschwemmungen bis 4.500 ml. Die Wirkungen auf den Kreislauf bestehen im Anstieg des systolischen, des diastolischen und des arteriellen Mitteldruckes sowie in einer, durch Barorezeptoren im rechten Vorhof ausgelösten, reflektorischen Bradykardie [2]. Der zentrale Venendruck steigt, am Anstieg des intrathorakalen Blutvolumens entsprechend, an [8]. Daß der zentrale Venendruck in Regionalanästhesie weniger ansteigt als in Allgemeinanästhesie, hat in der Hauptsache zwei Gründe: Durch Sympathikusblockade in den von der Anästhesie betroffenen Segmenten kommt es zu einer Vasodilatation und in deren Gefolge zu einer Erhöhung der Volumenkapazität dieses peripheren Gefäßabschnittes. Diese ist größer als bei der von uns angewendeten Methode der Allgemeinanästhesie. Die Erhöhung der Kapazität dieses ausgedehnten Gefäßbezirkes verhindert bei schneller Resorption großer Flüssigkeitsvolumina eine gefährliche Volumenbelastung des Herzens durch Blutpooling. Die zweite Ursache sehen wir im späteren Erkennen der Einschwemmung vor allem dann, wenn der zentrale Venendruck als Indikator für Änderungen des Blutvolumens nicht gemessen wird. Hierfür spricht auch, daß die maximalen Blutdruckanstiege, ebenfalls Indikator für die eingetretene Hypervolämie, in Allgemeinanästhesie im Mittel nach 43 min., dagegen in Regionalanästhesie bereits 33 min. nach Operationsbeginn gemessen wurden. Während in Allgemeinanästhesie unter anderem auch eine zu flache Narkose, Anstieg des pCO_2 oder Abfall des pO_2 differentialdiagnostisch zu erwägen sind, ist die Diagnose Einschwemmung während einer transurethralen Prostataresektion in Regionalanästhesie schneller gestellt. Eine Volumenüberlastung größeren Ausmaßes kann bei alten Patienten mit meist vorgeschädigtem Herzen [24] ein komplexes Schadensspektrum einleiten, an dessen Beginn eine Erhöhung des preload steht, die immer auch eine Erhöhung des myokardialen Sauerstoffverbrauchs nach sich zieht [14] und an dessen Ende über einen Anstieg des afterload das Lungenödem und Linksherzversagen stehen.

Kreislaufkomplikationen im Aufwachraum traten ausschließlich im Sinne von Hypotensionen auf und waren in beiden Gruppen annähernd gleich selten. Zumeist ließen sie sich auf eine überschießende Therapie des Einschwemmsyndroms mit Furosemid bis 80 mg und Sorbit 40%ig zurückführen. In keinem Fall war eine schwere Blutung, die Bluttransfusionen notwendig gemacht hätte, Ursache des Blutdruckabfalls.

Während intraoperativ keine Störungen von seiten der Atmung auftraten, zeigte das Verhalten der von uns gemessenen Ventilationsparameter im postoperativen Verlauf deutliche Veränderungen:

Die forcierte Vitalkapazität fiel bei beiden Anästhesieverfahren statistisch signifikant ab. Hierbei war der Abfall der Patienten, die in Allgemeinanästhesie operiert wurden, statistisch signifikant größer als bei Patienten, die eine Regionalanästhesie erhalten hatten ($p \leqslant 0{,}01$). Restriktive Veränderungen, als deren einfacher Parameter die Viralkapazität gelten darf [6, 26], finden sich demnach nach Allgemeinanästhesie in stärkerem Ausmaß als nach Leitungsanästhesie. Daß auch nach Spinal- und Periduralanästhesie Lungenfunktionsstörungen restriktiver Art auftreten, erklären wir im wesentlichen mit der intraoperativen Steinschnittlage, die über Zwerchfellhochstand und Einschränkung der Motilität insbesondere bei altersverändertem, starrem Thorax zu einer lagerungsbedingten Verminderung der Vitalkapazität führt [17]. Auch schmerz- und sedationsbedingte postoperative Schonatmung kann als pathogenetischer Faktor wirksam sein [5]. Inwieweit die Einschwemmung destillierten Wassers mit resultierender hyponatriämischer Hyperhydratation und Abfall der Osmolarität die Lungenfunktion im Sinne einer Restriktion verändert, können wir anhand der von uns gemessenen Parameter nicht aussagen.

Der maximale exspiratorische Atemstrom (peak flow) fiel nach Allgemeinanästhesie statistisch signifikant stärker ab als nach Leitungsanästhesie ($p \leq 0{,}01$). Nach Stein et al. [25] sowie Ross et al. [22] korreliert der reduzierte peak flow am engsten mit postoperativen Komplikationen. Die Größe des peak flow kann als Maß für einen effektiven Hustenstoß gesehen werden.

Der Abfall der absoluten Ein-Sekunden-Kapazität war nach Allgemeinanästhesie ebenfalls ausgeprägter als nach Regionalanästhesie, doch konnte dieser Unterschied nicht statistisch gesichert werden.

Entsprechend der Abnahme der forcierten Vitalkapazität und der absoluten Ein-Sekunden-Kapazität ändert sich die relative Ein-Sekunden-Kapazität, der sog. Tiffeneau-Wert, nicht. Dies entspricht auch den Ergebnissen von Diament und Palmer [7]; Klose et al. [13]; und Latimer et al. [15] und zeigt, daß obstruktive Lungenfunktionsstörungen hinter den beobachteten restriktiven Störungen in dieser frühen postoperativen Phase zurückstehen.

Veränderungen, die mit einem Verlust an belüftungsfähigem Parenchym einhergehen, stehen demnach im Vordergrund und sind nach Allgemeinanästhesie häufiger als nach Leitungsanästhesie. Die bei diesem Anästhesieverfahren ebenfalls ausgeprägtere Störung der Selbstreinigung der Lunge, wie sie sich in dem statistisch signifikanten Abfall des peak flow äußert, darf jedoch nicht übersehen werden. Der weitaus größere Abfall der forcierten Vitalkapazität und des maximalen exspiratorischen Atemstroms nach Intubationsnarkose kann über einen abgeschwächten Hustenstoß (reduzierter peak flow) nach unzureichender Inspiration (reduzierte Vitalkapazität) zur Sekretretention führen, die auf dem Boden schon bestehender Atelektasen nun zusätzlich zu Obstruktionen führt, die ihrerseits wieder die Ausbildung von Atelektasen fördern. Am Ende dieses circulus vitiosus steht die globale respiratorische Insuffizienz [13].

Von diesen pulmonalen postoperativen Funktionsstörungen sind nicht nur offensichtlich Lungenkranke, sondern auch Patienten betroffen, deren Lungenfunktionswerte präoperativ im Normbereich lagen. So kam es in unseren Untersuchungen bei 9 Patienten, die in Allgemeinanästhesie operiert wurden und präoperativ eine normale Vitalkapazität hatten, zu pathologischen Werten am 1. postoperativen Tag, während dies nach Regionalanästhesie nur in 4 Fällen beobachtet werden konnte.

Eine entsprechende Abnahme des peak flow fanden wir nach Allgemeinanästhesie in 6 Fällen, nach Regionalanästhesie bei nur 2 Patienten. Wir folgern hieraus, daß unabhängig von der präoperativen bronchopulmonalen Ausgangssituation zur Vermeidung postoperativer Lungenfunktionsstörungen, die nach Lutz et al. [18] nicht selten zum Tode führen, die rückenmarksnahen Leitungsanästhesien beim geriatrischen Patienten Vorteile gegenüber der Allgemeinanästhesie besitzen.

Auf Blutgasanalysen verzichteten wir vor allem deshalb, weil die Auswirkungen des Anästhesieverfahrens auf die Blutgase bereits hinlänglich oft beschrieben worden sind [10, 13] und wir unsere Patienten nicht zusätzlich belasten wollten.

Die intraoperativen Komplikationen von seiten des Kreislaufs sowie die postoperativen

Veränderungen der Atmung, in Allgemeinanästhesie zum Teil statistisch auffällig oder signifikant häufiger als in Regionalanästhesie, fanden ihren Ausdruck in der Häufigkeit kardiopulmonaler Komplikationen im postoperativen Verlauf, wobei die 28-Tage-Grenze nach Lutz et al. [18] zur Anwendung kam: zu schweren Komplikationen kam es nach Allgemeinanästhesie in 4 Fällen, wobei 2 Patienten während des Krankenhausaufenthaltes verstarben. Nach Regionalanästhesie kam es lediglich bei 1 Patienten zu einer nachweisbaren kardiopulmonalen Komplikation im Sinne einer Lungenembolie.

Zusammenfassend stellen wir fest, daß intra- und postoperative Komplikationen von seiten des Kreislaufs und der Atmung in und nach Allgemeinanästhesie häufiger auftreten als nach Regionalanästhesie; dies, obgleich die von uns verwendeten Verfahren der Allgemeinanästhesie als schonend bezeichnet werden können [4, 23]. Können wir den Anstieg des zentralen Venendrucks und die begleitende Hypertension als Ausdruck der Hypervolämie noch als operationsspezifisch betrachten, so müssen die übrigen beschriebenen Komplikationen im wesentlichen als anästhesiebedingt bezeichnet werden. Wir folgern hieraus, daß beim geriatrischen Patienten, unabhängig von der Art des Eingriffs, der Regionalanästhesie da, wo sie ausreichende Operationsbedingungen schafft, der Vorzug gegenüber dem von uns angewendeten Verfahren der Allgemeinanästhesie zu geben ist.

Summary

Intra- and postoperative cardiopulmonary complications were studied in geriatric patients, undergoing transurethral prostatectomy in general anesthesie (NLA) and regional anesthesia (EDA and spinal anesthesia). During anesthesia and operation severe hypotension and rise of central venous pressure were registered more often in general than in regional anesthesia ($p \leqslant 0.05$). Reduction of forced vital capacity and peak flow were also statistically significant in general anesthesia. Because cardiopulmonary complications are most frequently the reasons for intra- and postoperative mortality, regional anesthesia should be preferred for geriatric patients, whenever possible.

Literatur

1. Anderhub HP, Keller R, Herzog H (1974) Spirometrische Untersuchung der forcierten Vitalkapazität, Sekundenkapazität und max. Atemstromstärke bei 13.798. Dtsch Med Wochenschr 2:33
2. Aviado DM (1965) The lung circulation. Pergamon, London. p 878
3. Brandhauer K, Madersbacher H (1969) Früh- und Spätkomplikationen transurethraler Eingriffe an der Prostata. Urologe [A] 2:48
4. Bergmann H (1976) Die Auswahl der Anästhesiemittel und -methoden bei kardiopulmolatorischen Risikofaktoren. Klin Anaesth Intensivther 11:135-155
5. Bergmann H (1976) Pathophysiologie des postoperativen Lungenversagens. Klin Anaesth Intensivther 12:187-198
6. Comroe JH, Forster RE, Dubois AB, Briscoe WA, Carlsen E (1972) Die Lunge, klinische Physiologie und Lungenfunktionsprüfungen. Schattauer, Stuttgart
7. Diament MLKN, Palmer V (1966) Postoperative changes in gas tension of arterial blood and in ventilatory function. Lancet II:180
8. Eckert P (1976) Das Niederdrucksystem. Thieme, Stuttgart
9. Hamer P (1976) Allgemeine und spezielle Maßnahmen zur Verhütung und Beseitigung der postoperativen Atelektase. Klin Anaesth Intensivther 12:220-233
10. Helms U, Weihrauch H (1977) Veränderungen der Blutgase und des Säure-Basen-Haushaltes in der frühen postoperativen Phase nach Leitungs- und Intubationsanästhesie. Prakt Anaesth 4:259
11. Hutschenreuther K (1977) Anästhesieprobleme bei urologischen Eingriffen. Therapiewoche 27:5159

12. Iglesias JJ, Stams K (1975) Urologe [A] 14:287
13. Klose R, Osswald P, Lutz H (1977) Praeoperative spirometrische Beurteilung der Lungenfunktion und postoperativer Verlauf. Prakt Anaesth 4:297
14. Lappas DG, Powell WMJ, Dagget WM (1977) Cardiac dysfunktion in the perioperative period. Anesthesiology 47:117
15. Latimer RG, Dickmann M, Day WC, Gunn ML, Schmidt CD (1971) Ventilatory patterns and pulmonary complications after upper abdominal surgery determined by preoperative and postoperative computerized spirometrie and blood-gas analysis. Am J Surg 122:622
16. Leiners GC, Abramowitz S, Small MJ, Stenby VB, Lewis WA (1963) Exspiratory peak flow rate. Am Rev Respir Dis 88:644
17. Little DM (1960) Posture and Anaesthesia. Can Anaesth Soc J 7:2-15
18. Lutz H, Klose R, Peter K (1972) Untersuchungen zum Risiko der Allgemeinanästhesie unter operativen Bedingungen. Dtsch Med Wochenschr 97:1816
19. Marx GF (1975) Komplikationen in der transurethralen Chirurgie. Urologie 75:1-8
20. Morris JF, Koski A, Johnson LC (1971) Spirometric standards for healthy nonsmoking adults. Am Rev Respir Dis 103:57
21. Pulver KG, Otten M (1970) Die Allgemeinnarkose im Greisenalter. In: Anästhesie in extremen Altersklassen. Hutschenreuter K, Bihler K, Fritsche P (Hrsg) (Anaesthesiologie und Wiederbelebung, Bd 47, S. 114-122) Springer, Berlin, Heidelberg, New York
22. Ross BB, Gramiak R, Rahn H (1955) Physical dynamics of caugh mechanism. J Appl Physiol 8:264
23. Seitz W, Hempelmann G, Piepenbrock S (1977) Zur cardiovasculären Wirkung von Flunitrazepam (Rohypnol, Ro-5-4200). Anaesthesist 26:249
24. Stauch M (1974) Bedeutung altersbedingter Änderungen der Kreislauffunktion für die Anaesthesie. In: Anaesthesie im Alter. Ahnefeld FW, Halmágyi M (Hrsg) (Anaesthesiologie und Wiederbelebung, Bd 83, S. 23-31) Springer, Berlin, Heidelberg, New York
25. Stein M, Koota GM, Simon M, Frank HA (1962) Pulmonary evaluation of surgical patients. JAMA 181:765
26. Zeilhofer R, Eickeler R (1937) Möglichkeiten und Grenzen der Lungenfunktionsanalyse in der Praxis. Korrelation differenzierter und vereinfachter Parameter. Med Klin 68:237

Diskussion

Frage: Eine ganz allgemeine Frage: Wie würden Sie sich denn überhaupt verhalten, wenn Sie vor der Frage stehen, einen Patienten in schlechtem Allgemeinzustand für eine Prostataresektion anaesthesieren zu müssen? Würden Sie ihn der Spinal- oder der Allgemeinnarkose zuführen?
Tolksdorf: Der Periduralanaesthesie.

Influence of Different Methods for Postoperative Pain Relief on Pulmonary Function After Thoracic Surgery

C.P. Naumann

Postoperative pulmonary complications are most often seen after upper abdominal and thoracic surgery. Mild signs of retained secretions and pulmonary infection may be present in 50%-80% of these patients, but even without clinical signs a pronounced arterial hypoxaemia is usually seen in the postoperative period. P_aO_2 returns to preoperative levels 7-10 days after upper abdominal surgery; after thoracic surgery this may take up to 14 days.

Morbidity and mortality of postoperative pulmonary complications can be reduced by treating not only the **subjective** consequences of pain, but also the **objective** ones (Fig. 1).

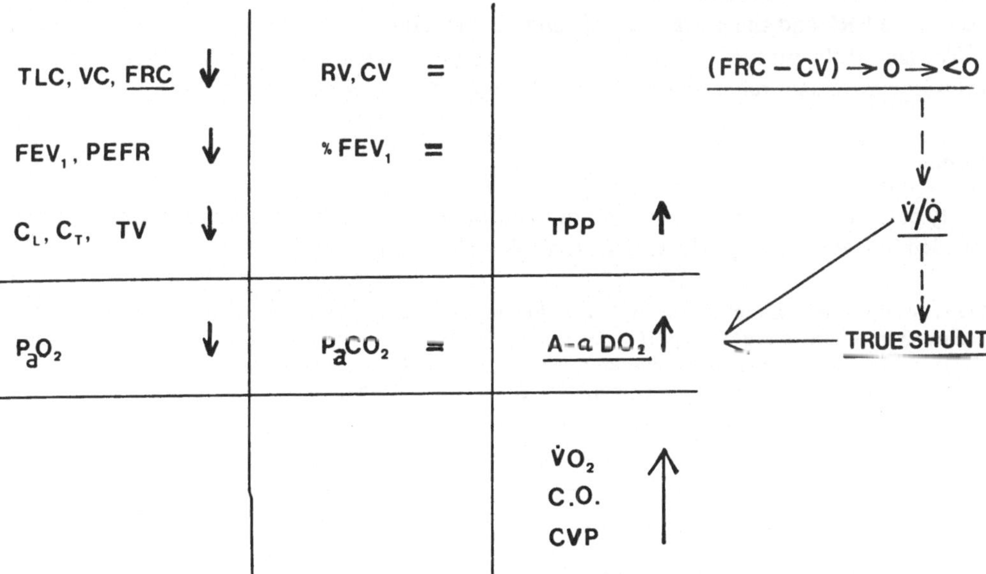

Fig. 1. The objective consequences of pain on lung volumes, ventilatory parameters, compliance, blood gases and circulation are shown. Postoperative hypoxaemia occurs in close correlation to decrease of FRC at constant CV. If CV exceeds FRC, *airway narrowing,* which causes ventilation/perfusion inequalities, *or airway closure,* which causes true shunt, will occur

Most lung volumes (with the exception of residual volume and closing volume) are decreased to 25%-50% of their preoperative levels; the postoperative change of ventilatory parameters (FVC, FEV_1, PEFR, MBC) is in the same range. $\%FEV_1$ is mostly unchanged, indicating the mainly restrictive nature of postoperative changes in pulmonary function.

The decrease of the FRC (while the closing volume (CV) is not altered), is of special significance: If the difference in FRC-CV approaches zero or becomes negative, airway closure will occur even under quiet breathing with normal tidal volumes. Small airways will be narrowed or closed, before expiration is finished and gas trapping distal of these airways will occur. The result will be an increase of A-a DO_2 because of ventilation/perfusion inequalities and also because of true shunt. There is a linear correlation between decrease of FRC-CV and increase of A-a DO_2 [2].

Another important factor is the rise of transpulmonary pressure (TPP), caused directly by the groaning respiration under pain and indirectly by the reduction in FRC. The elastic frame of the alveoli acts as a spring, which pulls both on the pleura visceralis and the bronchial walls and thus causes the negative intrapleural pressure and keeps the airways open. At lowered FRC the spring is less stretched, allowing the TPP to rise and the alveoli to narrow.

While the reduction of FRC and the resulting hypoxaemia are most marked during the first postoperative hours, when pain is worst, another causative mechanism for hypoxaemia and postoperative pulmonary complications plays an important role during the first postoperative days, which must partly be considered as side-effect of postoperative pain relief with centrally acting morphine-like analgesics. Respiration with low, constant tidal volumes without intermittent sighs, damage to the surfactant system and retention of secretions because of pain-inhibition of the cough reflex promote the development of miliary atelectasis, which tends to extend. Thus, the predominant aims of postoperative treatment should be the restoration of the preoperative FRC and the prevention of cough depression.

The aim of the present investigation was to compare the influence of different methods for postoperative pain relief on objective and subjective consequences of pain.

Methods

Seventy patients, who underwent lateral thoracotomies for elective lung surgery, were randomly divided into seven groups (I, II, IIIA, IIIB, IVA, IVB, V) (Table 1).

Table 1. Postoperative pain relief. The drugs used in Groups I-V and the method of administration (all Groups intermittent injections except Group IIIA: continuous injection) are listed in Column 1. The maximum allowed single dose and the maximum allowed number of doses/24 h can be seen.
Additional injections of Tilidin-Hcl (Valoron) were allowed for all groups

	Drug	Single Dose	Doses/24 Hrs.	Additional (If Needed)
Group I	Ketobemidon (Cliradon®)	0.1 mg/kg b.w.	max. 6	Tilidin (Valoron®) 25-50 mg s.c.
Group II	Etidocaine 1%	4-6-8 ml	max. 16	25-50 mg s.c.
Group III	Lidocaine 1% A Continuous B Intermittent	3 mg/kg bw/hr 12-15 ml	x 24 (+ Bolus) max. 24	25-50 mg s.c. 25-50 mg s.c.
Group IV	Bupivacaine 0.375% With Adrenaline A Start postop. B Start intraop.	8-10 ml	max. 16	25-50 mg s.c.
Group V	Bupivacaine 0.5% with Adrenaline + 2-Chloro-Procaine 3% 2/1	6-8 ml	max. 16	25-50 mg s.c.

The mean age of the patients was 57.3 years, 67% were operated for carcinoma bronchi, 55% of the patients had signs of chronic obstructive lung disease. There were no significant differences between the groups concerning these data and sex, weight and height.

Group I was to receive pain relief by parenteral injections of Ketobemidon (Cliradon), 0.1 mg/kg body wt; up to six doses during 24 h were allowed.

The patients of the Groups II-V had an epidural catheter inserted at T_5/T_6 interspace preoperatively and were to receive pain relief by sensory blockade with different local anaesthetic agents (see Table 1).

The first injections for pain relief were given 60-90 min postoperatively, when the patients were in severe pain and the first series of measurements (see below) had been calculated. Group IVB patients, however, had their first epidural injections intraoperatively, so there was no pain period postoperatively.

Pain medication was given by intermittent injections on demand, single doses and maximum number of injections, allowed per 24 h, are listed in table 1. Only Group IIIA patients had a continuous infusion of lidocaine by means of a motor syringe into the epidural space.

Additional injections of Tilidin-HCl (Valoron) were allowed for all groups, when a single dose had a bad effect or Group I patients had too many side-effects.

Serial pulmonary function tests and blood gas analyses (when the patients were brathing room air) were taken:

1. Preoperatively in supine position as control values ("preop.").
2. Postoperatively:
   a) 1 h after the end of anaesthesia, patients in pain ("postop. I").
   b) 2 h after the end of anaesthesia, when first pain medication had been given ("postop. II").
   c) six times at regular intervals up to 72 h postoperatively.

A-a DO_2 was calculated using the formula:

$$\text{A-a DO}_2 = P_AO_2 - P_aO_2 \quad (1), \quad \text{wherein}$$

$$P_AO_2 = P_IO_2 - \frac{P_aCO_2}{R} \quad (2).$$

R was assumed to be constant at 0.8[2].

The respiratory restoration factor (RRF) was calculated using this the following equation, given by Bromage [3]:

$$RRF = \frac{PEFR_{analg.} - PEFR_{pain}}{PEFR_{preop.} - PEFR_{pain}} \times 100.$$

The calculation of the RRF allows an *objective comparison* between the potency of different analgesics to abolish the objective consequences of pain, i.e. to restore preoperative pulmonary function.

The *subjective quality of analgesia*, as experienced by the patients and the nursing staff, was judged by using two scores: (Table 2). A subjective score was given, according to the patients' answers; a somewhat more objective score was given by the nursing staff, according to the ability to cough and take deep breaths. If the two scores did not correspond and the patient's score was 1, it was corrected to "0.5" or "1.5".

Table 2. Quality of analgesia in the postoperative period. A: Criteria for the subjective Score, as judged by the patients. B: Criteria for objective correction (as judged by the nursing staff) of the subjective score. This correction of the subjective scores was only made when the patients answer was Score 1

Postoperative Pain Relief	
Quality Of Analgesia In The Postoperative Period	
A Subjective Score	
0	= Pain-Free At Deep Inspiration
1	= Moderate Pain
2	= Severe Pain, Patient requested Supplementary Medication
B Subjective Score, Objective Correction	
1	= Moderate Pain, Inhibition Of Coughing
0,5	= Moderate Pain, No Coughing Inhibition
1,5	= Moderate Pain, Severe Coughing Inhibition

Results

Distinct differences have been found between the TEA Groups (II-V) and the MO Group (I), and also among the TEA Groups.

The results of the most different groups (Group I versus Groups IVA and B) will be presented in detail; the other results will only be mentioned summarily.

P_aO_2 (Fig. 2)

One hour postoperatively, when the patients were in pain, the arterial oxygen tension had decreased dramatically from 79.1 mmHg (± 3.3 s.e.) to 55.2 mmHg (± 2.2), i.e. a decrease of

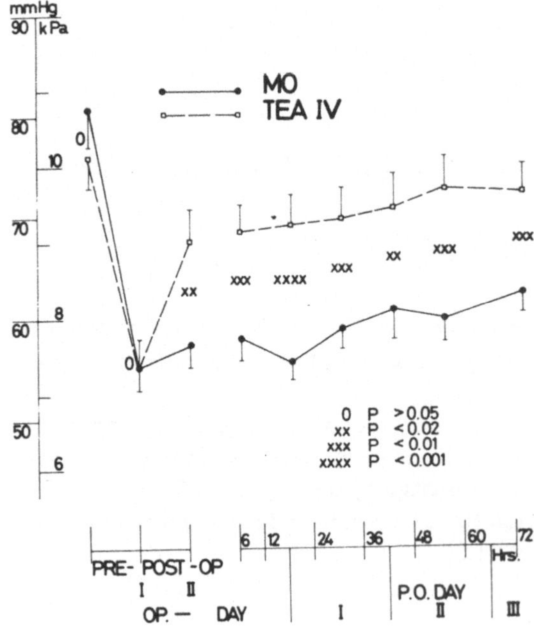

Fig. 2. The course of P_aO_2 during the 72 h postoperative ($\bar{x} \pm s_{\bar{x}}$). Preoperatively and 1 h postop. when the patients were in pain, there were no significant differences between Groups I and IV.
2 h postoperatively after the first pain medication, and during the following 72 h, there were significant differences for the restoration of P_aO_2 to preoperative levels

23.9 mmHg for all groups. Two hours postoperatively, after the first pain medication, however, significant differences between the groups were seen. P_aO_2 in Group IV patients rose significantly, while it showed only a slight, insignificant tendency to increase in Group I patients. The differences between the groups remained significant until the end of the 72-h observation period, when the values were 17.9 mmHg (± 2.4) (Group I), and 4.6 mmHg (± 1.1) (Group IV), below the preoperative levels.

P_aCO_2 (Fig. 3)

There were clear, but not significant tendencies towards **hyper**ventilation in the TEA Group IV and towards **hypo**ventilation in Group I. The differences between the Groups were significant over 48 h postoperative.

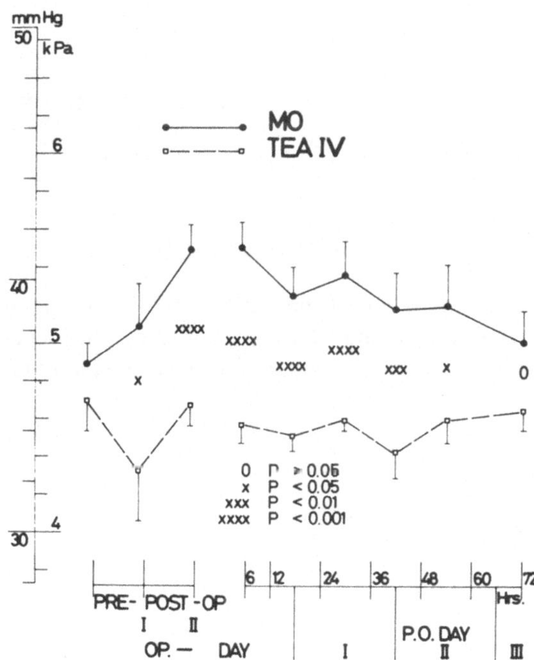

Fig. 3. The course of P_aCO_2 during the 72 h postoperative ($\bar{x} \pm s_{\bar{x}}$). Mild, but not significant hypoventilation in Group I. Mild, but not significant hyperventilation in Groups IV. The difference between Groups I and IV, however, were significant during the first 48 h

A-a DO_2 (Fig. 4)

To see whether the lower P_aO_2 values in Group I were caused by the relative hypoventilation, totally or in part, we calculated the A-a DO_2. One hour postoperatively the alveolo-arterial oxygen difference had increased in all patients (+ 24.2 mmHg ± 3.0) without significant differences between the groups.

Two hours postoperatively, when pain relief had been instituted, the A-a DO_2 was still 18.0 mmHg (± 1.8) higher than the preoperative level in Group I, but only 9.9 mmHg (± 1.2) over the preoperative level in Group IV patients. These significant differences were also present after 72 h (+ 16.8 mmHg ± 2.8 versus + 6.3 mmHg ± 1.4). This shows, that the relative hypo/hyperventilation is only to a minor degree responsible for the observed differences between the groups.

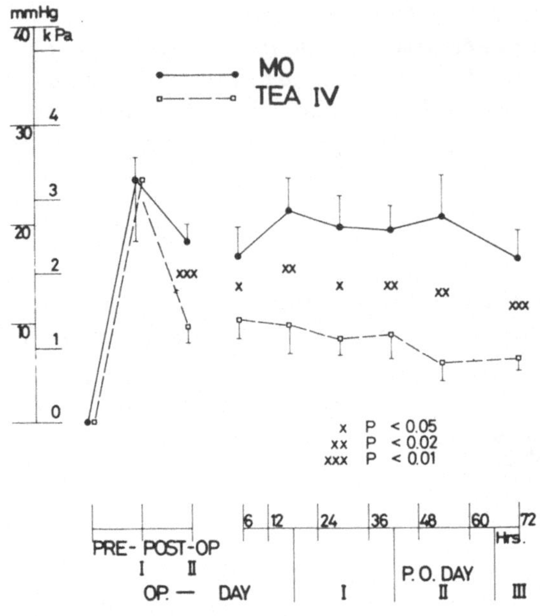

Fig. 4. The course of A-a DO_2 during the 72 h postoperative ($\bar{x} \pm s_{\bar{x}}$). Preoperatively and 1 h postoperatively, when the patients were in pain, there were no significant differences between Groups I and Group IV. 2 h postoperatively after the first pain medication, and during the following 72, there were significant differences for the restoration of A-a DO_2 to preoperative levels

Peak Expiratory Flow Rate (PEFR; Fig. 5)

The determination of the PEFR as ventilatory parameter was chosen, because it is in close correlation to FVC and FEV_1 [4], but is least influenced by the amount of lung tissue removed. Furthermore, it is a good indicator for the patients' ability to cough.

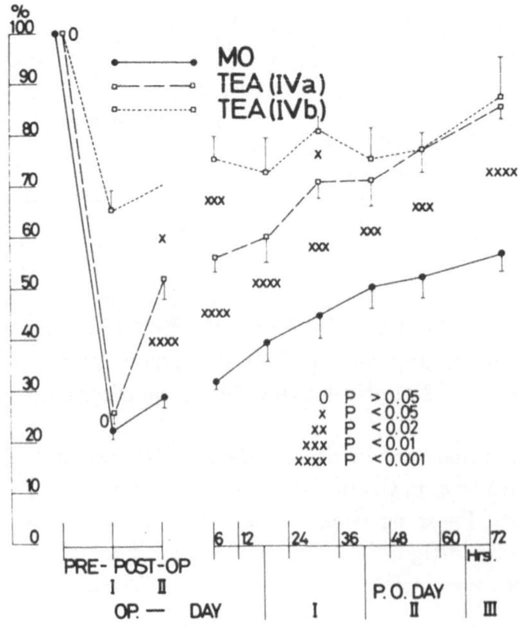

Fig. 5. The course of PEFR (% of control) during the 72 h postoperative ($\bar{x} \pm s_{\bar{x}}$).

1. Comparison between Groups I (MO) and IVA. The marked decrease in postoperative pain, the increase after pain medication (POSTOP II) and during the following 72 h shows significant differences for the restoration rates of preoperative PEFR between Groups I and IVA.
2. Comparison of the Groups IVA and IVB. Patients, who had not been in pain postoperatively (Group IVB), showed a smaller reduction in PEFR, than those having been in pain (Group IVA). The difference was significant up to 36 h postoperatively, but disappeared after this time

All patients, who were in pain 1 h postoperatively, (Groups I and IVA), showed a decrease to 23.1% (± 1.0) of the preoperative control values. Two hours postoperatively, however, Group IVA patients had improved to 52.2% (± 3.4), while Group I patients showed only a slight and not significant increase to 29.1% (± 2.0).

Seventy-two hours postoperatively Group IV patients had regained 86.9% (± 3.4) of their preoperative PEFR; MO patients (Group I) still 56.9% (± 3.2) ($p < 0.001$).

The critical level for PEFR (200 litres/min [7]), which may be necessary for effective cough, was still not reached after 72 h in Group I (189 litre/min ± 18.0); Group IV, patients however, reached it during the day of the operation.

Comparing Group IVA (start of TEA after initial pain period) to Group IVB (TEA started intraoperatively) (see Fig. 5), it is clear that the initial fall in PEFR is much less pronounced, when the patients have not been in postoperative pain (fall only to 67.1% of preoperative level).

Thirty-six hours postoperatively, however, this difference between Groups IVA and B had disappeared; so we do not know whether it is of practical importance.

RRF (Fig. 6) *Respiratory Restoration Factors*

In order to compare the potency of different analgesics to reverse the objective consequences of pain, we compared the RRF obtained from our Groups I - V 2 h postoperatively with those given in reports by Bromage [3] and Parbrook [6].

RRF for morphine-like analgesics range between 8-16. The combination of N_2O inhalations and analgesics of the morphine group has somewhat better results [1, 6]. The use of this method, however, is limited to 24 or 48 h because of the risk of bone marrow depression. I.V. infusion of lidocaine is also better than analgesics of the morphine group [3], but is not used because of the risk of toxic reactions. The RRF obtained in our TEA Groups varied widely; all but those of Group IIIA (lidocaine continuous administration) were significantly superior to those obtained with morphine derivates.

There was a good correlation between the RRF and the changes in A-a DO_2, and also with the clinical outcome.

Groups II, IV and V were not significantly different; etidocaine 1%, the mixture of bupivacaine 0.5% with adrenaline and 2-chloro-procaine 3% 2/1, and bupivacaine 0.375% with adrenaline alone are all suitable local anesthetic agents (Fig. 7). We prefer the latter agent, as the doses needed and the risk of toxic reactions are very low, the duration of action is reasonably long and a sensory blockade without apparent impairment of motory function is obtainable.

Subjective Pain Relief (Fig. 8 and Table 3)

The corrected pain scores are shown in Fig. 8 and their mean values are compared in Table 3.

Pain relief was estimated to be sufficient by Group I patients (for dosage of Ketobemidon see Fig. 9), but more satisfactory by Group IV patients. TEA patients were able to cough more effectively, and it was very impressive to see that these patients were much more cooperative in performing breathing exercises and interested in their own and each other's fates, while Group I patients tended to be drowsy and not at all cooperative.

Table 3. Mean values of corrected pain scores

Group	2	10	24	36	48	60	72 h postop.
I	1.0 ±0.1	0.8 ±0.1	0.9 ±0.1	0.8 ±0.1	0.6 ±0.1	0.7 ±0.2	0.6 ±0.1
IV	0.3 ±0.1	0.3 ±0.2	0.4 ±0.1	0.2 ±0.1	0.2 ±0.2	0.3 ±0.1	0.3 ±0.1

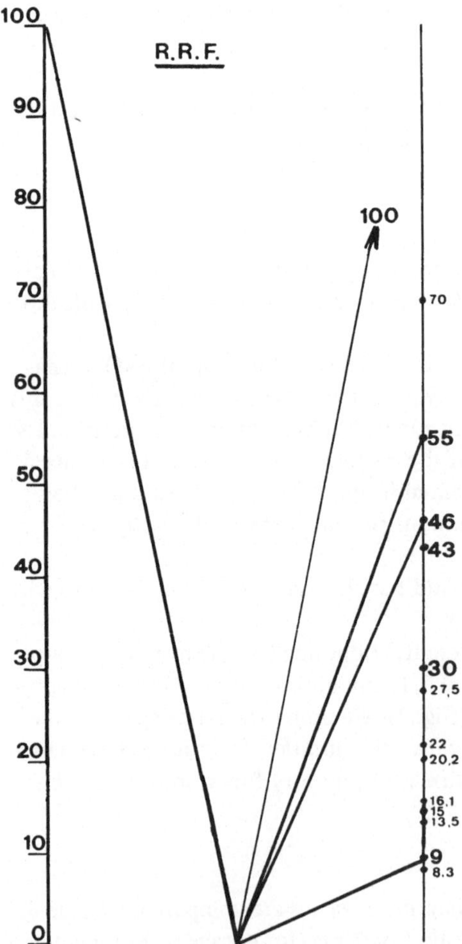

Fig. 6. Respiratory restoration factors were calculated for our Groups I (Ketobemidon) and II-V (TEA) for the PEFR values 2 h postoperatively and compared to those for different morphine-like analgesics, IV lidocaine infusion and a combination of N_2O inhalations with morphine derivates (see also 3, 6) [3, 6]

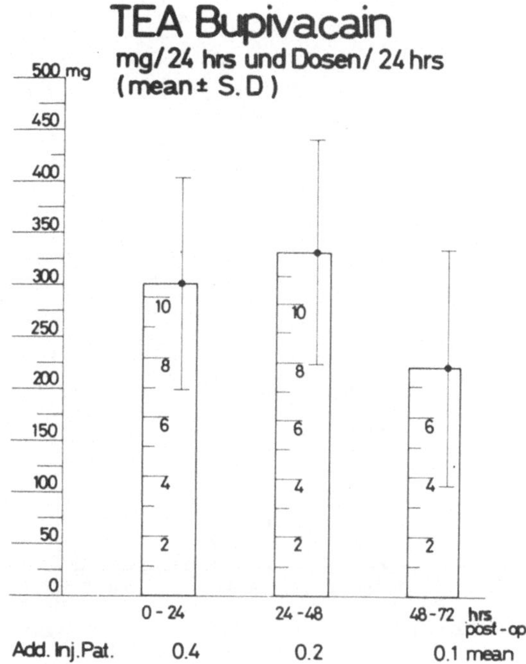

Fig. 7. Dosage of bupivacaine 0.375% with adrenaline in Groups IVA and B. The columns show the amount of the drug needed for the first, second and third 24 h periods in mg/24 h. The number of single doses is given inside the columns

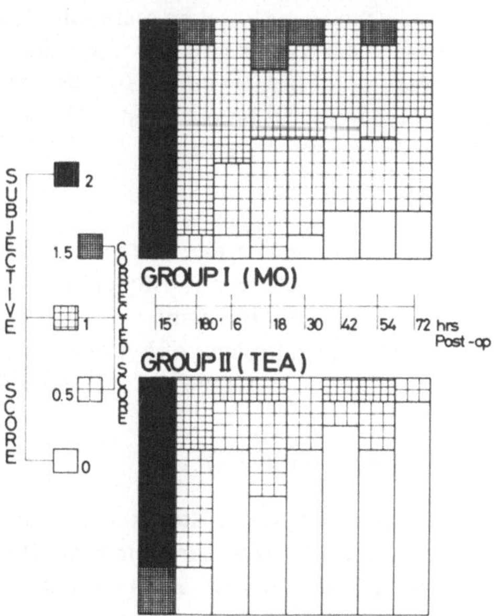

Fig. 8. Corrected pain scores in Groups I and II. The latter were comparable to those of Groups IVA and V

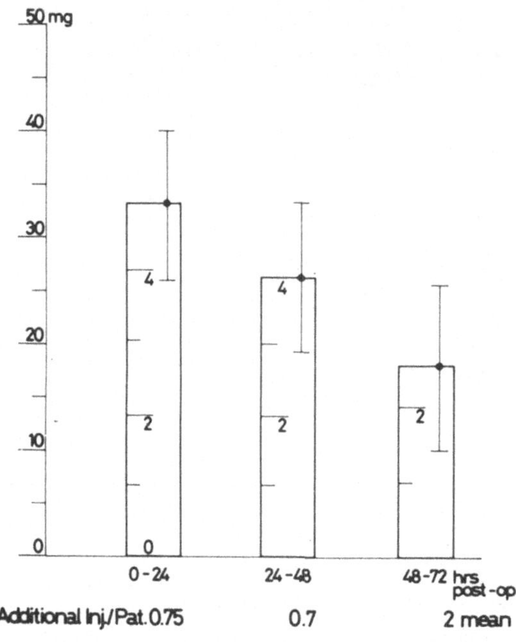

Fig. 9. Dosage of ketobemidon in mg/24 h and doses/24 h, $\bar{x} \pm s_{\bar{x}}$ in Group I. The number of injections and the single dosage is given inside the columns

Complications and Side-Effects

While the main side-effect in the morphine group (I) were the above mentioned lack of cooperation and a tendency to retain secretions, favoured by cough depression and breathing at low constant tidal volumes, the TEA patients also had a number of problems, which, however, usually were not of clinical importance and easy to manage.

One mild intoxication occurred in Group IIIA (the lidocaine continuous infusion group).

Hypotension (Table 4)

Mild or moderate hypotension was seen somewhat more often after epidural analgesia than after morphine-like analgesics, mostly at ambulation. It was, however, usually self-limiting; vasoconstrictor drugs had seldom and with decreasing frequency to be given and ambulation was almost never delayed because of hypotension. Paresis of lower extremity muscles was seen twice in Group II, but disappeared after reduction of dosage.

Urinary Retention (Table 5)

A common problem after postoperative epidural analgesia, even when only the upper thoracic segments are blocked, is urinary retention. It also occurred, to a lesser extent, in our morphine treated patients. Fortunately, most patients do not need a permanent urinary catheter, one single catheterisation is often enough and we were never forced to stop epidural analgesia because of urinary retention problems.

Table 4. Hypotension after pain medication. Comparison of Groups I and IVA. Mild or moderate hypotension was seen in both groups, somewhat more often in Group IVA, with decreasing frequency during the first, second and third 24 h periods. Ephedrine in doses of 25 or 50 mg sc was given on a few occasions, when the systolic blood pressure had not sponteneously risen to 100 mmHg within 10 min.

Group	$RR_{Syst.}$ (mmHg)	0-24 h	24-48 h	48-72 h
MO (I)	< 100 < 90	9 x (5 Patients) 2 x (1 Patient)	5 x (2 Patients) -- --	3 x (2 Patients) -- --
n = 10	Ephedrine (doses)	2	1	2
TEA (IVA)	< 100 < 90	12 x (6 Patients) 2 x (1 Patient)	1 x (1 Patient) -- --	2 x (2 Patients) -- --
n = 10	Ephedrine (doses)	3	1	1

Table 5. Comparison of the urinary retention between Groups I and IVA and the number of catheterisations. Urinary retention was seen rather often in Group IVA, but with decreasing frequency during the first, second and third 24 h periods. Urinary retention was also seen in Group I, perhaps because most of our patients were at an age where prostatic hypertrophy can occur

Group	0-24 h	24-48 h	48-72 h
MO (I) n = 10	2 x (2 Patients)	2 x (2 Patients)	2 x (1 Patient)
TEA (IVA) n = 10	7 x (7 Patients)	3 x (2 Patients)	1 x (1 Patient)

Tachyphylaxie

Under two conditions tachyphylaxie was evident. Firstly, during the second and third 24-h-periods, the number of blocked segments decreased when the same dose of the local anesthetic agent was given (Table 6). In Group IV patients it was, however, always possible to compensate for this phenomenon by increasing the dose from 1 ml/segment to 1.2 or 1.5 ml/segment.

Secondly, marked signs of tachyphylaxis were seen in Group IIIA when the continuous administration of lidocaine into the epidural space was used. In Fig. 10 the dosages of lidocaine needed for a rather unsatisfactory analgesia by continuous drip infusion are compared to those given for a better analgesia by intermittent injections. According to our experience, continuous drip infusions into the epidural space are not suitable for pain relief after thoracic surgery.

Discussion

One main factor in the etiology of early postoperative hypoxaemia, predisposing to postoperative pulmonary complications, is the reduction in FRC, caused by pain, muscle spasms and, may be, by the side-effects of centrally acting analgesics. Generally, the aim of postoperative pain treatment is simply to give the patient subjective pain relief. It must be stressed, that it is

Table 6. The number of blocked segments in Group IV, 2-72 h postoperatively with the same dose, decreased steadily, so the doses had to be increased after 24 h from 1 ml/segment to 1.2 up to 1.5 ml/segment. This phenomenon is believed to be a sign of tachyphylaxis

Hours Postoperatively	2	10	24	36	48	60	72
Segments	8.7 ±0.3	7.4 ±0.4	7.1 ±0.4	7.1[a] ±0.4	7.2[a] ±0.3	6.9[a] ±0.7	6.8 ±0.3
Number Of Patients With Increased Dosage (+ 2 ml/Dose)	--	--	--	2	5	7	7

[a] Increased Dosage

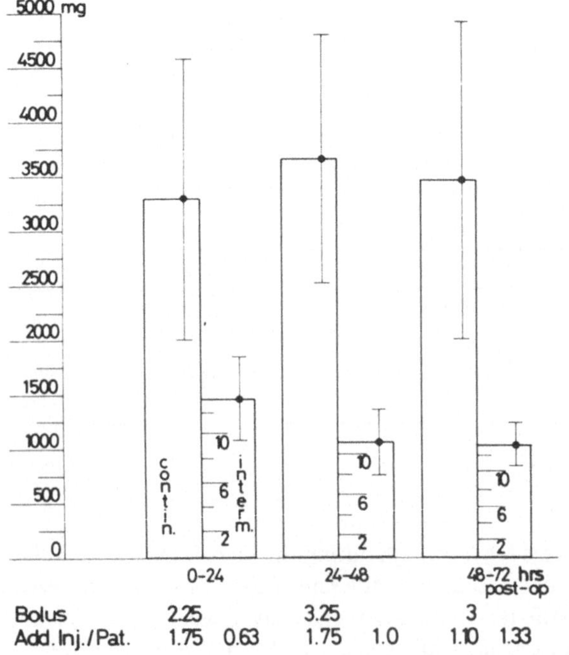

Fig. 10. Dosage of 1% lidocaine (mg/24 h and doses/24 h; $\bar{x} \pm s_{\bar{x}}$) in Group IIIA (lefthand column shows the continuous infusion) and Group IIIB (righthand columns shows the number of single doses given intermittently)

even more important to treat the objective consequences of pain, and primarily, to restore as soon as possible normal FRC.

For this purpose, centrally acting analgesics are not very effective. Epidural analgesia is not ideal, its RRF is less than 100, but it is the most effective treatment known. For practical reasons it is not suitable for routine use, except in intensive care units. It is to be recommended for high risk patients after thoracic and upper abdominal surgery. We have used this method for more than 250 patients for up to 22 days and we have seen no major complications. The method can be considered save, when the following requirements are met:

1. The epidural space in the center of the segments to be blocked should be punctured. The dosage can thereby be reduced and the risk of toxic reactions and of side-effects like hypotension is diminished.

2. A long-acting local anaesthetic agent with low toxicity and in a suitable concentration to achieve sensory block without impairment of motor function should be used. According to our experience, bupivacaine with adrenaline in a 0.375% solution is a highly suitable agent; the results using 1% etidocaine are nearly as good. The mixture of 0.5% bupivacaine with adrenaline and 3% 2-chloro-procaine (2/1) is advantageous only because of its short onset time and if tachyphylaxis becomes a serious problem; motor function however, seems to be adversely affected.
3. The method should only be used when careful supervision of the patients can be guaranteed, e.g. in an intensive care unit, or with specially trained nursing staff.
4. The anaesthesiologist should be well experienced and familiar with the techniques for epidural puncture.

Zusammenfassung

In einer randomisierten Studie an 70 Patienten nach elektiver Lungenchirurgie wird der Verlauf von P_aO_2, P_aCO_2, A-a DO_2 und der PEFR während 72 Stunden postoperativ untersucht. Die Patienten der Gruppe I erhielten zur Schmerzbehandlung das Morphinderivat Ketobemidon. Die übrigen 6 Gruppen erhielten eine thorakale Epidural-Analgesie (Th 5/Th 6) mit verschiedenen Lokalanästhetika (II: Etidocain 1%, IIIA: Lidocain kontinuierlich, IIIB: Lidocain intermittierend, IVA: Bupivacain 0.375% mit Adrenalin, Start postoperativ, IVB: Bupivacain 0.375%, Start intraoperativ, V: Mischung Bupivacain 0.5% und 2-Chloroprocain 3% im Verhältnis 2/1).

Die subjektive Wirkung der Analgesiemethoden wurde nach einem „Schmerz-Score" bewertet.

1 Stunde postoperativ unter Schmerzwirkung zeigte sich bei allen Patienten eine ausgeprägte Hypoxämie (P_aO_2-Abfall um 23.9 mmHg), bei Normokapnie und eine Abnahme der PEFR auf 23.3% des Ausgangswertes.

2 Stunden postoperativ nach der ersten Schmerzbehandlung und während der folgenden 72 Stunden normalisierten sich alle Parameter in den TEA-Gruppen II-V (mit Ausnahme von IIIA) signifikant schneller als in Gruppe I (Ketobemidon).

Auch in der subjektiven und klinischen Wertung war die Schmerzbehandlung mit thorakaler Epidural-Analgesie der mit Ketobemidon deutlich überlegen.

Die postoperative Epidural-Analgesie wird als wertvolle Alternative zur Schmerzbehandlung für Patienten mit erhöhtem Risiko, vor allem nach zwerchfellnahen Operationen, betrachtet.

References

1. Alexander JI, Spence AA (1973) Apparent improvement in postoperative lung volumes by using the Entonox apparatus. Br J Anaesth 45:90
2. Alexander JI, Spence AA, Parikh RK, Stuart B (1973) The role of airway closure in postoperative hypoxemia. Br J Anaesth 45:34
3. Bromage PR (1955) Spirometry in assessment of analgesia after abdominal surgery. A method of comparing analgesic drugs. Br Med J II:589
4. Collins CD, Darke CS, Knowelden J (1968) Chest complications after upper abdominal surgery: Their anticipation and prevention. Br Med J I:401
5. Ellison LT, Duke JF, Strickland GW (1966) Oxygen requirements in the early postoperative period (48 hours) ventilation and respiratory exchange. Ann Surg 163:559
6. Parbrook GD (1966) Post-operative pain relief: Comparison of methadone and morphine, when used concurrently with nitrous-oxide analgesia. Br Med J II:616
7. Stein M, Cassara EL (1970) Preoperative pulmonary evaluation and therapy for surgery patients. JAMA 211:787

Diskussion

Frage: May I make a comment on your results in that I agree with the restoration of lung function in patients who had both epidural anesthesia intraoperatively and the epidural analgesia postoperatively?
Naumann: I think that it is known that after surgery under epidural anesthesia the lung volumes are unchanged as long as the epidural block is effective. The lung volumes decrease and the arterio-alveolar oxygen differences increase from the moment the block becomes ineffective.

Modifying Effects of Anaesthesia on the Postoperative Pulmonary Function in Patients Undergoing an Aorto-Femoral Bypass Operation. Comparison Between Neuroleptanaesthesia, Halothane, and Continuous Thoracic Epidural Anaesthesia

H.J. Wüst, E. Godehardt, D. Günter, W. Sandmann und L. Zumfelde

Impairments of the pulmonary function after upper abdominal surgery in high risk patients are the most common complications. In 60%-70% of these cases a hypoxaemia complicates the postoperative course [11, 16].

It has been shown that pulmonary complications can be prevented by the use of continuous epidural anaesthesia for postoperative pain release [9, 11]. However the effects of the anaesthetic techniques – neuroleptanaesthesia (NLA), halothane and continuous epidural anaesthesia – in combination with the acute intraoperative haemodilution on the postoperative pulmonary function have not yet been discussed in detail.

Therefore the effects of three standard anaesthetic regimen and acute haemodilution on the incidence of postoperative pulmonary complications were studied.

Patients and Methods

For this purpose 68 patients, classified in risk groups I-IV (ASA), were anaesthetised in a randomized order either with neuroleptanaesthesia Type II, halothane or continuous thoracic epidural anaesthesia in combination with diazepam sleep. The patients were undergoing aorto-femoral bypass (AFB) operations.

Apart from the specific drugs necessary for the anaesthetic technique (for details see Table 1), all patients were treated in the same way.

Table 1. Aorto-femoral bypass operation – duration of operation and medication in the three anaesthetic groups

Number		NLA 23	SD	Halothane 22	SD	Epidural 23	SD
Duration of anaesthesia	h	5.45	± 0.99	5.47	± 1.18	4.97	± 1.07
DHBP Induction	mg/kg	0.18	± 0.02				
Fentanyl total	mg/kg	0.049	± 0.013				
Hexobarbital inducation	mg/kg			4.667	± 2.24		
Diazepam total	mg/kg					0.981	± 0.31
Succinylcholine induction	mg/kg	1.0		1.0		1.0	
Pancuronium total	mg/kg	0.205	± 0.054	0.186	± 0.05		
Halothane	vol% vapor			0.91	± 0.54		

After endotracheal intubation the patients were ventilated artificially with 108.4 ± 9.4 ml/min/kg. The $F_I O_2$ was 0.5. For fluid replacement 4200 ml isotonic electrolyte solutions and 2000 ml blood and protein solutions were infused. After a mean duration of 317 min under anaesthesia the patients were extubated in the operating theatre. For postoperative pain release a sensory epidural analgesia between T_5 and L_3 was started 4-5 h after the end of operation. 8 ml bupivacaine 0.125% was injected via a preoperatively introduced epidural catheter, lying between the eight and ninth thoracic interspinal spaces. The analgesia was maintained by a continuous injection (perfusor Braun-Melsungen) of 6-11 ml/h bupivacaine 0.125%.

The physical examination of the pulmonary function [4], namely FVC and FEV_1 measurements and arterial pH and blood gas analyses, were made prior to operation. On the first, second and third days after the operation the control of blood gases was repeated. An X-ray of the chest was also taken before the operation and routinely on the first, second and third postoperative days.

After the operation the patients received no oxygen treatment. Only if hypoxaemia was evident, i.e. if the postoperative arterial PO_2 was lower than 70% of the preoperative control, did we increase the inspiratory oxygen concentration. Therefore, we took for each patient a quotient between the preoperative control and the arterial PO_2 on the first and second postoperative days, referred to as PO_2 Qu_1 and PO_2 Qu_2 in the following. In patients whose $F_I O_2$ was 0.4 or more the quotient was censored to 0.7. For the initial examination the Wilcoxon, Man-Whitney test was used.

Results

Blood Gases

On the morning of the first postoperative day the inspiratory oxygen concentration had to be increased in 10 of 23 patients after NLA and in 6 of 23 patients after epidural anaesthesia. In the halothane group 7 of 22 patients needed this treatment. The PO_2 quotient was censored to 0.7 in these patients.

While the median of the PO_2 quotient changed after epidural and halothane anaesthesia by 12% on the first postoperative day, it decreased after NLA by 28% (Table 2). It increased only slightly on the second postoperative day.

Table 2. Medians of the PO_2 $quotient_1$ and $quotient_2$ $\frac{\text{preop. Pa } O_2}{\text{postop. Pa } O_2}$

Number	NLA 23	SD	Halothane 20	SD	Epidural 23	SD
Q_1 1st postop. day	0.715	± 0.145	0.897	± 0.134	0.871	± 0.179
Q_2 2nd postop. day	0.7564	± 0.203	0.8854	± 0.1542	0.8815	± 0.1968

The sums of ranks in the Wilcoxon, Man-Whitney test showed a significantly lower arterial PO_2 on the first postoperative day after NLA (($p < 0.05$), (Table 3)). At the same time there

Table 3. Aorta-femoral operation – Sums of ranks $\frac{\text{preop. } PO_2}{\text{postop. } PO_2}$

	Epidural	NLA
Number	23	23
Sums of ranks	619	462*
	Halothane	**NLA**
n	20	23
Sums of ranks	516	430*

* $p < 0.05$

was a significantly higher PCO_2 of 42 ± 5 torr in the NLA group compared with 36 ± 4 torr in the other two groups.

Findings in the Chest X-ray

Corresponding to the hypoxaemia after NLA 16 of 23 patients showed infiltrations of 1-3 lobes in the chest X-ray. After halothane and epidural anaesthesia 7 and 5 patients respectively showed a pathological infiltration (Table 4). The reason for this can be seen in the amounts of cristalloid solutions given (Table 5).

Table 4. Findings in the chest X-ray on the first postoperative day

	NLA	Halothane	Epidural
Number	23	22	23
Infiltrations	16	7	5
Normal	7	15	18

Table 5. Aorta-femoral operation – Infiltrations in the chest X-ray in relation to infusion therapy

	X-ray	No.	Cristalloid Solutions ml sd	Volume Replacement ml sd
NLA	Normal	7	3217 ± 973	1417 ± 492
	Infiltrations	16	4218 ± 1354	2382 ± 756
Halothane	Normal	15	4061 ± 1182	2007 ± 674
	Infiltrations	7	3163 ± 2284	2663 ± 666
Epidural	Normal	18	4414 ± 1330	1956 ± 607
	Infiltrations	5	5512 ± 1564	2100 ± 652

The patients operated under epidural anaesthesia, tolerated the highest amount of electrolyte solutions and blood replacement without any pathological findings in the chest X-ray. After NLA the patients showed infiltrations after the same infusion and transfusion volume and only if these patients were less infused and transfused, could no pathology in the chest X-ray be cited.

The high standard deviation and low mean value of the cristalloid solution in the patients with infiltrations under halothane anaesthesia was caused by three patients. They needed sympatho-mimetic drugs intraoperatively, because of haemodynamic difficulties.

Discussion

In this prospective randomized study a significant influence of the anaesthetics on the incidence of postoperative pulmonary complications was found. Thus the decrease in arterial PO_2 by 28% and the infiltrations in the chest X-ray, seen in 16 of 23 patients on the first postoperative day after NLA, indicated a higher rate of complications than in the other two groups of patients, undergoing reconstructions of the abdominal aorta under halothane or continuous epidural anaesthesia. In these groups the arterial PO_2 decreased by 10% and 13% respectively and only 7 and 5 patients respectively showed infiltrations in the chest X-ray.

These results are in accordance with those of other investigators, who showed that the postoperative pulmonary function is maintained better after regional anaesthetic techniques than after general anaesthesia [7]. However, in contrast to the present investigation their patients were awake and spontaneously breathing.

Hypoxaemia after general anaesthesia has been attributed to changes of the pulmonary function due to controlled ventilation [2, 10]. From this Spence et al. [11] suggested that the beneficial effects of regional anaesthetic techniques on the postoperative pulmonary function were inhibited by artificially controlling ventilation. This point of view was not supported in the present study.

While Thompson et al. [12, 13] could not show any effect of the intraoperatively fluid regimen on the postoperative pulmonary function, the infiltration rate in the chest X-rays of our patients is related to the amount of cristalline solutions infused intraoperatively. Thus the tolerance to this treatment was lower in the NLA than in the epidural group and somewhat lower than in the halothane group. But in 7 patients of the latter group pathological findings occurred with a more restrictive fluid regimen. In 3 of these patients anaesthesia was complicated by a myocardial insufficiency.

NLA was recommended as the anaesthetic method of choice in respiratory risk patients by other investigators, who did not find any residual effects of the narcotic fentanyl on respiration in the immediate postoperative period [3, 5, 8].

In contrast to this the arterial PCO_2 in the present series of NLA indicated the long lasting effect of fentanyl on spontaneous respiration. It should be noted, however, that in the present study larger doses of fentanyl were used than in the previous reports. This might explain the different results.

Conclusion

After neuroleptanaesthesia Type II a higher incidence of postoperative pulmonary complications and a lower PO_2 was found than after epidural and halothane anaesthesia. These poor results in the present series under NLA were attributed to the intraoperative haemodilution and to the residual depressant effects of fentanyl on respiration.

References

1. Beecher HK (1933) Effect of laparatomy on lung volume. Demonstration of a new type of pulmonary collapse. J Clin Invest 12:651
2. Bendixen HH, Hedley-Whyte J, Laver MB (1963) Impaired oxygenation in surgical patients during general anesthesia with controlled ventilation. N Eng J Med 269:991
3. Bergmann H (1967) Indikation und Kontraindikation zur Neuroleptanalgesie. Wien Med Wochenschr 117:673
4. Bromage PR (1955) Spirometry in assessment of analgesia after abdominal surgery. Br Med J II:589
5. Gemperle M, Grueninger B (1964) Blutgasanalyse nach Neuroleptanalgesie Typ II. Anaesthesist 13:6
6. Hansen G, Drabloes PA, Steinert R (1977) Pulmonary complications, ventilation and blood gases after upper abdominal surgery. Acta Anaesthesiol Scand 21:211
7. Helms U, Weihrauch H (1977) Veränderungen der Blutgase und des Säurebasen-Haushaltes in der frühen postoperativen Phase nach Leitungs- und Intubationsnarkose. Prakt Anaesth 12:259
8. Hollmen A, Hakalehto J, Lauritsalo K, Mattila MAK (1966) A comparison of postoperative acid-base-equilibrium and respiratory adequacy after two types of neuroleptanalgesia. Br J Anaesth 38:191
9. Muneyuki M, Ueda J, Urabe N, Takashita H, Inamoto A (1968) Postoperative pain relief and respiratory function in man: Comparison between intermittent intravenous injections of meperidine and continuous lumbar epidural analgesia. Anesthesiology 29:304
10. Nunn JF (1967) Hypoxaemia after general anaesthesia. Lancet II:631
11. Spence AA, Smith G (1971) Postoperative analgesia and lung function: A comparison of morphine with extradural block. Br J Anaesth 43:144
12. Thompson JE, Vollmar RW, Austin DJ, Kartchner MM (1968) Prevention of hypotensive and renal complications of aortic surgery using balanced salt solution. Thirteen-year experience with 670 cases. Ann Surg 167:767
13. Thompson JE, Hollier LH, Patman RD, Perssen AV (1975) Surgical management of abdominal aortic aneurysms: Factors influencing mortality and morbidity – A 20-year experience. Ann Surg 181:654

Diskussion

Frage: Wie erklären Sie den Unterschied zwischen der NLA-Gruppe und der Halothangruppe. Sind die Patienten völlig in Ruhe gelassen worden nach der Operation?

Wüst: Nein. Die Ärzte und Schwestern auf der Intensivstation wußten nicht Bescheid, welche Narkose durchgeführt worden war. Das hat zwar teilweise zu sehr großen Verwirrungen geführt. Es wurden teilweise Narkoseverfahren für Veränderungen angeschuldigt, die sie gar nicht hervorgerufen hatten; aber dadurch wurde gewährleistet, daß die postoperative physikalische Therapie bei allen Patienten einheitlich durchgeführt wurde. Sie begann, sobald die Patienten wach und kooperativ waren, mit einem zweistündlichen Aufsitzen und Abhusten, zweistündlichen Atemübungen mit der Blasflasche und einer dreimal täglichen Inhalationstherapie. Außerdem wurden die Patienten ab dem Morgen des 1. postoperativen Tages dreimal für je eine halbe Stunde auf die Bettkante bzw. in den Sessel gesetzt.

Frage: Gibt es irgendwelche Erklärungsmöglichkeiten unabhängig jetzt von den postoperativen Maßnahmen für diese Unterschiede zwischen Halothan- und Neuroleptanaesthesie?

Wüst: Wie ich im Vortrag gestern ausgeführt habe, kommt es ja zu einer Druck- und Widerstandsentlastung während der Halothan-Narkose und das kann, obwohl das Blutvolumen sich gegenüber praeoperativ nicht geändert hat, eine Ursache sein. Eine weitere mögliche Erklärung ist die Tatsache, daß unter Neuroleptanaesthesie die Pulmonalisdrucksteigerung höher ausfällt als in den anderen Narkoseverfahren.

The Benefits of Intraoperative Epidural Anaesthesia Prolonged into the Postoperative Period with Main Emphasis on Pulmonary Function

J. Modig

While improved methods of anaesthesia during surgery have reached a high degree of reliability with minimal disturbance of physiological functions intraoperatively, the relief of pain in the postoperative period has not developed to the same level. Postoperative pain relief is a badly neglected facet of surgical care, and the fact that centrally-acting analgesics – prescribed in a stereotyped pattern – still comprise the method most widely used only reflects lack of interest in pain relief and unfamiliarity with nerve-blocking techniques.

It has long been known that after surgery patients have arterial oxygen tensions that are lower than their preoperative values [7, 15, 35, 37, 43]. Such hypoxaemia may persist for several days after surgery [26, 37, 38], and has been attributed to a failure adequately to aerate the lungs [4, 6]. However, studies have shown, using chest radiography alone, that no evidence of atelectasis can be found even when the arterial oxygenation is severely impaired [3, 17]. Considerable evidence has accumulated pointing to a disturbance of the relation between lung ventilation and perfusion. This means that in some parts of the lungs – preferentially the dependent regions – the ventilation to alveoli is low or zero, while the perfusion is intact.

This postoperative impairment of ventilatory function is dependent upon several factors, such as the site and extent of surgery. A reduction in arterial oxygen tension is to be expected after thoracic or abdominal surgery, due to mechanical interference with ventilation, but it may also follow peripheral limb surgery [11]. Thus after surgery there is a reduction in functional residual capacity, which is more pronounced following upper abdominal than lower abdominal or peripheral limb surgery [1]. Major interference with ventilatory mechanics may also be caused by the intraoperative anaesthetic technique. Thus Renck [39] found that in patients undergoing transvesical prostatectomy under general anaesthesia there was a significant impairment of the peak expiratory flow rate within 1 h after operation, compared with patients under lumbar epidural or spinal anaesthesia. From Renck's study it was further shown that patients given lumbar epidural or spinal anaesthesia did not react with a decrease in PaO_2 immediately after the operation, in contrast to patients given intraoperative general anaesthesia, who had a significant PaO_2 decrease. Similar findings concerning ventilatory and blood-gas data have been made by Wulff et al. [47], who noted a significant decrease in functional residual capacity and PaO_2 after total hip replacement performed under general anaesthesia, but not following hip arthroplasty under lumbar epidural analgesia. Impairment in arterial oxygenation after various surgical procedures performed under general anaesthesia, in contrast to those under spinal or epidural anaesthesia, has also been reported by other authors [44]. Thus in the early postoperative period muscle power and ventilatory ability may be impaired by the residual effects of muscle relaxants potentiated by the depression of the central nervous system induced by the anaesthetic drugs or the inhalation anaesthetics. This is in sharp contrast to the situation in patients given intraoperative epidural or spinal anaesthesia, who remain conscious and alert with no or only minor respiratory muscle impairment and thus better alveolar ventilation. Another important cause of ventilatory derangement in patients operated on under general anaesthesia is the reduction in functional residual capacity [19, 27], which probably predisposes to alveolar closure and atelectasis in the postoperative course. Such a reduction is not seen following induction of epidural analgesia [29, 45]. A number of other factors may also impede the ventilatory mechanics and functional residual capacity in the postoperative patient. These include the supine posture, restrictive bandaging, and a distended abdomen due to bowel distension and pneumoperitoneum. Further, increasing age, heavy smoking, preexisting lung disease, obesity, a postoperative naso-gastric tube or postoperative wound infection are predisposing factors for pulmonary complications [18].

Pain, especially after upper abdominal surgery, is a potent cause of decreased respiratory performance. Pain causes spasm of the abdominal muscles. This results in a rapid shallow type of breathing and reluctance to take deep breaths, and coughing tends to be suppressed, with retention of bronchial secretions and eventually atelectasis. Centrally-acting analgesics used for postoperative pain relief reduce the pain subjectively, but give only a minor or no increase in ventilatory performance. Epidural nerve blockade, unlike narcotics, provides complete analgesia without depression of the central nervous system and thus facilitates better lung expansion [5, 40]. Epidural analgesia used for postoperative pain relief has two important advantages over other nerve-blocking techniques: (1) it can be repeated intermittently or given continuously trough a catheter thus maintaining a constant analgesic state [16] and (2) it can be given at the appropriate segments to relieve both somatic and visceral pain.

Sjögren and Wright [41] studied the physiological effects of continuous epidural anaesthesia with both the thoracic and lumbar techniques for postoperative pain relief in cholecystectomised patients. In a representative period of analgesia on the first day after surgery the following changes were noted compared with the preoperative measurements. Dynamic tests of ventilatory capacity such as forced vital capacity and forced expiratory volume in 1 s showed, on average, a 50% decrease. During postoperative pain when the epidural drip was discontinued, the ventilatory function deteriorated further by about 20% compared with the pain-free state. Similar detrimental effects of pain after upper abdominal surgery on the functional residual capacity and vital capacity, and variable restoration towards normal preoperative values following induction of epidural analgesia, have been reported by other authors [5, 40, 46]. Sjögren and Wright [41] also found that the arterial oxygen tension was only moderately decreased, by about 11%, in the pain-free state on the morning after surgery. This is in agreement with the finding of Spence and Smith [42] of a decrease in PaO_2 of about 13% on the first day after upper abdominal surgery in patients given thoracic epidural blockade for postoperative pain relief. In another group of their patients treated with conventional doses of morphine by IM injection on demand, a more pronounced fall in PaO_2 of 25% was observed. Of special interest in their study was that hypoxaemia still persisted on the fifth postoperative day in patients receiving morphine, in sharp contrast to those treated with epidural blockade. Muneyuki et al. [34] noted a significant improvement in PaO_2 on the first day after upper abdominal surgery when an epidural blockade was given for pain relief, while the reverse was found, with a significant decrease in PaO_2, when pain was treated with narcotics.

It is of special interest in this context to extract certain data from the report of Hollmén and Saukkonen [24] on patients undergoing cholecystectomy. In the immediate postoperative period, when the patient began to complain of pain, this was relieved with either parenteral analgesics or thoracic epidural blockade. In the former group a significant drop in PaO_2 occurred due to a low ventilation/perfusion ratio; while the true shunt, i.e. perfusion of non-ventilated alveoli, remained unchanged. Miller et al. [32], who also examined patients after cholecystectomy, found that pain relieved with an epidural blockade resulted in a significantly greater vital capacity 3-4 h postoperatively compared with parenteral analgesics. This early difference in ventilatory mechanics probably led to the significantly higher PaO_2 and lower $PaCO_2$ in the epidural group observed on the morning after surgery, compared with the narcotic group.

In order to study more closely the postoperative differences in arterial oxygenation between two types of analgesic regimens used for postoperative pain relief, Modig [33] investigated 31 cardio-respiratorily healthy patients with a mean age of 62.5 years subjected to total hip replacement under continuous lumbar epidural analgesia. Such hypoxaemia-predisposing factors as direct mechanical interference with ventilation caused by the surgical procedure, and general anaesthesia, were thus eliminated, permitting an investigation of the exclusive influence of continuous lumbar epidural analgesia versus parenteral analgesics on postoperative arterial oxygenation.

The intraoperative epidural analgesia was maintained until the first postoperative measurement period, about 2.5 h after surgery. The patients were subsequently divided into three groups. One group comprised 10 patients who were given pentazocine (Fortalgesic) IM, on demand, for analgesia. A second group (plain lidocaine) of 14 and a third group (lidocaine with adrenaline: 4 μg/ml) of 7 patients received continuous lumbar epidural analgesia for 3 days via an epidural catheter; for this 0.4% lidocaine (Xylocain) was given as a drip infusion [16]. The continuous drip infusion, which was preceded by a single injection of 2% lidocaine, was administered by an infusion pump, and the upper level of analgesia extended, on average, to the tenth thoracic segment. Occasionally supplementary injections of 2% lidocaine were given in addition to the continuous infusion to maintain the level of analgesia.

All patients were nursed semi-recumbent in a 30° head-up position, and had the same type of chest and limb physiotherapy twice a day postoperatively. In order to achieve almost complete postoperative pain relief, with better cooperation in the routine limb exercise programme, the pentazocine-treated patients were given rather large doses of analgesics, especially at the time when the epidural blockade wore off. Complete and constant pain relief, which still left the patient alert, cooperative and with almost unaffected motor function in the legs, was obtained in the epidural groups.

No notable changes were found in PaO_2 2.5 h after operation (Fig. 1). This confirms the observation by other authors [39, 47] that epidural analgesia used for different kinds of surgery – where control of ventilation is not essential – does not cause a decrease in arterial oxygenation. PaO_2 was, however, significantly influenced by the type of analgesic regimen used in the later postoperative period. Patients treated with a continuous epidural blockade throughout the first 3 days postoperatively did not have any decrease in arterial oxygenation (see Fig. 1), thus differing significantly from the pentazocine-treated patients. In this age group the latter type of analgesic regimen caused a highly significant decrease in PaO_2 which persisted throughout days 1-3. On the 7th day after surgery when the patients had been actively mobilized and no analgesics were needed, PaO_2 returned to the preoperative level. In patients given an epidural blockade the $PaCO_2$ values tended to lie in the hyperventilatory range postoperatively contrary to those receiving parenteral analgesics (see Fig. 1), in whom they lay in the normal range. Hollmén and Saukkonen [23] made essentially the same findings concerning $PaCO_2$ in patients subjected to transvesical prostatectomy under lumbar epidural analgesia prolonged into the postoperative period.

The breathing pattern in the pentazocine and epidural groups differed. Patients in the epidural groups had greater tidal volumes and lower respiratory frequencies after surgery than those in the "narcotic" group. Further, in the nitrogen-washout curves (during true shunt determinations), occasional spontaneous deep breaths were observed in patients who were given an epidural blockade, but these were absent in patients receiving pentazocine. Elimination of the sigh mechanism after parenteral analgesics has also been reported by other authors [13].

The significant decrease in PaO_2 in the pentazocine group during the first 3 days postoperatively was due to the highly significant increase in total venous admixture – which includes

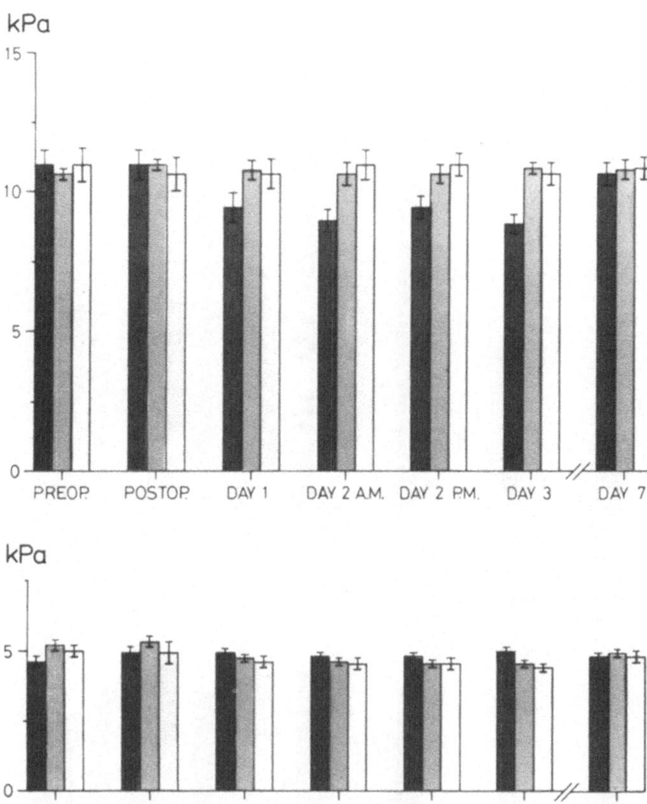

Fig. 1. Above, PaO_2 (kPa; mean ± SE), and below, $PaCO_2$ (kPa; mean ± SE) during the different measurement periods in three groups of patients. One group was given pentazocine IM on demand (n = 10; dark columns), while the other two groups received continuous epidural blockade with 0.4% lidocaine with (n = 7; light columns) or without (n = 14; medium coloured columns) adrenaline

the true shunt and the shunt-like effect resulting from a low ventilation/perfusion ratio (Fig. 2). By subtracting the true shunt (which was also significantly increased in these patients in days 1-3) from the total venous admixture [20], it was found that about 50% of the total venous admixture was due to the shunt-like effect of a low ventilation/perfusion ratio. No significant changes were observed either in total venous admixture or in true shunt in patients given continuous epidural analgesia during the first 3 postoperative days. Thus, during these days the total venous admixture was significantly greater in patients receiving pentazocine than in those who were given an epidural blockade. An important reason for this difference was the low ventilation/perfusion ratio found in the "narcotic" group. Better postoperative oxygenation of arterial blood due to a more even distribution of the ventilation in relation to perfusion in the lung has also been observed by Hollmén and Saukkonen [22] in patients given epidural analgesia, compared with those treated with narcotics.

Airway closure [12, 31] explains the nature of the two shunt components, i.e. that due to atelectatic but perfused alveoli, and that due to alveoli underventilated in relation to perfusion. It occurs when the net forces acting on small airways are sufficiently strong to induce their collapse; and the lung volume at which airway closure starts to occur is called for con-

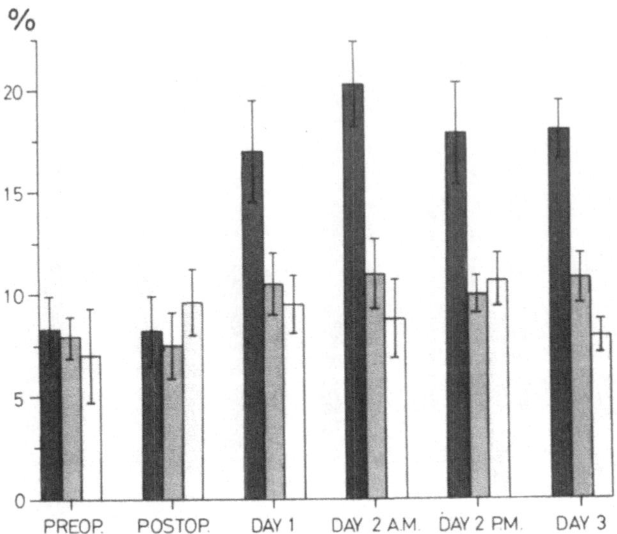

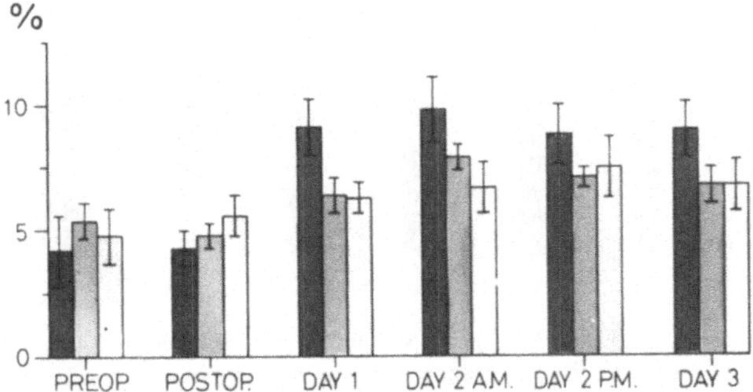

Fig. 2. Above, total pulmonary venous admixture (%; mean ± SE), and below, "true" pulmonary shunting (%; mean ± SE) during the different measurement periods in the three groups of patients. Symbols as in Fig. 1

venience the "closing capacity". In normal young subjects airway closure occurs only at lung volumes well below the functional residual capacity. Decreasing elastic properties and loss of airway integrity, as in heavy cigarette smoking, bronchitis and in the ageing lung, explain the observation of increased airway closure resulting in a closing capacity exceeding the functional residual capacity [2, 8, 21, 28]. Factors reducing the functional residual capacity, such as obesity, a supine posture, abdominal distension, or spasm of the abdominal muscles caused by pain, also make the closing capacity exceed the functional residual capacity.

In patients who were given regular injections of pentazocine the chest radiographs showed a "high diaphragm", which was not the case in the epidural groups. This difference was probably due to the inhibitory effect of pentazocine on the gastro-intestinal motility, causing bowel distension [10], whereas epidural blockade has a stimulating effect on gastro-intestinal propulsion [14] due to the sympathetic blockade and increased vagal tone [36]. The high position of the diaphragm interferes considerably with the respiratory mechanics, especially in elderly, semi-recumbent patients, resulting in a further decrease in functional residual capacity and significant airway closure during parts of or throughout the respiratory cycle. Airway closure occurs initially in the dependent lung regions, as the intrapleural pressure becomes progressively higher down the lung [9]. Since the same regions are the most richly perfused, airway closure profoundly influences the arterial oxygen tension. Patients given epidural blockade had a greater functional residual capacity and also a larger tidal volume, with occasional spontaneous deep breaths, and thus airway closure occurred during only a small part of the respiratory cycle.

Another question of importance is how epidural blockade influences the circulation. On the first day after gall-bladder surgery, when epidural blockade of both the lumbar and thoracic approaches was given for pain relief, Sjögren and Wright [41] found a tendency to a hyperkinetic circulation. That is, cardiac output increased proportionately more than oxygen uptake, which gives a favourable situation of oxygen transport; and this was accomplished without an increase in cardiac work, due to a reduction in total peripheral resistance with a resultant decrease in systemic blood pressure.

Essentially the same circulatory findings were made by Modig [33] in patients subjected to total hip replacement under epidural analgesia prolonged into the postoperative period. Comparisons were made with patients treated with pentazocine for pain relief after surgery. Postoperatively there was a significant increase in cardiac index in both the pentazocine and epidural groups. However, the tendency towards a hyperkinetic circulation was more pronounced in patients given an epidural blockade, which was also manifested in an increased mixed venous oxygen tension in these groups throughout the postoperative study period.

Factors contributing to the larger increase in cardiac index in the epidural groups include a compensatory adjustment due to peripheral vasodilatation caused by the sympathetic blockade, the effects of systemic lidocaine on the circulation [25, 30] and a somewhat larger supply of fluid. The incorporation of adrenaline into the anaesthetic solution has a role of its own. After vascular uptake adrenaline will have a dose-related effect on the cardiovascular dynamics.

The conclusions drawn from the investigations described above concerning especially pulmonary but also circulatory functions thus favour intraoperative epidural analgesia prolonged into the postoperative period as against general anaesthesia and parenteral analgesics, particularly in patients with pre-existing cardiopulmonary disease. Furthermore, when controlled ventilation is essential intraoperatively, epidural blockade is superior to parenteral analgesics postoperatively with respect to both pulmonary and circulatory functions and subjective pain relief.

Summary

Based on a series of physiological investigations the beneficial effects on pulmonary function of intraoperative epidural blockade maintained into the postoperative period, as against intraoperative general anaesthesia with postoperative administration of parenteral analgesics are emphasized. The cardiopulmonary advantages of continuous lumbar epidural blockade as postoperative pain relief after major hip surgery, compared with parenteral analgesics, are described in more detail.

References

1. Alexander JI, Spence AA, Parikh RK, Stuart B (1973) The role of airway closure in postoperative hypoxaemia. Br J Anaesth 45:34
2. Anthonisen NR, Dauson J, Robertson PC, Ross WRD (1969/70) Airway closure as a function of age. Respir Physiol 8:58
3. Bendixen HH, Hedley-Whyte J, Chir B, Laver MB (1963) Impaired oxygenation in surgical patients during general anesthesia with controlled ventilation. A concept of atelectasis. N Engl J Med 269:991
4. Bromage PR (1955) Spirometry in assessment of analgesia after abdominal surgery. A method of comparing analgesic drugs. Br Med J II:589

5. Bromage PR (1967) Extradural analgesia for pain relief. Br. J Anaesth 39:721
6. Cleland JGP (1949) Continuous peridural and caudal analgesia in surgery and early ambulation. Northwest Med (Seattle) 48:26
7. Conway CM, Payne JP (1963) Post-operative hypoxaemia and oxygen therapy. Br Med J I:844
8. Craigh DB, Wahba WM, Don HF, Couture JG, Becklake MR (1971) "Closing volume" and its relationships to gas exchange in seated and supine positions. J Appl Physiol 31:717
9. Daly WJ, Bondhurst S (1963) Direct measurement of respiratory pleural pressure changes in normal man. J Appl Physiol 18:513
10. Danhof JE (1967) Pentazocine effects on gastrointestinal motor functions in man. Am J Gastroenterol 48:295
11. Diament ML, Palmer KNV (1969) Postoperative changes in gas tensions of arterial blood and in ventilatory function. Lancet II:180
12. Dollfuss RE, Milic-Emili J, Bates DV (1967) Regional ventilation of the lung, studied with boluses of ^{133}Xenon. Respir Physiol 2:234
13. Egbert LD, Bendixen HH (1964) Effect of morphine on breathing pattern. A possible factor in atelectasis. JAMA 188:485
14. Gelman S, Feigenberg Z, Dintzman M, Levy E (1977) Electroenterography after cholecystectomy. Arch Surg 112:580
15. Gordh T, Linderholm H, Norlander O (1958) Pulmonary function in relation to anaesthesia and surgery evaluated by analysis of oxygen tension of arterial blood. Acta Anaesthesiol Scand 2:15
16. Green R, Dawkins M (1966) Post-operative analgesia. The use of continuous drip epidural block. Anaesthesia 21:372
17. Hamilton WK, McDonald JS, Fischer HW, Bethards R (1964) Postoperative respiratory complications. A comparison of arterial gas tensions, radiographs and physical examinations. Anesthesiology 25:607
18. Hansen G, Drabløs PA, Steinert R (1977) Pulmonary complications, ventilation and blood gases after upper abdominal surgery. Acta Anaesthesiol Scand 21:211
19. Hedenstierna G, McCarthy G, Bergström M (1976) Airway closure during mechanical ventilation. Anesthesiology 44:114
20. Hedstrand UE, Modig J (1974) Measurement and calculation of pulmonary physiological parameters. Med Progr Technol 3:25
21. Holland J, Milic-Emili J, Macklem PT, Bates DV (1968) Regional distribution of pulmonary ventilation and perfusion in elderly subjects. J Clin Invest 47:81
22. Hollmén A, Saukkonen J (1969) Zur postoperativen Schmerzausschaltung nach Oberbauchoperationen. Narkotica, Intercostalblockade und Epiduralanaesthesie und deren Einfluß auf die Atmung. Anaesthesist 18:298
23. Hollmén A, Saukkonen J (1971) Effect of epidural or general anaesthesia on the arterial acid-base balance, oxygenation and venous admixture in prostatectomy patients. Ann Clin Res 3:168
24. Hollmén A, Saukkonen J (1972) The effects of postoperative epidural analgesia versus centrally acting opiate on physiological shunt after upper abdominal operation. Acta Anaesthesiol Scand 16:147
25. Kao FF, Jalar UH (1959) The central action of lignocaine and its effect on cardiac output. Br J Pharmacol 14:522
26. Knudsen J (1970) Duration of hypoxaemia after uncomplicated upper abdominal and thoraco-abdominal operations. Anaesthesia 25:372
27. Laws AK (1968) Effects of induction of anaesthesia and muscle paralysis on functional residual capacity of the lungs. Can Anaesth Soc J 15:325
28. Leblanc P, Ruff F, Milic-Emili J (1970) Effects of age and body position on "airway closure" in man. J Appl Physiol 28:448
29. McCarthy GS (1976) The effect of thoracic extradural analgesia on pulmonary gas distribution, functional residual capacity and airway closure. Br J Anaesth 48:243
30. McWhirter WR, Schmidt FH, Fredrickson EL, Steinhaus JE (1973) Cardiovascular effects of controlled lidocaine overdosage in dogs anesthetized with nitrous oxide. Anesthesiology 39:398
31. Milic-Emili J, Henderson JAM, Dolovich MB, Trop D, Kaneko K (1966) Regional distribution of inspired gas in the lung. J Appl Physiol 21:749
32. Miller L, Gertel M, Fox GS, MacLean LD (1976) Comparison of effect of narcotic and epidural analgesia on postoperative respiratory function. Am J Surg 131:291
33. Modig J (1976) Respiration and circulation after total hip replacement surgery. A comparison between parenteral analgesics and continuous epidural block. Acta Anaesthesiol Scand 20:225

34. Muneyuki M, Ueda Y, Urabe N, Kato H, Shirai K, Inamoto A (1972) Oxygen breathing and $\dot{Q}_s/\dot{Q}_t$ during postoperative pain relief in man. Can Anaesth Soc J 19:230
35. Nunn JF, Payne JP (1962) Hypoxaemia after general anaesthesia. Lancet II:631
36. Öhrn PG (1976) Postoperative gastrointerstinal propulsion. The role of sympathoadrenal activity studied in the rat. Acta Univ. Upsaliensis Abstracts of Uppsala Dissertations from the Faculty of Medicine. Vol. 242
37. Palmer KNV, Gardiner AJS (1964) Effect of partial gastrectomy on pulmonary physiology. Br Med J 1:347
38. Palmer KNV, Gardiner AJS, McGregor MH (1965) Hypoxaemia after partial gastrectomy. Thorax 20:73
39. Renck H (1969) The elderly patient after anaesthesia and surgery. Acta Anaesthesiol Scand [Suppl] 34
40. Simpson BR, Parkhouse J, Marshall R, Lambrechts W (1961) Extradural analgesia and the prevention of postoperative respiratory complications. Br J Anaesth 33:628
41. Sjögren S, Wright B (1972) Circulation, respiration and lidocaine concentration during continuous epidural blockade. Acta Anaesthesiol Scand [Suppl] 46
42. Spence AA, Smith G (1971) Postoperative analgesia and lung function: A comparison of morphine with extradural block. Br J Anaesth 43:144
43. Stephen CR, Talton J (1965) Hypoxaemia in the postoperative period. JAMA 191:139
44. Thompson DS, Eason CN (1970) Hypoxaemia immediately after operation. Am J Surg 120:649
45. Wahba WM, Craig DB, Don HF, Becklake MR (1972) The cardio-respiratory effects of thoracic epidural anaesthesia. Can Anaesth Soc J 19:8
46. Wahba WM, Don HF, Craig DB (1975) Post-operative epidural analgesia: effects on lung volumes. Can Anaesth Soc J 22:519
47. Wulff K, Arborelius M, Rosberg B (1975) Regional lung function following prosthetic hip replacement surgery. Eur J Intensive Care Med 1:129

Diskussion

Frage: There is one question I would like to address to all speakers. Have you observed any signs of pulmonary congestion or interstitial pulmonary edema when the epidural anesthesia was ended?
Modig: We have not investigated this phenomenon because such studies are extremely difficult. Clinically we have not observed any signs of pulmonary congestion after ending the epidural blockade.

Tachyphylaxis During Postoperative Peridural Analgesia of Long Action

H. Renck

In epidural analgesia (EA) the injection of a local anaesthetic agent is made into an area where the target nerves are entrenched behind the barriers of the dura mater and the pia-arachnoidea; in addition blood flow inflicts heavy losses on the advancing local anaesthetic. In contrast to spinal anaesthesia the resulting effects of local anaesthetics are weak. Further, the possibility of providing prolonged pain relief by means of continuous EA is limited by the tendency for patients to develop a form of tolerance, repeated injections being less effective: the phenomenon of tachyphylaxis. Although tachyphylaxis in EA is a much talked-of phenomenon, comparatively little information can be obtained from current literature.

The purpose of the present paper – based on personal experience and available data – is to summarize:

1. The magnitude of tachyphylaxis in EA,
2. Underlying mechanisms,
3. Modifying factors,
4. Therapeutic suggestions that can reduce its effects in clinical practice.

According to Bromage [3] tachyphylaxis in EA is manifested by a decay in both time and space, so that for a given dose the area of segmental blockade, intensity and duration, diminish in an exponential manner with successive injections. Conventionally [1] segmental spread or [2] segmental spread and duration of the block are employed in the delineation of tachyphylaxis while [3] intensity of the blockade is usually excluded, being difficult to quantify. As will be further discussed, a fourth factor – accumulation of local anaesthetics in the plasma – bears a certain relationship to tachyphylaxis and should therefore be evaluated in parallel with the other three.

Employing various short-acting local anaesthetic agents of the amide type in lumbar epidural analgesia (LEA) Bromage et al. [4] found that in widely spaced injections each dose has to be increased by 25%-30% of the previous one in order to achieve the same spread and duration of the blockade. Using long-acting local anaesthetics of the amide type for prolongation of thoracic epidural analgesia (TEA) evident signs of tachyphylaxis have been noted. During prolongation with 3-5 ml of etidocaine given every 3 h after an initial dose of 5 ml, consecutive reductions of the segmental spread occurred in groups of postoperative patients [12]. During continuous epidural administration of 1.0% bupivacaine by means of a constant injection pump, segmental spread could be maintained by increments of the injection rate but the quality of the blocks deteriorated with time [13]. In that study further dose increments resulted in widened segmental spread but not in any appreciable improvement in the intensity of the blocks. Based on experience (1978) it is suggested that any successful prolongation of TEA with amide type drugs over 24-36 h in postoperative patients is inhibited by the effect of tachyphylaxis. On the other hand, TEA has been prolonged over considerable periods of time in patients with chronic pain with subjectively satisfying results [1; Renck and Skole, 1974, unpublished work].

Tachyphylaxis with local anaesthetics is apparently a phenomenon that exclusively occurs in the intact animal and man [8]. As to the underlying mechanisms there are two hypotheses

[14]: a true reduction in effect at the receptor level, or that the dose reaching the receptors declines drastically with successive injections. The latter could involve a structural derangement of the epidural space resulting in a different distribution and uptake of the drug. The most popular concept, however, is that tachyphylaxis is related to a reduction of the amount of penetrant free base owing to a progressive decrease in the local pH [5]: Local anaesthetic agents are lipidsoluble bases; the non-ionized form is able to penetrate cell membranes while the ionized form acts on receptor sites. Since these bases are water-insoluble, they are marketed as water-soluble ionized salts of strong acids. These solutions have a low pH. The relative amounts of the agent present in non-ionized and ionized forms are dependent on the pKa of the agent and the pH of the solution, according to the Henderson-Hasselbach formula:

$$\log \frac{\text{ionized}}{\text{non-ionized}} = \text{pKa} - \text{pH}$$

This means that at a pH below pKa ionization is more complete, while in an alkaline medium the agent is present chiefly in the non-ionized form.

In the cerebrospinal fluid (CSF) the buffer capacity is low so that after administration of acidic solutions the uptake of local anaesthetics by nerve cells is restricted. In the study by Cohen et al. [5] repeated injections of conventional solutions of local anaesthetics in the subarachnoid space were followed by incremental decreases in CSF pH. This was not the case when THAM-buffered solutions of procaine were employed. A "slowed" cellular uptake of the drug results in an increased vascular uptake leading to accumulation in plasma, if the agent has a slow metabolic degradation. This is the reason why accumulation, in addition to variations in onset and duration, spread and intensity of the blockade, must be kept in mind in the total evaluation of tachyphylaxis in EA.

How then, from a practical point of view, could the problem of tachyphylaxis in EA be reduced? It is the author's opinion that at present there is no way in which we can totally abolish this problem by employing solutions of commercially available local anaesthetic agents. The use of modified solutions could mean an important step forward, but is in many countries restricted by law. The "experimental" application of "home-made", modified solutions in man should generally be avoided as little is known about their side-effects. In addition, alternative methods for prolonged pain-relief are available so no absolute indication for "experimentation" can be presented. A very strong need for animal investigation is thus emphasized.

In the discussion about the practical management of continuous EA aiming at reduction of the effects of tachyphylaxis the following can be stressed:

Dosage Interval and Mode of Administration of the Local Anaesthetic Agent

Bromage et al. [4] showed that the timing of a succeeding dose is critical in determining whether attenuation or augmentation of the resulting block will be produced. A progressive decrease in duration and spread of analgesia was observed when the time interval between the return of cutaneous sensation and the subsequent injection of local anaesthetics was increased above 10 min, reaching a constant degree when the non-analgesic interval exceeded 60 min. When the non-analgesic interval was shorter than 10 min a tendency towards wider segmental spread was found but also that the intensity of the resulting block was augmented on some occasions.

These findings indicate that prolongation by means of constant, slow-rate administration of a local anaesthetic agent should result in a better quality of blockade than that from intermittent administration. Favourable reports of the effects of drip infusion EA have been given by Dawkins and Steel [6] and Holmdahl et al. [7]. Based upon experience of about 200 cases in which TEA was prolonged in the postoperative course by means of drip infusion of unbuffered solutions of 0.4% lidocaine, 0.4% mepivacaine, 0.1% bupivacaine or constant injection of 1.0% bupivacaine, it is the author's opinion that the characteristics of the blocks prolonged by this method are no better than those resulting from intermittent administration of these agents [10, 12, 13]. By constant administration it is possible to maintain a constant spread but the intensity of the blockade declines in spite of dose increments. In the evaluation of tachyphylaxis we must therefore consider the intensity of the block which, however, is very difficult to quantify objectively in postoperative patients. The above concept must therefore be viewed with some reservation.

Properties of the Local Anaesthetic Agent/Solution

The more long-acting the agent/solution one employs the less frequent are the top-up doses needed to maintain analgesia over a given period, with a consequent reduction in the influence of tachyphylaxis. When compared with short-acting agents, long-acting, such as bupivacaine or etidocaine, prolong cutaneous analgesia in LEA to a degree, while in TEA it is considerable. However, in postoperative TEA a discrepancy exists in that subjective wound pain returns before cutaneous sensation to pin-prick [11]. Thus long-acting agents are not as ideal as some data concerning duration of action might suggest. The continuous administration of these agents in TEA produces no neurological side-effects [10] while in a small series of patients etidocaine for LEA caused a high incidence of prolonged sensory and motor block after termination of administration of the agent [9]. The prolonged block was interpreted as the effect of local precipitation of this poorly soluble agent in the epidural space.

In this connection, it deserves to be pointed out that according to Tucker and Mather [14] the calculated plasma accumulation rate is slower for long-acting than for short-acting agents.

A potentially increased duration of action can be accomplished by the addition of epinephrine to the local anaesthetic solution. In order to improve the stability and prolong the shelf-life of these solutions they are commercially dispensed with a low pH which adversely affects the ability of the drug to penetrate cell membranes. By mixing adrenaline to the local anaesthetic solution just prior to administration the anaesthesiologist can reduce this problem and achieve a less prolonged onset time of the block, reduce the influence of pH at the site of injection and reduce the vascular uptake of the agent.

In order to favour a rapid uptake of the local anaesthetic agent by the nerve cells the pKa of the agent should be as close as possible to the pH at the site of administration producing a low degree of extracellular ionization. Receptor affinity is related to the degree of intracellular ionization and is thus increased by intracellular acidosis. Considering these factors Bromage [2] suggested the use of carbon dioxide salts of local anaesthetics. In these preparations the drug is initially available in a bicarbonate form which is very rapidly converted to the non-ionized form when the PCO_2 of the solution falls to that of the tissues. A rapid diffusion of carbon dioxide into the cells occurs and causes a fall in intracellular pH. Employing such solutions the onset time of EA was reduced and the intensity of the blockade improved as compared to the effects of the hydrochloride salts of local anaesthetics. Dose requirements in obstetrical LEA prolonged over 12 h were reduced by 25%-35% [2].

Neither carbon dioxide salt nor buffered solutions of local anaesthetics are commercially available in most countries.

Accumulation in plasma of long-acting local anaesthetic agents occurs regulary in continuous TEA [9, 12, 13]. After 24 h continuation plasma concentrations reach levels similar to continuous LEA which by comparison involves three times the quantity of drug [10]. The reason behind this difference between TEA and LEA is not known but most likely it has to do with the vascularisation in various parts of the epidural space. No clear signs of toxicity in TEA has been observed by the author, but mild degrees of toxicity are difficult to differentiate from the drowsiness or mild confusion that sometimes is present in the early postoperative period. However, accumulative absorption from continuous epidurals over a prolonged period is generally better tolerated than a sudden overdosage [3] so the danger of toxicity should perhaps not be over-emphasized. According to the results of Cohen et al. [5] it is reasonable to assume that prolonged administration of buffered solutions is followed by less pronounced rises in plasma concentrations of the local anaesthetic.

It can be summarized that tachyphylaxis and accumulation are very evident in continuous TEA and that these factors limit the duration of successful prolongation in postoperative patients. Consecutive dose increments, the use of long-acting agents/solutions and short analgetic intervals between doses can reduce the effect of tachyphylaxis, while carbon dioxide salts or buffered solutions of local anaesthetic agents may further reduce the rate of development of tachyphylaxis and thus accumulation of local anaesthetics in plasma.

References

1. Brandt M, Kvisselgaard N (1972) Erfaringer med kontinuerlig torakal, epidural analgesi. Dan Med Bull 134:2378
2. Bromage PR (1965) A comparison of the hydrochloride and carbon dioxide salts of lidocaine and prilocaine in epidural analgesia. Acta Anaesthesiol Scand [Suppl] 16:55
3. Bromage PR (1967) Physiology and pharmacology of epidural analgesia. Anesthesiology 28:592
4. Bromage PR, Pettigrew RT, Crowell DE (1969) Tachyphylaxis in epidural analgesia: I. Augmentation and decay of local anesthesia. J Clin Pharmacol 9:30
5. Cohen EN, Levine DA, Colliss JE, Gunther RE (1968) The role of pH in the development of tachyphylaxis to local anesthetic agents. Anesthesiology 29:994
6. Dawkins CJ, Steel GC (1971) Thoracic extradural (epidural) block for upper abdominal surgery. Anaesthesia 26:41
7. Holmdahl M Hison, Sjögren S, Ström G, Wright B (1972) Clinical aspects of continuous epidural blockade for postoperative pain relief. Ups J Med Sci 77:47
8. Poppers PJ (1977) Tachyphylaxis to local anesthetic agents. In: Advances in Regional Anaesthesia. Proceedings of the International Symposium on local Anaesthetics and Regional Anaesthesia. p 77 Ed. Poppers, van Dijk. The Hague
9. Renck H (1975) Clinical experience with long-acting local anaesthetic agents. Acta Anaesthesiol Scand [Suppl] 60:125
10. Renck H (1978) Thoracic epidural analgesia in the management of postoperative pain. Acta Anaesthesiol Scand [Suppl] 70:43
11. Renck H, Edström H (1975) Thoracic epidural analgesia I. A double-blind study between bupivacaine and etidocaine. Acta Anaesthesiol Scand [Suppl] 57:89
12. Renck H, Edström H (1976) Thoracic epidural analgesia III. Prolongation in the early postoperative period by intermittent injections of etidocaine with adrenaline. Acta Anaesthesiol Scand 20:104
13. Renck H, Edström H, Kinnberger B, Brandt G (1976) Thoracic epidural analgesia II. Prolongation in the early postoperative period by continuous injection of 0.1% bupivacaine. Acta Anaesthesiol Scand 20:47
14. Tucker GT, Mather LE (1975) Pharmacokinetics of local anaesthetic agents. Br J Anaest 47:213

Ketamin-Valium als Adjuvans zur Periduralanaesthesie bei Erwachsenen

K. Korttila und J. Levänen

Das mögliche Auftreten von Halluzinationen und Sehstörungen im Anschluß an die Narkose hat den Einsatz von Ketamin als Narkoseeinleitungshilfe besonders bei jungen und mittelalterlichen Erwachsenen begrenzt [1]. Die post-anaesthetischen Wirkungen von Ketamin in analgetischer oder unterschwelliger Dosierung sind jedoch bisher nicht so eingehend untersucht worden wie die Wirkungsweise bei höherer Dosierung. Die vorliegende Studie wurde durchgeführt, um die Nebenwirkungen von Ketamin in Kombination mit Diazepam zu erforschen, und zwar als Adjuvans zur Leitungsanaesthesie, besonders bei Epiduralblockaden. Die Untersuchungen wurden durchgeführt bei jungen und mittelalterlichen Erwachsenen.

Methode

56 junge und 29 mittelalterliche Erwachsene, bei denen ein chirurgischer Eingriff im unteren Abdominal- oder Anorektalbereich, bzw. an den Extremitäten in Epidural-, Sakral- oder Brachialplexusblockade durchgeführt wurde, erhielten intravenös Analgesie- oder Anaesthesiedosen von Ketamin in Kombination mit Diazepam direkt vor Beginn der Operation. 41 Patienten erhielten keine zusätzlichen Medikamente zur Leitungsanaesthesie und wurden in zwei Kontrollgruppen geteilt.

Am ersten postoperativen Tag wurden die Patienten über ihre postanaesthetischen Reaktionen und die Verträglichkeit der Narkosetechnik befragt. Das Pflegepersonal äußerte sich zu dem Aufwand an Arbeit und Überwachung, den die Patienten zur postoperativen Versorgung benötigten.

Ergebnisse

Die Verabreichung von Ketamin in der Dosierung 0,5 mg/kg kombiniert mit Diazepam 0,15 mg/kg an junge oder mittelalterliche Patienten hatte keine größeren Nebenwirkungen als in den Kontrollgruppen. Ebensowenig benötigten diese Patienten verstärkte postoperative Pflege und Überwachung. Demgegenüber verursachte die Verabreichung von Ketamin 1,5 mg/kg, bzw. 3,0 mg/kg, kombiniert mit 0,15 mg/kg bzw. 0,3 mg/kg Diazepam signifikant ($p < 0{,}05$) häufigere postoperative Angst- und Verwirrungszustände. Entsprechend größer war der Bedarf an postoperativer Pflege und Überwachung als in den Kontrollgruppen (Abb. 1).

Diskussion

Da die Patienten dieser Studie zu den Altersgruppen gehörten, die auf Ketamin die heftigsten Reaktionen zeigen, benutzten wir Ketamin nicht allein. Wir verabreichten stattdessen Diazepam als Schlafmittel am Abend vor der Operation zur Praemedikation und i.v. zur Sedierung in Kombination mit Ketamin, da es die Fähigkeit hat, hypertensive Reaktionen und Ketamin-bedingte Halluzinationen zu vermindern [1]. Es kann gefolgert werden, daß bei jungen und mittelalterlichen Patienten die Unterstützung der Leitungsanaesthesie durch Ketamin 0,5 mg/kg

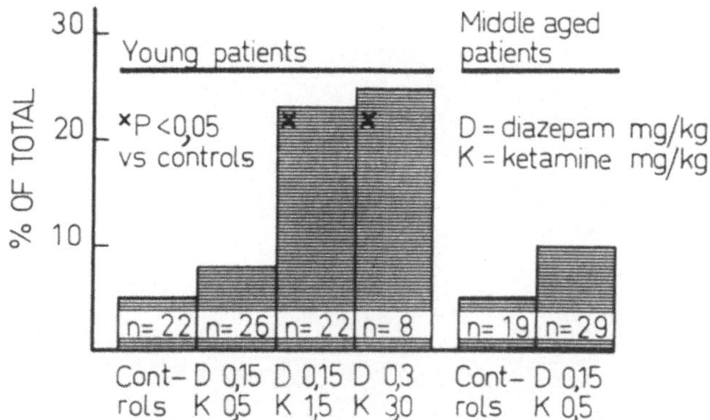

Abb. 1. Extra postoperative work and supervision

und Diazepam 0,15 mg/kg keine Nebenwirkungen hervorruft. Bei der Dosierung von 1,5 mg/kg oder höher muß dagegen mit Komplikationen gerechnet werden.

Literatur

1. Bovill JG, Clarce RSJ, Dundee JW, Pandit SK, Moore J (1971) Clinical studies of induction agents XXXVIII: Effect of premedication and supplements on ketamine anaesthesia. Br J Anaesth 43:600

Sachverzeichnis

Anaesthesiologie und Intensivmedizin Anaesthesiology and Intensive Care Medicine

95 Mobile Intensive Care Units
Advanced Emergency Care Delivery Systems
Edited by R. Frey, E. Nagel, P. Safar
Assistant Editors: P. Rheindorf, P. Sands
1976. 67 figures. XV, 271 pages
(61 pages in German)
ISBN 3-540-07561-5

98 Intraaortale Ballongegenpulsation
Experimentelle Untersuchungen zur Frage des Wirkungsspektrums und der klinischen Indikation
Von E. R. de Vivie
1976. 42 Abbildungen, 8 Tabellen. X, 96 Seiten
ISBN 3-540-07776-6

100 Anaesthesie und ärztliche Sorgfaltspflicht
Von H. W. Opderbecke
1978. 1 Tabelle. IX, 124 Seiten
ISBN 3-540-08976-4

101 Myokarddurchblutung und Stoffwechselparameter im arteriellen Blut bei Hämodilutionsperfusion
Von D. Regensburger
1976. 20 Abbildungen, 14 Tabellen. VII, 75 Seiten
ISBN 3-540-07877-0

102 Coronarinsuffizienz, Pathophysiologie und Anaesthesieprobleme bei der Coronarchirurgie
Bericht des Workshops am 23. und 30. Juni 1975 in Düsseldorf/Amsterdam
Herausgegeben von M. Zindler, R. Purschke
1977. 79 Abbildungen, 19 Tabellen.
XIII, 166 Seiten
ISBN 3-540-08015-5

103 Fettemulsionen in der parenteralen Ernährung
Symposion im Juni 1976 in Stockholm
Herausgegeben von A. Wretlind, R. Frey, K. Eyrich, H. Makowski
1977. 95 Abbildungen, 33 Tabellen. X, 222 Seiten
ISBN 3-540-08104-6

104 Die akute normovolämische Hämodilution in klinischer Anwendung
Von A. J. Coburg
1977. 21 Abbildungen, 17 Tabellen. XI, 89 Seiten
ISBN 3-540-08025-2

105 Lungenveränderungen während Dauerbeatmung
Von H. Reineke
1977. 26 Abbildungen, 7 Tabellen. VII, 56 Seiten
ISBN 3-540-08101-1

106 Etomidate
An Intravenous Hypnotic Agent
First Report on Clinical and Experimental Experience
Edited by A. Doenicke
1977. 59 figures, 16 tables. XI, 155 pages
ISBN 3-540-08485-1

107 Die kontrollierte Hypotension mit Nitroprussidnatrium in der Neuroanaesthesie
Von K. Huse
1977. 9 Abbildungen, 38 Tabellen. IX, 98 Seiten
ISBN 3-540-08218-2

108 Transcutane Sauerstoffmessung
Methodik und klinische Anwendung
Von K. Stosseck
1977. 31 Abbildungen, 6 Tabellen. VIII, 68 Seiten
ISBN 3-540-08481-9

109 20 Jahre Fluothane
Herausgegeben von E. Kirchner
1978. 151 Abbildungen, 56 Tabellen.
XVIII, 343 Seiten. (18 Seiten in Englisch)
ISBN 3-540-08602-1

110 Neue Untersuchungen mit Gamma-Hydroxibuttersäure
Herausgegeben von R. Frey
1978. 63 Abbildungen, 34 Tabellen. XIII, 149 Seiten
(79 Seiten in Englisch)
ISBN 3 540 08724-9

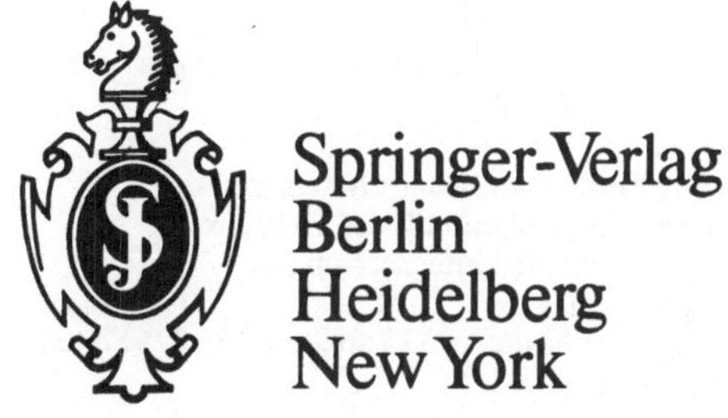

Anaesthesiologie und Intensivmedizin Anaesthesiology and Intensive Care Medicine

111 Anaphylaktoide Reaktionen
nach Infusion natürlicher und künstlicher Kolloide
Von J. Ring
Geleitwort von K. Messmer und R. Frey
1978. 65 Abbildungen, 84 Tabellen. XV, 202 Seiten
ISBN 3-540-08753-2

112 Kreislaufproblematik und Anaesthesie bei geriatrischen Patienten
Von G. Haldemann
1978. 24 Abbildungen, 3 Tabellen. VIII, 55 Seiten
ISBN 3-540-08785-0

113 Regionalanaesthesie in der Geburtshilfe
Unter besonderer Berücksichtigung von Carticain
Herausgegeben von L. Beck, K. Strasser, M. Zindler
1978. 19 Abbildungen, 24 Tabellen. IX, 94 Seiten
ISBN 3-540-08828-8

114 Zur funktionellen Beeinflussung der Lunge durch Anaesthetica
Von B. Landauer
Geleitwort von E. Kolb
1979. 53 Abbildungen, 61 Tabellen. XV, 155 Seiten
ISBN 3-540-09042-8

115 Zum Problem der Aspiration bei der Narkose
Intraluminales Druckverhalten im Oesophagus-Magen-Bereich
Von G. Sehhati-Chafai
1979. 27 Abbildungen, 55 Tabellen. X, 99 Seiten
ISBN 3-540-09162-9

116 Acute Care
Based on the Proceedings of the Sixth International Symposium on Critical Care Medicine
Edited by B. M. Tavares, R. Frey
1979. 133 figures, 100 tables. XVI, 345 pages
ISBN 3-540-09210-2

117 Der Einfluß von Anaesthetica auf die Kontraktionsdynamik des Herzens
Tierexperimentelle Untersuchungen
Von K.-J. Fischer
1979. 181 Abbildungen, 33 Tabellen. XII, 276 Seiten
ISBN 3-540-09143-2

118 Dobutamin
Eine neue sympathomimetische Substanz
Herausgegeben von H. Just
1978. 56 Abbildungen, 6 Tabellen. XI, 81 Seiten
ISBN 3-540-09077-0

119 Sympathico-adrenerge Stimulation und Lungenveränderungen
Von G. Metz
1979. 40 Abbildungen, 11 Tabellen. VIII, 90 Seiten
ISBN 3-540-09168-8

120 Äthylenoxid-Sterilisation
Von E. G. Star
1979. 2 Abbildungen, 4 Tabellen. VIII, 43 Seiten
ISBN 3-540-09294-3

121 Zur Herzwirkung von Inhalationsanaesthetica
Der isolierte Katzenpapillarmuskel als Myokard-Modell
Von H. P. Siepmann
1979. 14 Abbildungen, 5 Tabellen. VIII, 63 Seiten
ISBN 3-540-09230-7

122 Coronare Herzkrankheit
Physiologische, kardiologische und anaesthesiologische Aspekte
Weiterbildungskurs für Anaesthesieärzte am 10. Juni 1978 in Wuppertal
Herausgegeben von J. Schara
1979. 61 Abbildungen, 15 Tabellen. IX, 97 Seiten
ISBN 3-540-09416-4

123 Pathologische pulmonale Kurzschlußperfusion
Theoretische, klinische und tierexperimentelle Untersuchungen zur Variabilität
Von H. Kämmerer, K. Standfuss, E. Klaschnik
1979. 23 Abbildungen, 8 Tabellen. VIII, 71 Seiten
ISBN 3-540-09498-9

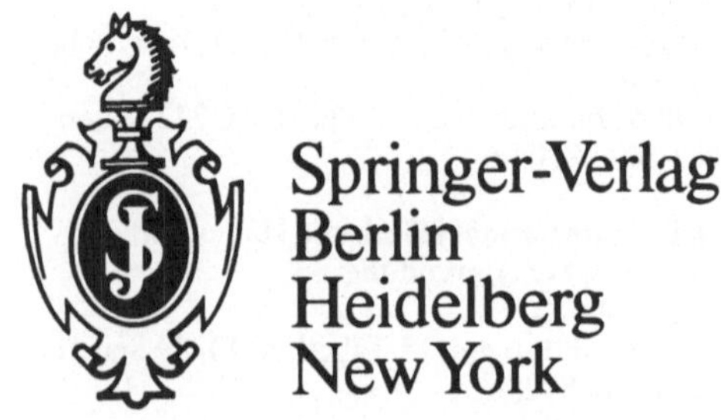